Imaging of Bone Tumors in Axial Bones

Xiaoguang Cheng • Yongbin Su
Mingqian Huang

Imaging of Bone Tumors in Axial Bones

Springer

中国协和医科大学出版社
Peking Union Medical College Press

Xiaoguang Cheng
Department of Radiology
Beijing Jishuitan Hospital, Capital
Medical University
Beijing, Beijing, China

Yongbin Su
Department of Radiology
Beijing Jishuitan Hospital, Capital
Medical University
Beijing, Beijing, China

Mingqian Huang
Department of Diagnostic, Molecular
and Interventional Radiology
Mount Sinai Health System
New York, NY, USA

ISBN 978-981-95-2261-3 ISBN 978-981-95-2262-0 (eBook)
https://doi.org/10.1007/978-981-95-2262-0

Jointly published with Peking Union Medical College Press
The print edition is not for sale in China (Mainland). Customers from China (Mainland) please order the print book from: Peking Union Medical College Press.

This Springer imprint is published by the registered company Springer Nature Singapore Pte Ltd.
The registered company address is: 152 Beach Road, #21-01/04 Gateway East, Singapore 189721, Singapore

Foreword

Beijing Jishuitan Hospital has a long history and experience in the diagnosis and treatment of various orthopedic diseases. Despite this abundant experience, the diagnosis of bone tumors remains difficult because of the low morbidity of this condition. Professor Song Xian-wen, known as the father of Chinese bone tumors, recalled the establishment of the Chinese bone tumor treatment team in the 1970s and said that "After we had done a lot of clinical work and treated hundreds of orthopaedic patients, we found the complexity of bone tumors… the diagnosing of bone tumors needed the combination of clinical, radiological test and pathological result…." The diagnosis of bone tumors is difficult because bone tumors are a type of orthopedic disease and also have imaging features that are common to other orthopedic diseases such as congenital abnormalities and degenerative bone disease. Furthermore, there are similarities between bone tumors and metabolic bone diseases, and even between the different subtypes of bone tumors.

The World Health Organization's classification system for bone tumors has undergone a transition from being based on histoembryology to histogenesis. The introduction of bone tumor "radiomics" has also further revealed the complexity of bone tumors. The complexity of bone tumors necessitates a combination of clinical, radiological, and pathological findings for accurate diagnosis.

One point that requires special emphasis is that even though some people think that pathological diagnosis is the "gold standard" in combination diagnosis, imaging is actually more reliable than pathology for diagnosing some types of bone tumors. Therefore, in general, we believe that imaging should be the basis for the final diagnosis of bone tumors.

The study of bone tumors requires strong integration of theories and practice. These theories are only fully assimilated after continuous practice. Thus, the importance of practice is endorsed by many famous professors in Beijing Jishuitan Hospital. Professor Song Xian-wen from the Department of Bone Tumors and Professor Wang Yun-zhao from the Department of Radiology have done a lot of work in determining the correlations between histology and radiology.

I recall Professor Wang Yun-zhao holding an imaging meeting in a small room that was about 6 m^2; this meeting was so popular that most of the doctors had to listen from outside the room. This tradition of discussing imaging and the thirst for practical knowledge drives us all. The good news is that this tradition has been inherited by the Department of Radiology in Beijing

Jishuitan Hospital. The writing of this series of books is the cumulative product of continuous practice and imaging meetings that have been held over the past several decades.

This series of books contains high-quality images, which will increase the ability of clinicians to use imaging to diagnose bone tumors. I believe that there are at least two important benefits to be gained from this series of books. The first one is the provision of examples of typical radiological findings of bone tumors, which can be consulted as needed. The second one is the description of the analysis process used in bone tumor imaging diagnosis. This describes a real practice that can help the reader to train, verify, and improve his or her diagnostic skills and finally become a "master of bone tumor imaging diagnosis."

In conclusion, this series of books is a crystallization of collective wisdom that contains rich content and detailed information that is both scientific and practical. This series of books provides doctors and students with a valuable reference related to bone tumors, which is important in increasing the ability of clinicians to use imaging to diagnose bone tumors.

I am pleased to write the foreword for this series of books and hope that its publication aids in the development of bone tumor radiology in China and the world.

Niu Xiaohui

Department of Orthopaedic Oncology
Surgery, Beijing Jishuitan Hospital,
Capital Medical University
Beijing, China
November 1, 2020

Preface

The correct diagnosis of bone tumors and tumor-like lesions is challenging due to their low prevalence, lack of features, and the variety of bone tumors. The close teamwork of orthopedists, radiologists, and pathologists is the key to meeting this challenge.

The Bone Tumor Department of Beijing Jishuitan Hospital, founded in 1984, was the first center to specialize in bone tumor treatment in China and is well regarded both in China and abroad. Professor Wang Yun-zhao, the most famous musculoskeletal radiologist in China, established the Department of Radiology and performed extensive radiology–pathology correlation studies on bone tumors. He was very good at the diagnosis of bone tumors and accumulated a rich database of case studies. Fellows from all over China participated in the bone tumor training course in the department every year. However, we found a lack of books about bone tumors, particularly books with a case-based approach. Therefore, a few years ago we started to collect this series of bone tumors, with carefully selected cases that included comprehensive X-ray, CT, and MRI studies. We present the cases in the way of the morning roundtable discussion at Jishuitan Hospital, pointing out the key features of each case.

One of the features of this series of books is that we document the real roundtable discussion of cases in our department. Usually, a young radiologist presents the case with medical history, then the residents or fellows read the images and propose possible differential diagnoses, followed by the attending radiologist, pros and cons of the opinion of the residents, and then one of the most experienced professors, Xiaoguang Cheng, presents his opinion on the case. Finally, the pathological finding is presented and carefully correlated with the radiological findings to find the pros and cons of the diagnosis. In some cases, if the pathological finding was inconsistent with radiology or orthopedics, then the case was sent to the pathology department with a request for a review. Finally, the treatment and follow-up of the patients by the orthopedist is an important part of the discussion. This series of books exemplifies the close teamwork required between radiologists, orthopedists, and pathologists.

We greatly appreciate the hard work of graduates and fellows in sorting out the cases and documentation. We are especially grateful to M.D. Yangdong Liu for her excellent secretarial work. *Imaging of Bone Tumors in Axial Bones* is the last one in our series of books about imaging of bone tumors. The publication of this first edition of our book would not have been possible without the help of the Peking Union Medical College Press and Lei Nan in particular.

Beijing, China	Xiaoguang Cheng
New York, NY, USA	Mingqian Huang
Beijing, China	Yongbin Su
May 16, 2025	

Acknowledgments

To my wife, Kejia, thank you for your endless love and support, especially during that time you carried our dear son, Yihang.

To my friends and coauthors, Ruopei and Yandong, I deeply appreciate your dedication and hard work.

Yongbin Su

For my family, my husband, Wilson, and my kids, Penelope and Oliver. Thank you for your unwavering love and support.

To my grandmother, you are my role model and inspiration.

Mingqian Huang

Contents

Authors and Collaborators

Authors

Xiaoguang Cheng, MD Department of Radiology, Beijing Jishuitan Hospital, Capital Medical University, Beijing, Beijing, China

Yongbin Su, MD Department of Radiology, Beijing Jishuitan Hospital, Capital Medical University, Beijing, Beijing, China

Mingqian Huang, MD Department of Diagnostic, Molecular and Interventional Radiology, Mount Sinai Health System, New York, NY, USA

Contributors

Wei Cai Department of Radiology, Beijing Jishuitan Hospital, Capital Medical University, Beijing, People's Republic of China

Guangming Cao Department of Radiology, Yan'an University Affiliated Hospital, Yan'an, Shanxi, People's Republic of China

Xiangshu Chen Department of Radiology, Beijing Jishuitan Hospital, Capital Medical University, Beijing, People's Republic of China

Yi Ding Department of Pathology, Beijing Jishuitan Hospital, Capital Medical University, Beijing, People's Republic of China

Qiangqiang Feng Department of Radiology, Beijing Jishuitan Hospital, Capital Medical University, Beijing, People's Republic of China

Jian Geng Department of Radiology, Beijing Jishuitan Hospital, Capital Medical University, Beijing, People's Republic of China

Lihua Gong Department of Pathology, Cancer Hospital Chinese Academy of Medical Sciences, Beijing, People's Republic of China

Zhe Guo Department of Radiology, Beijing Jishuitan Hospital, Capital Medical University, Beijing, People's Republic of China

Xue Hou Department of Radiology, Beijing Jishuitan Hospital, Capital Medical University, Beijing, People's Republic of China

Meiyu Hu Department of Radiology, The Sixth Affiliated Hospital of Sun Yat-sen University, Guangdong, People's Republic of China

Yanping Hu Department of Medical Imaging, Kaifeng People's Hospital, Henan, People's Republic of China

Pengju Huang Department of Radiology, Beijing Anding Hospital, Capital Medical University, Beijing, People's Republic of China

Shanqiang Huang Department of Radiology, Taizhou Hospital of Zhejiang Province, Zhejiang, People's Republic of China

Kai Li Department of Radiology, Beijing Jishuitan Hospital, Capital Medical University, Beijing, People's Republic of China

Qing Li Department of Radiology, The first Affiliated Hospital of Soochow University, Zhejiang, People's Republic of China

Wugen Li Department of Radiology, The Second Affiliated Hospital of Nanchang University, Nanchang, Jiangxi, People's Republic of China

Xinmin Li Department of Radiology, Beijing Jishuitan Hospital, Capital Medical University, Beijing, People's Republic of China

Xintong Li Department of Radiology, Beijing Jishuitan Hospital, Capital Medical University, Beijing, People's Republic of China

Ying Li Department of MRI, The First Affiliated Hospital of Zhengzhou University, Zhengzhou, Henan, People's Republic of China

Baoyue Liu Department of Pathology, Beijing Jishuitan Hospital, Capital Medical University, Beijing, People's Republic of China

Weifeng Liu Department of Orthopaedic Oncology, Beijing Jishuitan Hospital, Capital Medical University, Beijing, People's Republic of China

Yandong Liu Department of Radiology, Beijing Jishuitan Hospital, Capital Medical University, Beijing, People's Republic of China

Luxin Lou Department of Radiology, Beijing Jishuitan Hospital, Capital Medical University, Beijing, People's Republic of China

Kangkang Ma Department of Orthopedics, Handan Iron and Steel Hospital, Handan, Hebei, People's Republic of China

Yimin Ma Department of Radiology, Beijing Jishuitan Hospital, Capital Medical University, Beijing, People's Republic of China

Zhanhua Qian Department of Radiology, Beijing Jishuitan Hospital, Capital Medical University, Beijing, People's Republic of China

Tao Wang Department of Orthopaedic Oncology, Beijing Jishuitan Hospital, Capital Medical University, Beijing, People's Republic of China

Changmin Xu Department of Radiology, The Second Affiliated Hospital of Nanchang University, Nanchang, Jiangxi, People's Republic of China

Hairong Xu Department of Orthopaedic Oncology, Beijing Jishuitan Hospital, Capital Medical University, Beijing, People's Republic of China

Li Xu Department of Radiology, Beijing Jishuitan Hospital, Capital Medical University, Beijing, People's Republic of China

Xiaoming Xu Department of Radiology, Beijing Jishuitan Hospital, Capital Medical University, Beijing, People's Republic of China

Dong Yan Department of Radiology, Beijing Jishuitan Hospital, Capital Medical University, Beijing, People's Republic of China

Huili Zhan Department of Radiology, Beijing Jishuitan Hospital, Capital Medical University, Beijing, People's Republic of China

Wenshuang Zhang Department of Radiology, Beijing Jishuitan Hospital, Capital Medical University, Beijing, People's Republic of China

Jialong Zhao Department of Radiology, Second Hospital of Zhangjiakou, Zhangjiakou, Hebei, People's Republic of China

Fengyun Zhou Department of Radiology, Chongqing University Cancer Hospital, Chongqing, People's Republic of China

Yuhong Zuo Department of Radiology, Guizhou Provincial Orthopedics Hospital, Guiyang, Guizhou, People's Republic of China

1 Aneurysmal Bone Cyst: Case 1

1.1 Medical History

Patient is a 15-year-old male. He was seen at an outpatient clinic for cervical spine axis lesion.

1.2 Physical Examination

Not done.

1.3 Imaging Findings

1.3.1 Radiograph (Figs. 1.1 and 1.2)

Radiographs of the cervical spine showed malalignment between C1 and C2 with expansile bony destructive changes at C2 vertebral body.

1.3.2 CT Imaging (Figs. 1.3, 1.4, 1.5, 1.6, 1.7, 1.8, 1.9, 1.10, and 1.11)

CT images of the cervical spine demonstrated expansile bone destructive changes of C2 with internal traces of mineral and fluid-fluid levels.

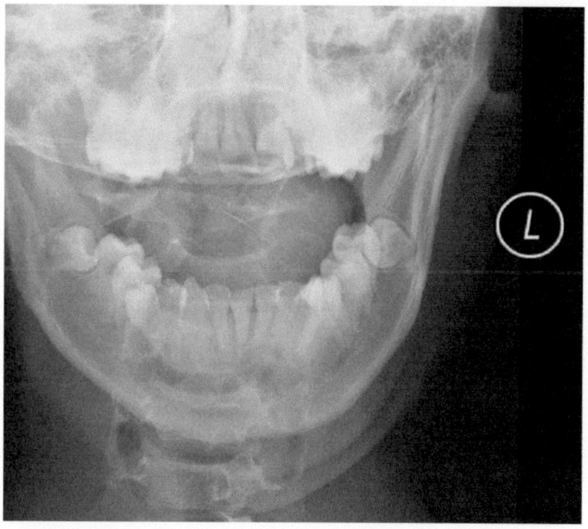

Fig. 1.1 Open mouth view of cervical spine

There was noncontinuous peripheral sclerosis. Heterogeneous avid enhancement was noted. There was compression of the spinal canal at the level.

X. Cheng et al., *Imaging of Bone Tumors in Axial Bones*,
https://doi.org/10.1007/978-981-95-2262-0_1

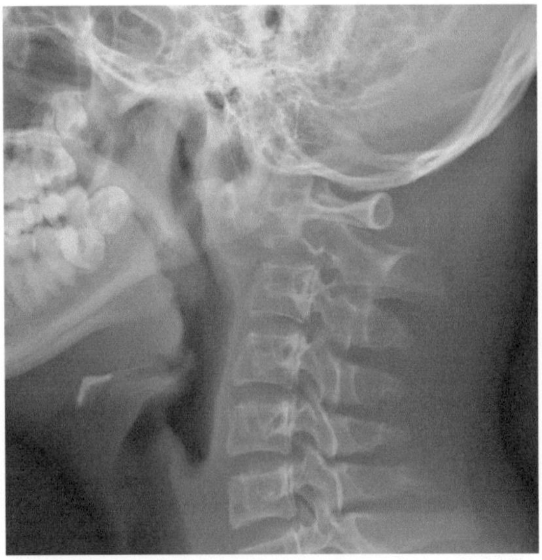

Fig. 1.2 Lateral view of cervical spine

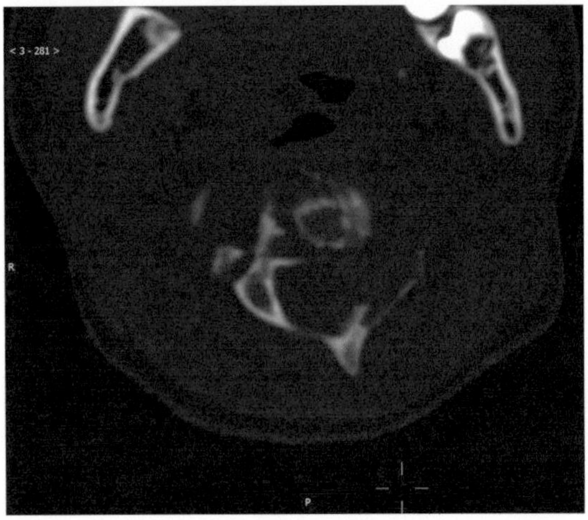

Fig. 1.3 Axial CT image of the cervical spine in bone window (C2 level)

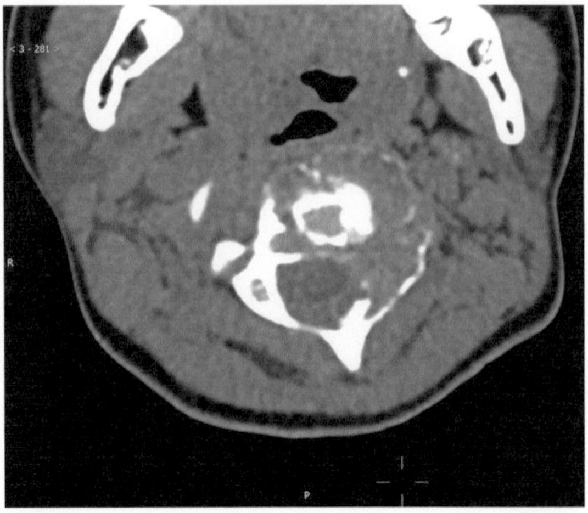

Fig. 1.4 Axial CT image of the cervical spine in soft tissue window (C2 level)

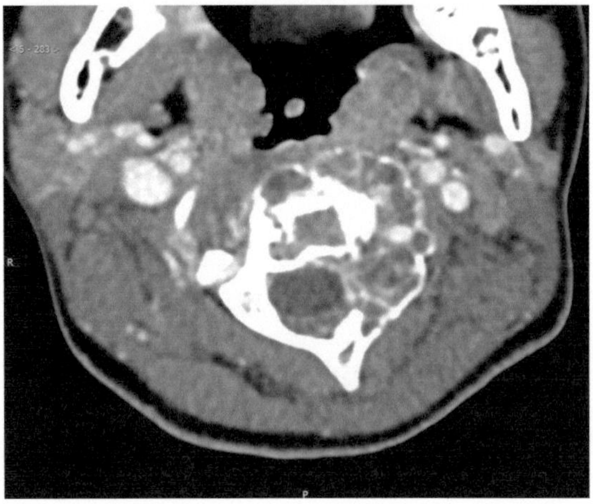

Fig. 1.5 Axial post-contrast CT image of the cervical spine in soft tissue window (C2 level)

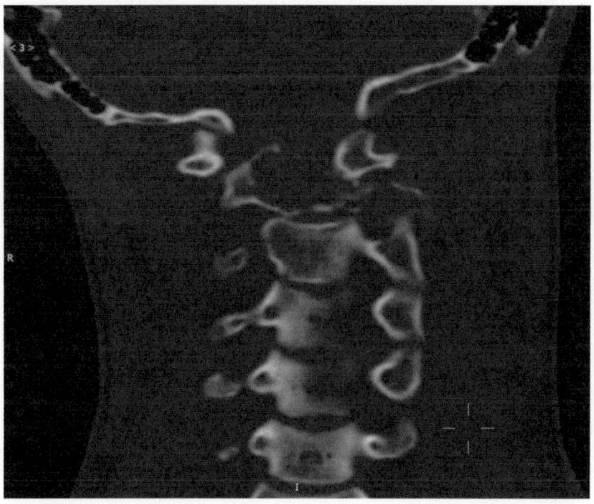

Fig. 1.6 Coronal CT image of the cervical spine in bone window

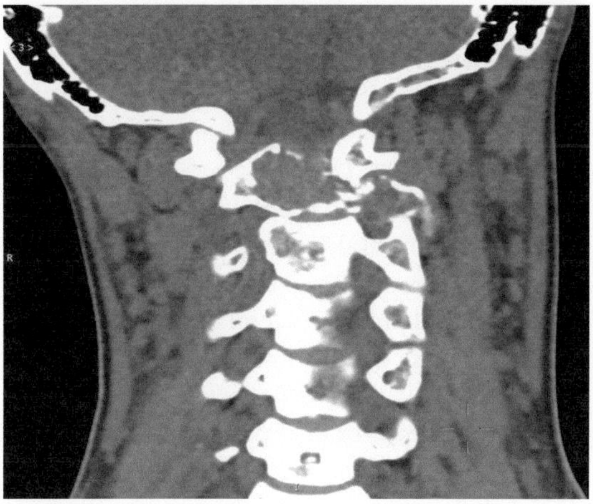

Fig. 1.7 Coronal CT image of the cervical spine in soft tissue window

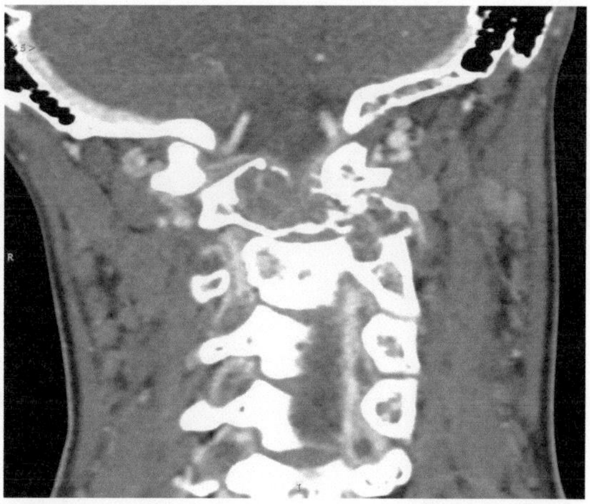

Fig. 1.8 Coronal post-contrast CT image of the cervical spine in soft tissue window

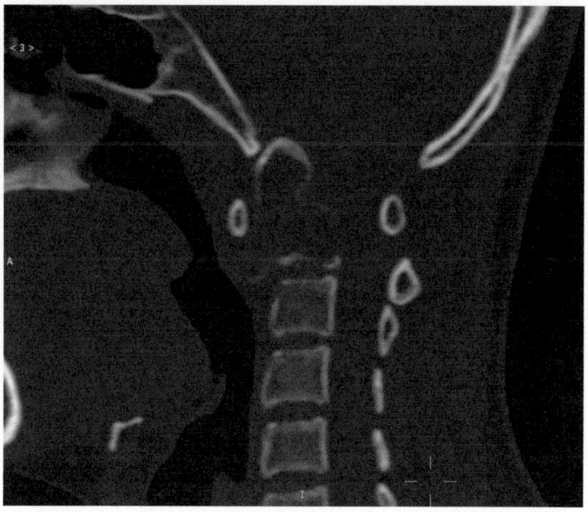

Fig. 1.9 Sagittal CT image of the cervical spine in bone window

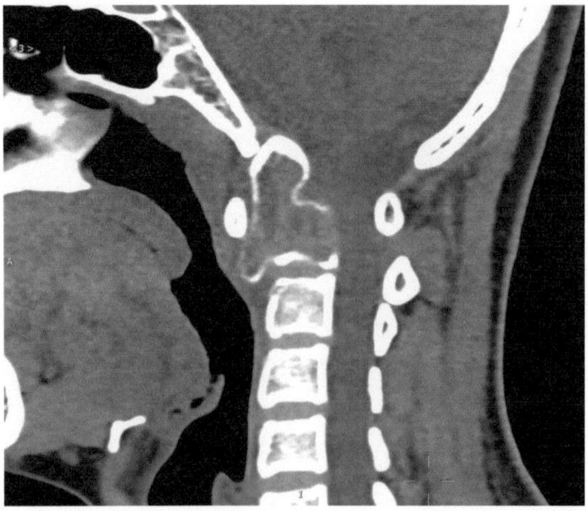

Fig. 1.10 Sagittal CT image of the cervical spine in soft tissue window

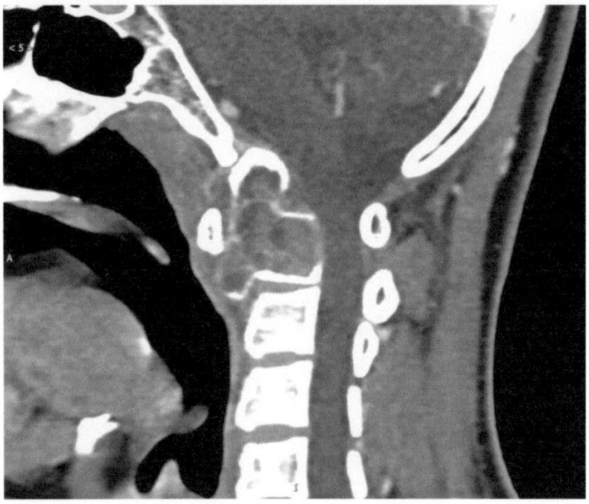

Fig. 1.11 Sagittal post-contrast CT image of the cervical spine in soft tissue window

1.4 Description and Discussion from Residents

Radiographs of the cervical spine show decreased density at the left part of C2 with clear margin. On CT scan images, odontoid process and left lateral part and vertebral arch show expansile bone destruction with internal heterogenous densities and fluid-fluid levels. There was a thin peripheral osseous shell without soft tissue mass. Avid septation-like enhancement noted. Since vertebral elements are small, cortical destruction cannot be used as a sign to make judgment on the aggressiveness of the lesion. Additionally, there was involvement at the facet joints of C3. However, with narrowed space at the facet joints and strong adjacent ligaments, spinal lesions tend to extend along the joint; this can't be the focus for differential diagnosis. The vertebral body and elements expansile lesion with internal fluid-fluid levels of adolescent; our top consideration is aneurysmal bone cyst (ABC). Giant cell tumor with ABC-like changes is in the differential diagnosis. Giant cell tumors usually affect older patients, and with solid components more common in the lesion, not consistent with the current case.

1.5 Analysis and Comments from Professor Cheng Xiao-Guang

Radiographs of the cervical spine show lesion around C1 and C2. There was anterior translation of anterior arch of atlas with overlapping of the C1 and C2 vertebral bodies, suggesting subluxation, and focus of our diagnosis. CT images show odontoid process, lateral part, and elements expansile bone destruction with heterogeneous internal densities and no punctate calcifications or soft tissue mass or disruption of the peripheral bone shell. There was multicystic-like enhancement noted. Given the patient's age, the top consideration is aneurysmal bone cyst. Giant cell tumor with ABC-like changes is in the differential diagnosis.

1.6 Diagnosis

Aneurysmal bone cyst.

Suggested Reading

Ariyaratne S, Jenko N, Iyengar KP, et al. Primary benign neoplasms of the spine. Diagnostics (Basel). 2023;13(12):2006.

Novais EN, Rose PS, Yaszemski MJ, et al. Aneurysmal bone cyst of the cervical spine in children. J Bone Joint Surg Am. 2011;93(16):1534–43.

2 Osteoid Osteoma: Case 2

2.1 Medical History

Patient is a 15-year-old male. He experienced neck pain with limited range of motion for 4 months.

2.2 Physical Examination

There is a palpable mass deep at the posterior neck, measuring about 3.0 cm × 2.0 cm × 2.0 cm with clear margin, rubbery, smooth, and with point tenderness which radiates.

2.3 Imaging Findings

2.3.1 Radiograph (Figs. 2.1 and 2.2)

Radiographs of the cervical spine show increased density around the elements of the C3 on the right.

2.3.2 CT Imaging (Figs. 2.3, 2.4, 2.5, 2.6, 2.7, and 2.8)

CT images of the cervical spine demonstrated lucent lesion in a semioval shape around the right elements of C3, measuring about 1.0 cm with internal punctate high densities and peripheral osseous sclerosis.

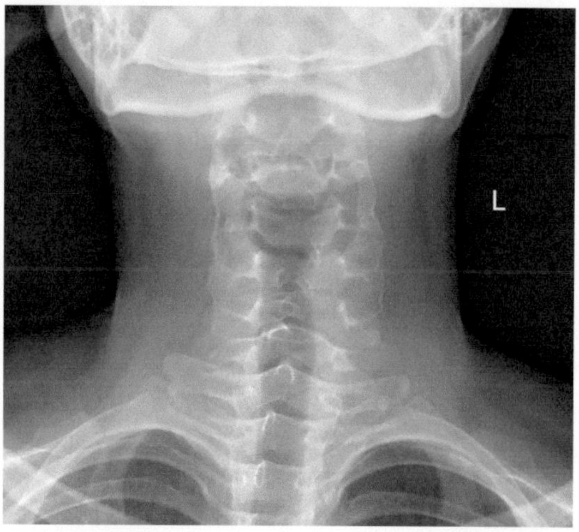

Fig. 2.1 Frontal view of cervical spine

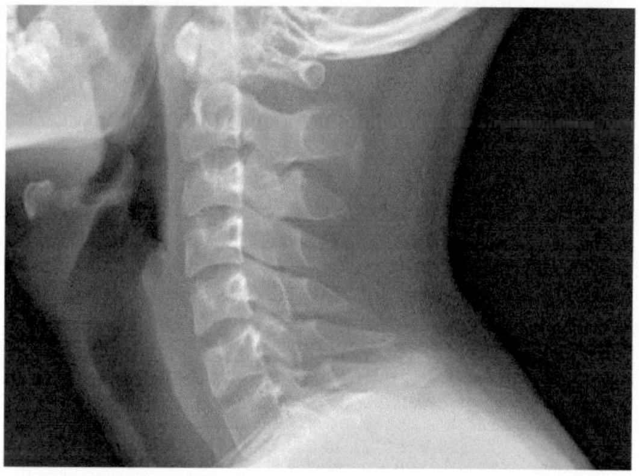

Fig. 2.2 Lateral view of cervical spine

X. Cheng et al., *Imaging of Bone Tumors in Axial Bones*,
https://doi.org/10.1007/978-981-95-2262-0_2

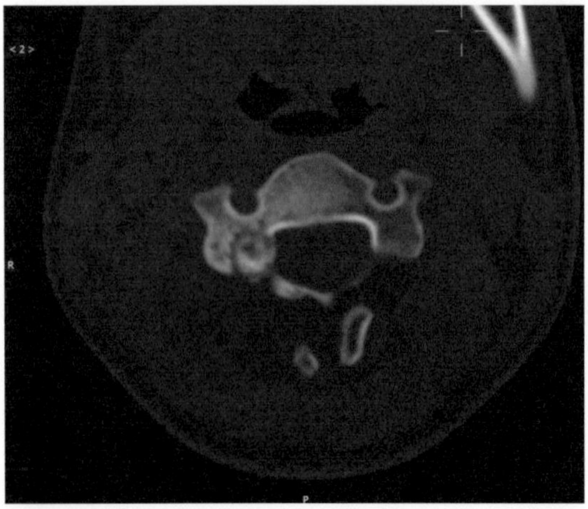

Fig. 2.3 Axial CT image of the cervical spine in bone window (C3 level)

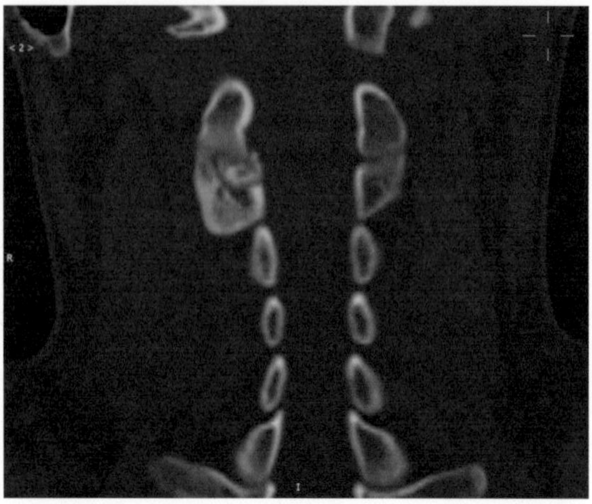

Fig. 2.5 Coronal CT image of the cervical spine in bone window

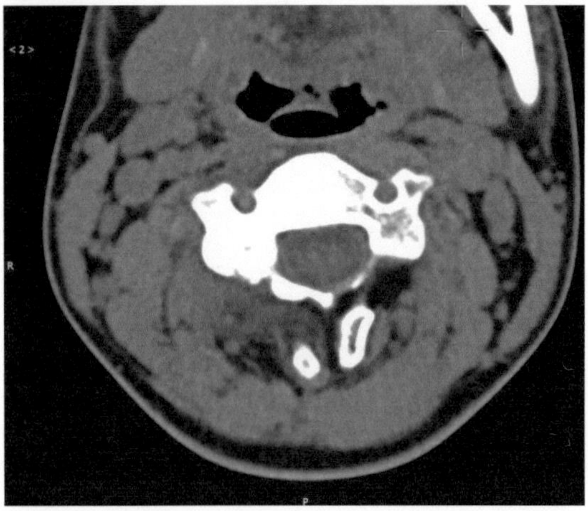

Fig. 2.4 Axial CT image of the cervical spine in soft tissue window (C3 level)

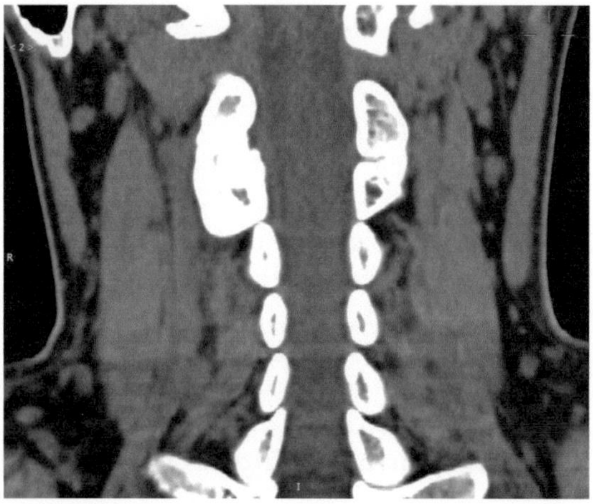

Fig. 2.6 Coronal CT image of the cervical spine in soft tissue window

2.3.3 MR Imaging (Figs. 2.9, 2.10, 2.11, 2.12, and 2.13)

MR images of the cervical spine demonstrated bone destruction around the posterior elements of C3 on the right with surrounding marrow edema and soft tissue edema. No soft tissue mass noted. No abnormal signal of the adjacent intervertebral disc or spinal cord.

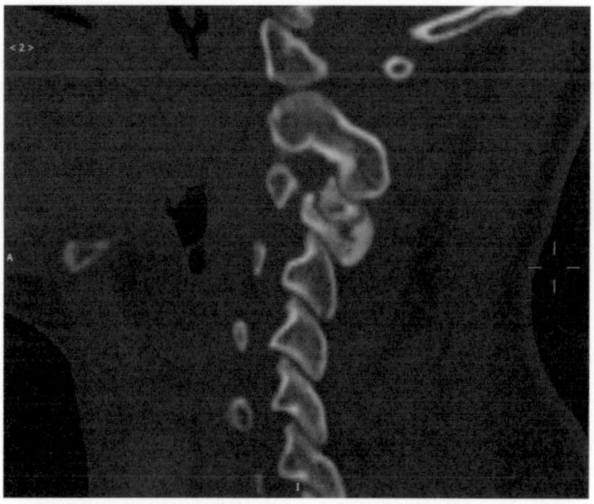

Fig. 2.7 Sagittal CT image of the cervical spine in bone window

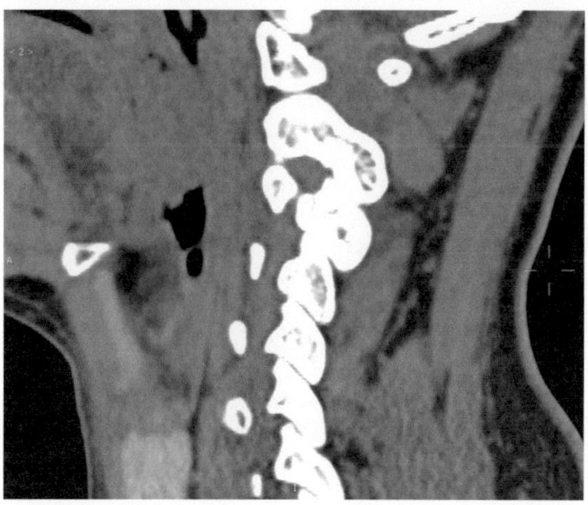

Fig. 2.8 Sagittal CT image of the cervical spine in soft tissue window

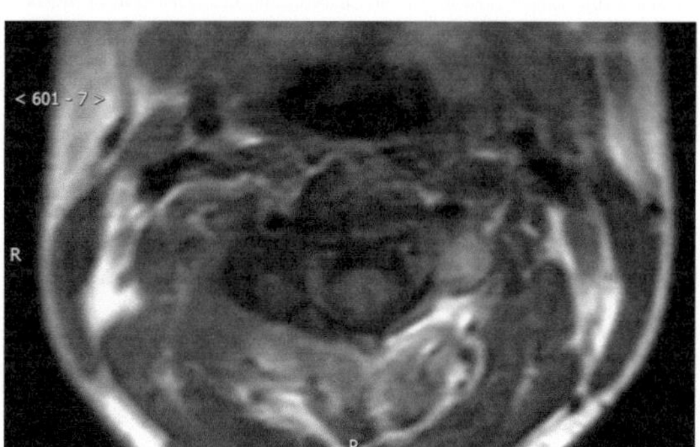

Fig. 2.9 Axial T1-weighted MR image of the cervical spine

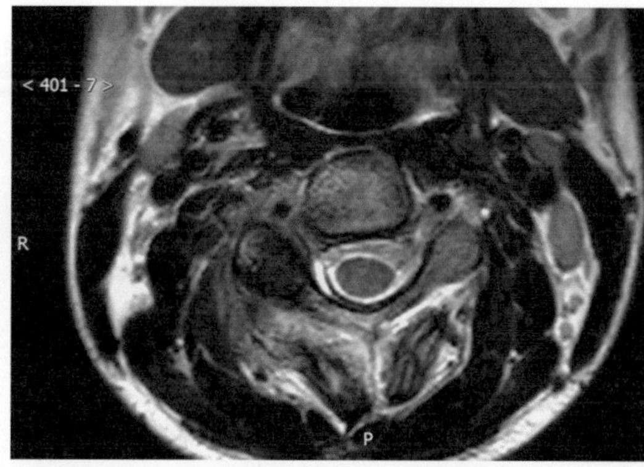

Fig. 2.10 Axial T2-weighted MR image of the cervical spine

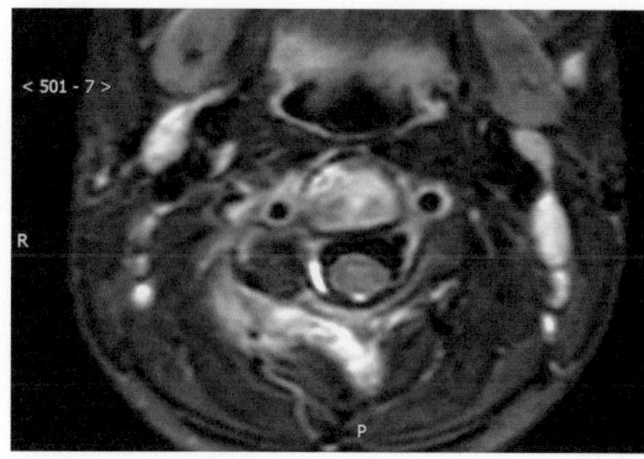

Fig. 2.11 Axial STIR MR image of the cervical spine

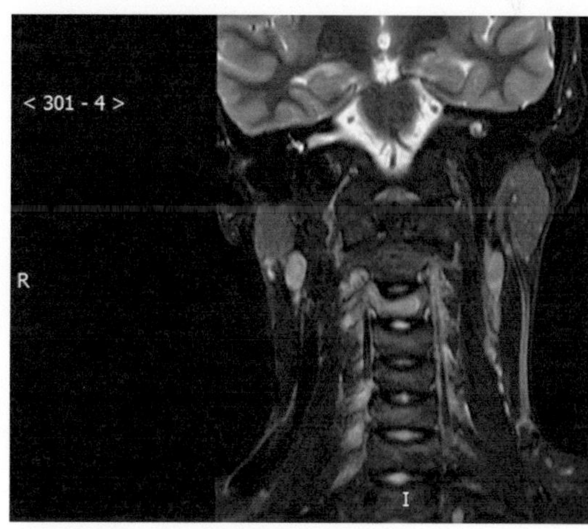

Fig. 2.12 Coronal STIR MR image of the cervical spine

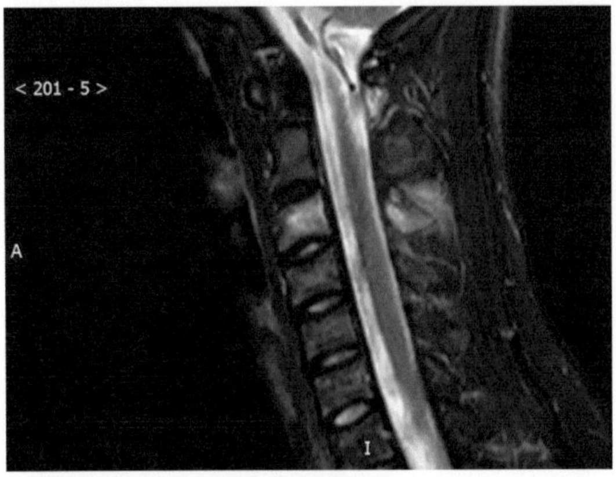

Fig. 2.13 Sagittal STIR MR image of the cervical spine

2.4 Description and Discussion from Residents

Radiographs of the cervical spine showed high density around the right C3 articular process. On the CT images, there was low density lesion around right C3 transverse process and superior articular process, about 1 cm in size with internal calcification and peripheral sclerosis and adjacent soft tissue edema. Low signal noted of the lesion on MR images with extensive edema of the adjacent soft tissue and bone, typical for osteoid osteoma. Contrast enhanced MR images have advantage of showing the characteristic findings of osteoid osteoma. The area of nidus with rich vascular supply and usually demonstrated as circular avid enhancement surrounding the calcification. This is usually not well depicted on CT images with contrast.

2.5 Analysis and Comments from Professor Cheng Xiao-Guang

The patient is an adolescent. There was increased density around lamina and spinous process of C3 on radiographs. On the CT images, there was destruction around the elements of C3 on the right (nidus) with internal calcification with peripheral reactive sclerosis. Apparent surrounding bone marrow edema and soft tissue edema noted on the MR images, typical of osteoblastoma/osteoid osteoma. Osteoblastoma and osteoid osteoma are identical on pathology. Our imaging diagnosis is based on size of the lesion: the nidus of osteoblastoma >2 cm, while osteoid osteoma usually <1.5 cm or 2 cm. Additionally, some of the lesions of osteoblastoma are not as regular in shape when compared to osteoid osteoma, and the internal calcification can be irregular or not present. However, the peripheral sclerosis is usually more apparent.

2.6 Diagnosis

Osteoid osteoma.

Suggested Reading

Gadiya A, Shah K, Patel P, et al. Osteoid osteoma of cervical spine: a case report and review of literature. J Orthop Case Rep. 2019;9(1):78–81.

Levine AM, Boriani S, Donati D, et al. Benign tumors of the cervical spine. Spine (Phila Pa 1976). 1992;17(10 Suppl):S399–406.

Osteoblastoma: Case 3

3

3.1 Medical History

Patient is a 40-year-old male. He presented with neck pain without clear cause and radiates to the left upper arm with mild limited range of motion. He had an open biopsy.

3.2 Physical Examination

There is protuberance along the spinous process of C7 on the left with palpable and rubbery mass noted. The mass did not appear to be adhered to adjacent structures but with point tenderness.

3.3 Imaging Findings

3.3.1 Radiograph (Figs. 3.1 and 3.2)

Radiographs of the cervical spine demonstrated degenerative changes without radiographic evidence of bone destruction.

3.3.2 CT Imaging (Figs. 3.3, 3.4, 3.5, 3.6, 3.7, and 3.8)

CT images of the cervical spine demonstrated expansile bone destruction along the left C7, with the cross-section area measuring about 1.3 cm × 1.6 cm with clear margin and no peripheral sclerosis. Avid enhancement was noted.

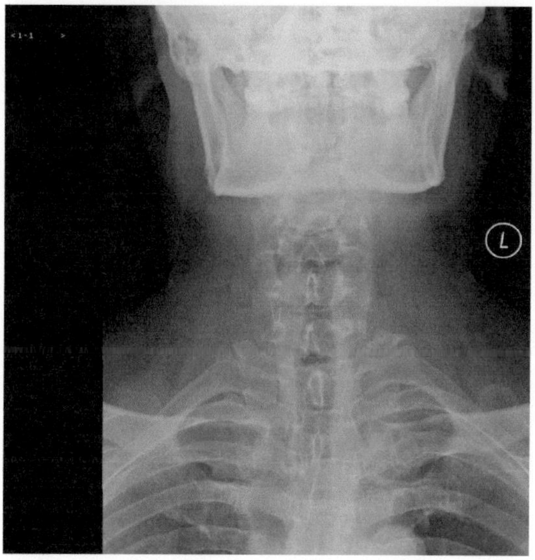

Fig. 3.1 Frontal view of cervical spine

X. Cheng et al., *Imaging of Bone Tumors in Axial Bones*,
https://doi.org/10.1007/978-981-95-2262-0_3

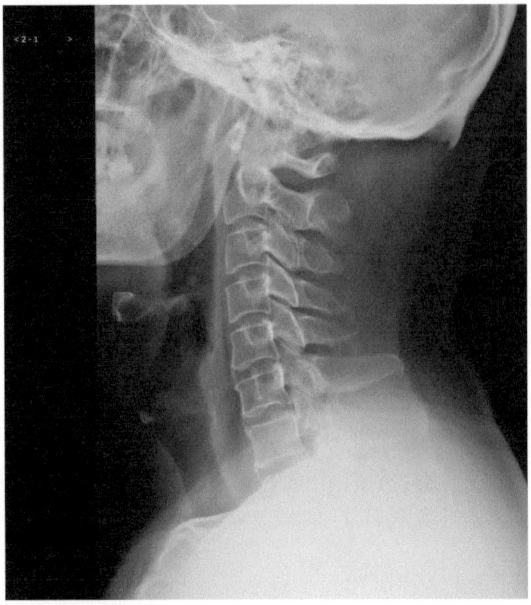

Fig. 3.2 Lateral view of cervical spine

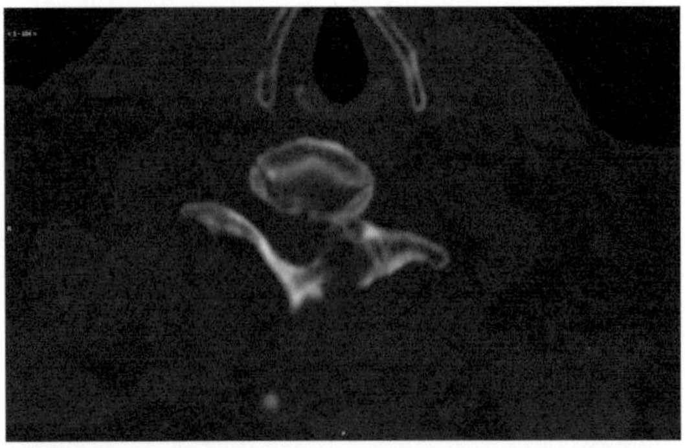

Fig. 3.3 Axial CT image of the cervical spine in bone window (C7 level)

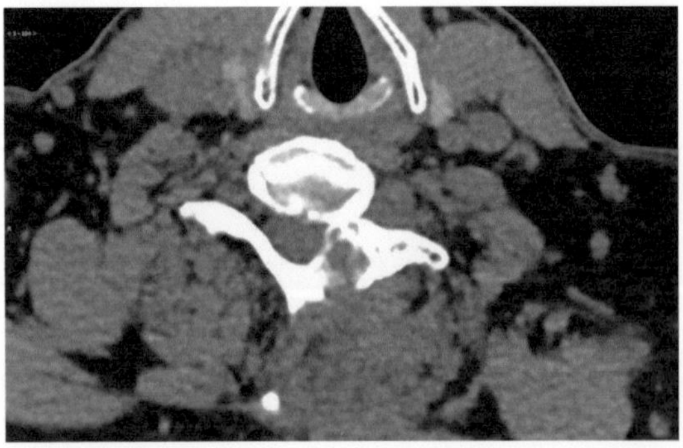

Fig. 3.4 Axial CT image of the cervical spine in soft tissue window (C7 level)

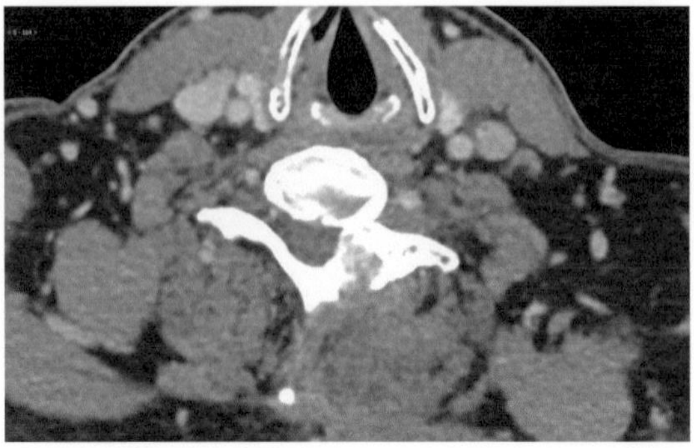

Fig. 3.5 Axial post-contrast CT image of the cervical spine in soft tissue window (C7 level)

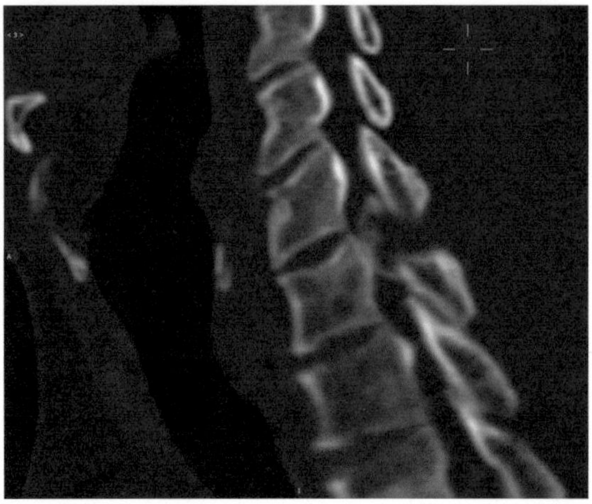

Fig. 3.6 Sagittal CT image of the cervical spine in bone window

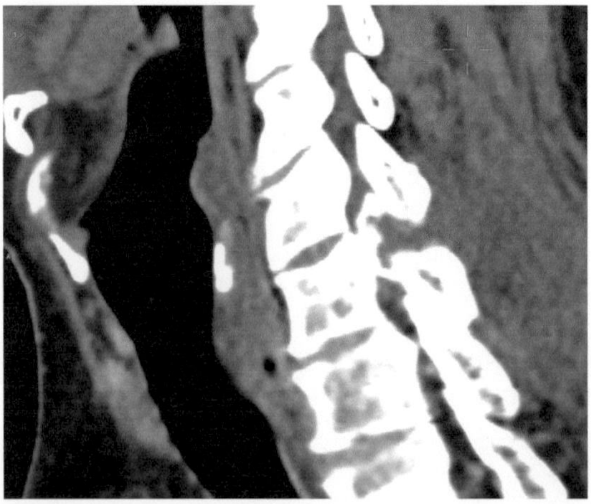

Fig. 3.7 Sagittal CT image of the cervical spine in soft tissue window

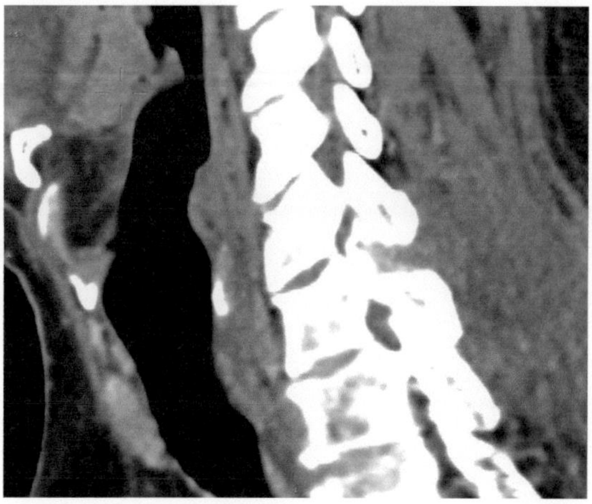

Fig. 3.8 Sagittal post-contrast CT image of the cervical spine in soft tissue window

3.4 Description and Discussion from Residents

Radiographs of the cervical spine showed no clear bone destruction. CT scan showed bone destruction around the left lamina and articular process of C7. There was mild expansile appearance of the anterior cortex with clear margin and no peripheral sclerosis. There was soft tissue density internally without calcification or fragments with avid enhancement. There was soft tissue swelling along the left posterior aspect to the lesion without enhancement, likely edema from postoperative changes. Overall, we favor a benign process. Based on the location of the lesion, our top consideration is osteoblastoma. However, there usually is more sclerosis, which is not typical of this case. Fibrous or chondroid lesions are in the differential diagnosis. However, the enhancement pattern is not consistent with the current case. Infection is also in the differential diagnosis. Bone destruction and periosteal reactions are common with infection but infection is rare with expansile changes.

3.5 Analysis and Comments from Professor Cheng Xiao-Guang

Patient is a middle-aged male. Radiographs showed no apparent abnormalities. CT images showed bone destruction around the C7 posterior elements on the left. The lesion is very focal with clear margin and mild expansion anteriorly. This is accompanied by narrowing of the left neuroforamen, consistent with the symptoms. Soft tissue swelling in the left posterior region noted. Avid enhancement noted of the lesion without enhancement of the soft tissue swelling, suggestive of postoperative changes. A nonaggressive process involves the posterior elements; my top consideration is osteoblastoma.

3.6 Diagnosis

Osteoblastoma.

Suggested Reading

Chai BB, Charles H, Cho CH. Cervical spine mass imaging: MRI or CT. Spine J. 2013;13(6):713–4.

Kan P, Schmidt MH. Osteoid osteoma and osteoblastoma of the spine. Neurosurg Clin N Am. 2008;19(1):65–70.

4 Epithelioid Sarcoma: Case 4

4.1 Medical History

Patient is a 27-year-old male. He was seen at outpatient clinic for cervical spine pain starting about 3 months ago.

4.2 Physical Examination

Not done.

4.3 Imaging Findings

4.3.1 CT Imaging (Figs. 4.1, 4.2, 4.3, 4.4, 4.5, 4.6, 4.7, 4.8, and 4.9)

CT images of the cervical spine demonstrated bone destruction along the left lateral C3 and C4 involving the pedicle and lamina with associated soft tissue mass with heterogeneous density. There is extension to the prevertebral soft tissue with mass affect upon the pharyngeal wall. There is posterior extension with mass effect upon the central canal and compression the thecal sac. There is involvement of the left neuroforamen with mass effect upon the left vertebral artery. Avid heterogeneous enhancement was noted.

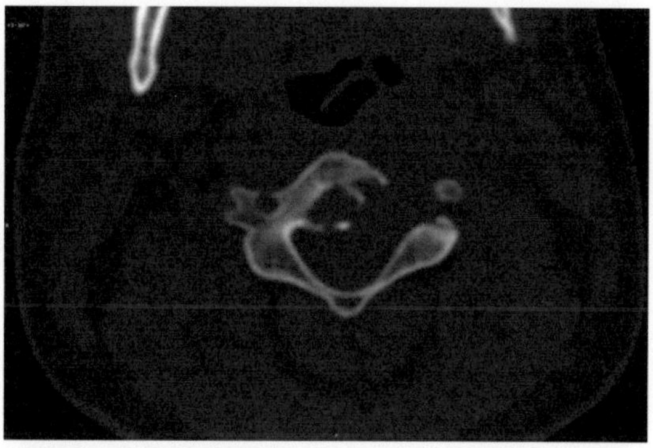

Fig. 4.1 Axial CT image of the cervical spine in bone window (C3 level)

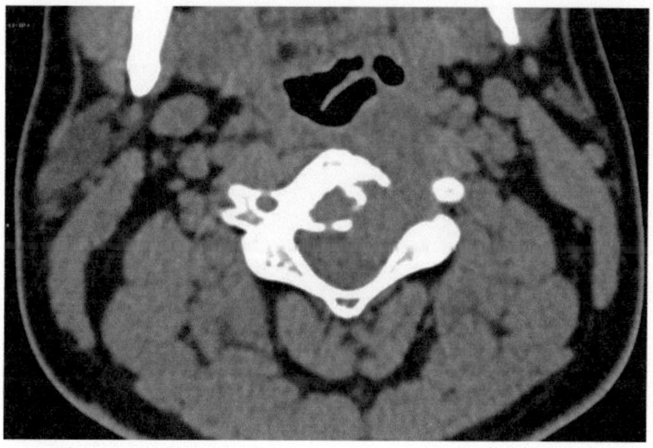

Fig. 4.2 Axial CT image of the cervical spine in soft tissue window (C3 level)

X. Cheng et al., *Imaging of Bone Tumors in Axial Bones*,
https://doi.org/10.1007/978-981-95-2262-0_4

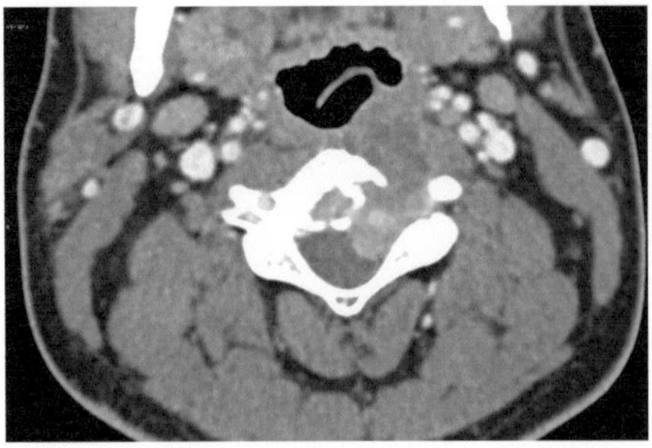

Fig. 4.3 Axial post-contrast CT image of the cervical spine in soft tissue window (C3 level)

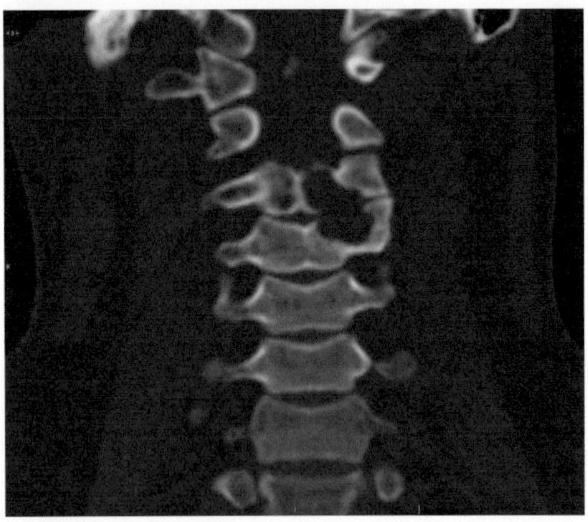

Fig. 4.4 Coronal CT image of the cervical spine in bone window

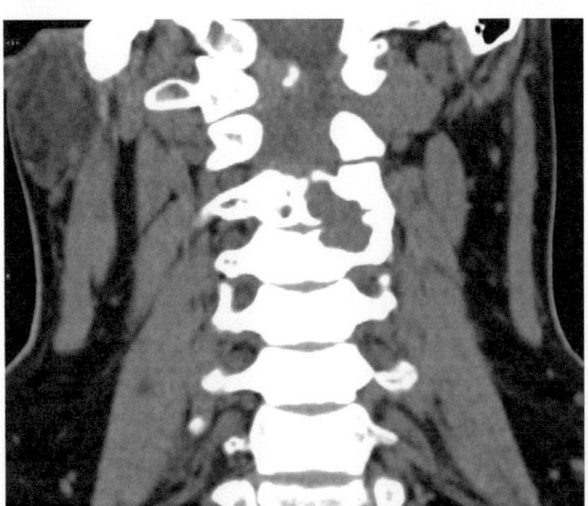

Fig. 4.5 Coronal CT image of the cervical spine in soft tissue window

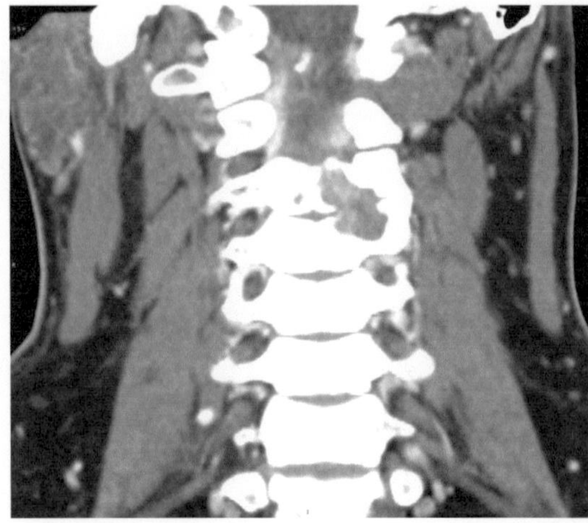

Fig. 4.6 Coronal post-contrast CT image of the cervical spine in soft tissue window

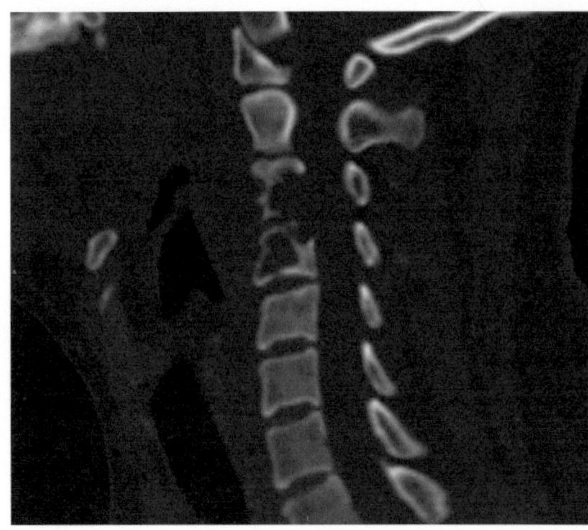

Fig. 4.7 Sagittal CT image of the cervical spine in bone window

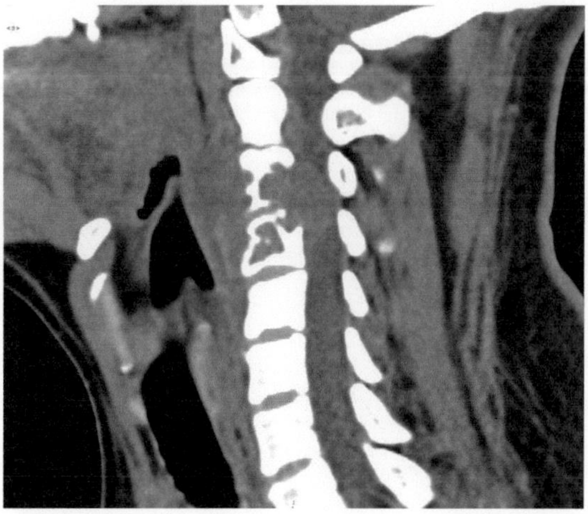

Fig. 4.8 Sagittal CT image of the cervical spine in soft tissue window

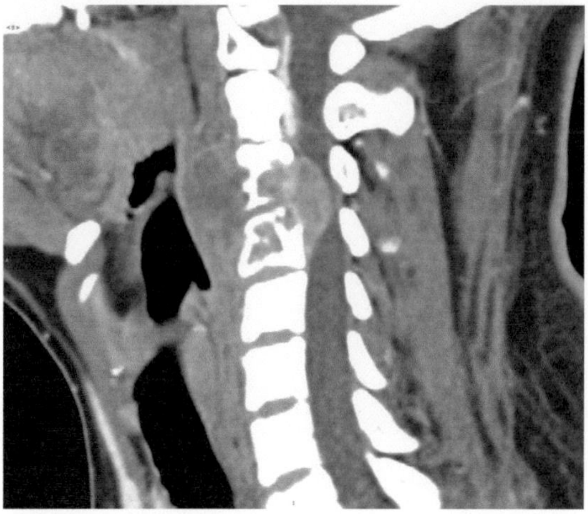

Fig. 4.9 Sagittal post-contrast CT image of the cervical spine in soft tissue window

4.4 Description and Discussion from Residents

On CT scan images, there was bone destruction along the vertebral body, pedicle, and lamina of C3 and C4 without peripheral sclerosis and with associated soft tissue mass. The anterior extension demonstrated indistinct border from the posterior pharyngeal wall. There was posterior extension with mass effect upon the central canal and involved the neuroforamen. Mild increased density noted adjacent to the vertebral body with narrowing of the intervertebral disc space. Avid heterogeneous enhancement was noted. Our differential diagnosis includes (1) infectious causes, such as tuberculosis. The process involved two vertebral bodies with peripheral soft tissue mass supporting the diagnosis. However, lack of significant disc space narrowing and the enhancement pattern was not consistent with infection. (2) Eosinophilic granuloma (Langerhans cell histiocytosis, LCH) usually manifests as bone destruction of vertebral body with soft tissue mass. However, LCH usually not affecting adjacent vertebral bodies and the soft tissue mass usually with homogeneous density, not consistent with the current case. (3) Metastatic lesion. This can affect multiple vertebral bodies with a variety of manifestations. Based on the imaging findings of the current case, we favor metastatic lesion in the central canal and invading the vertebral body. But the patient is young, unlikely with metastatic disease. (4) Peripheral nerve sheath tumor, it can affect two vertebral segments with soft tissue mass in and outside of the central canal. But the too mild expansion of the neuroforamen of the current case is not consistent with peripheral nerve sheath tumor.

4.5 Analysis and Comments from Professor Cheng Xiao-Guang

The patient is a young male. CT images show bone destruction of C3 and C4 with mild compression of C3 and with surrounding soft tissue mass with relatively low density. Avid heterogeneous enhancement was noted in the soft tissue mass. Disc space change is critical at differentiating spinal infection from tumor. No significant disc space change of the current case is not suggestive of infection, and enhancement pattern is also not consistent with infection. With eosinophilic granuloma affecting the spine, there is usually collapse of the vertebral body, not consistent with current case. Overall, I favor aggressive tumor, such as metastatic lesion, lymphoma, or multiple myeloma.

4.6 Diagnosis

Epithelioid sarcoma.

Suggested Reading

Lee C, Choe WJ, Nara Kim N. Epithelioid sarcoma in the cervical spine: a case report. Korean J Spine. 2015;12(3):165–8.

Sudhir G, Jayabalan SV, Ram A, et al. Epithelioid sarcoma of lumbar spine: a rare mesenchymal tumor masquerading as infection. Asian J Neurosurg. 2021;16(1):191–5.

Chondrosarcoma: Case 5

5

5.1 Medical History

Patient is a 49-year-old male. He had intermittent neck pain with right-hand pain and numbness for about 6 months.

5.2 Physical Examination

Nothing significant.

5.3 Imaging Findings

5.3.1 Radiograph (Figs. 5.1 and 5.2)

Radiographs of the cervical spine show increased density mass around the spinous processes of C5 and C6 without clear margin.

5.3.2 CT Imaging (Figs. 5.3, 5.4, 5.5, 5.6, 5.7, 5.8, and 5.9)

CT images of the cervical spine demonstrated bone destruction around the spinous process of C5 with soft tissue mass. The lesion showed internal low and intermediate densities and internal multiple irregular calcifications. There is mass effect to the surrounding osseous structures with avid peripheral enhancement.

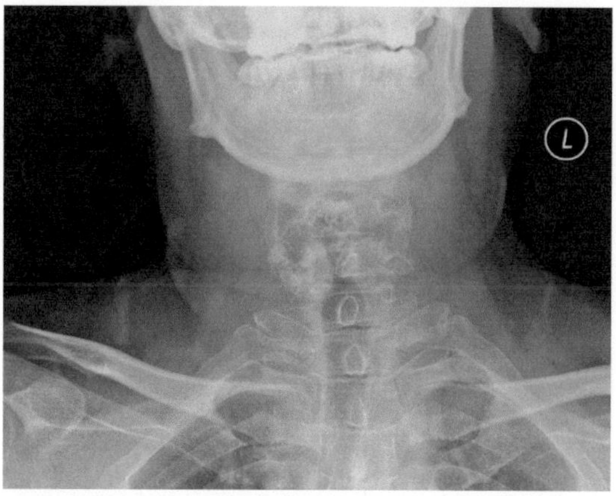

Fig. 5.1 Frontal view of cervical spine

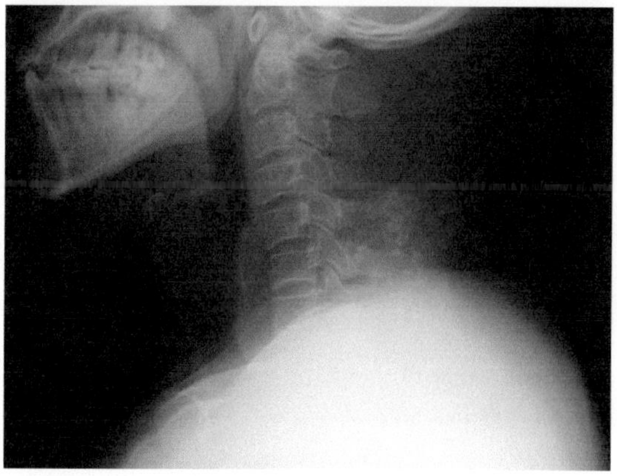

Fig. 5.2 Lateral view of cervical spine

X. Cheng et al., *Imaging of Bone Tumors in Axial Bones*,
https://doi.org/10.1007/978-981-95-2262-0_5

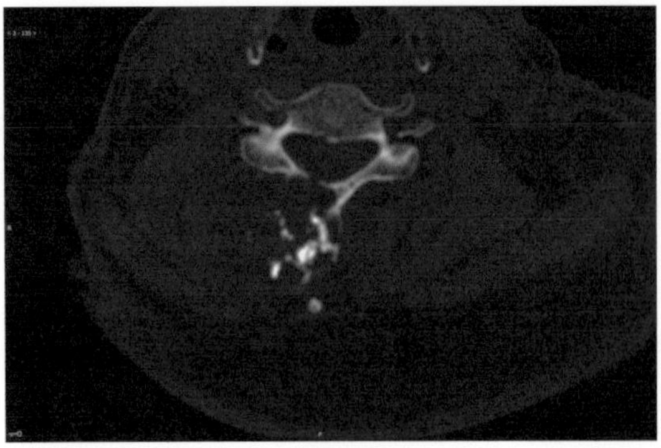

Fig. 5.3 Axial CT image of the cervical spine in bone window

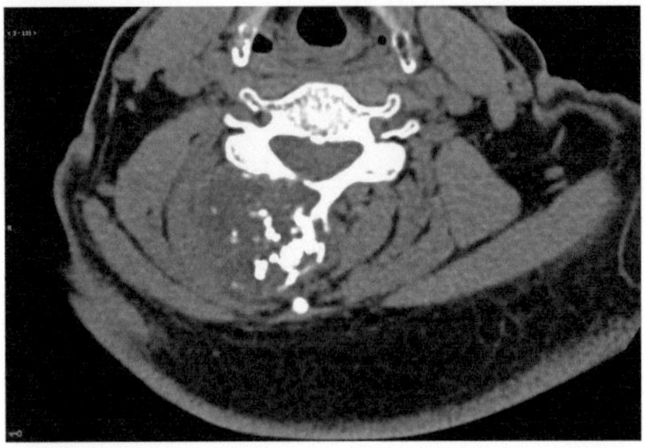

Fig. 5.4 Axial CT image of the cervical spine in soft tissue window

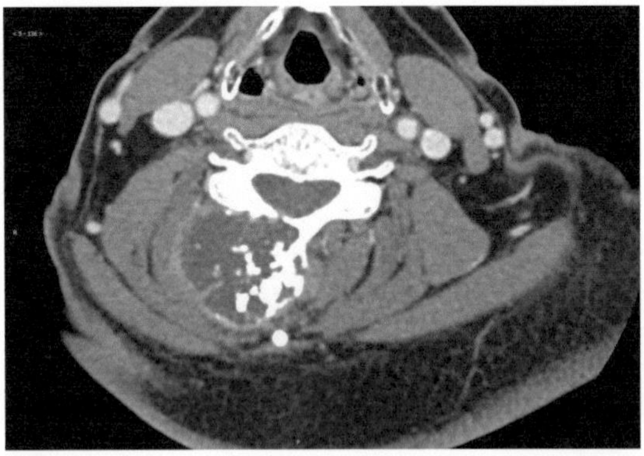

Fig. 5.5 Axial post-contrast CT image of the cervical spine in soft tissue window

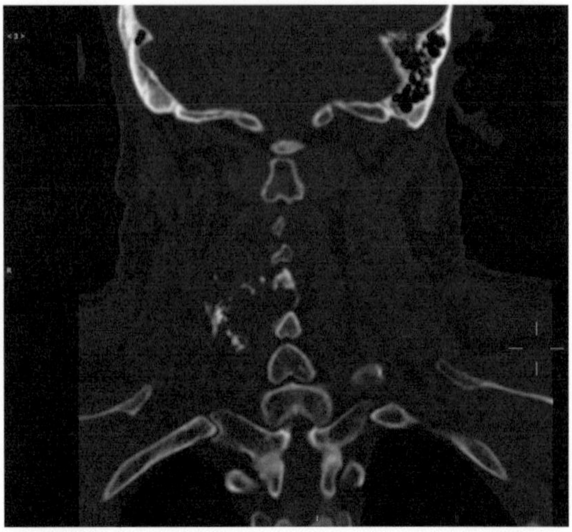

Fig. 5.6 Coronal CT image of the cervical spine in bone window

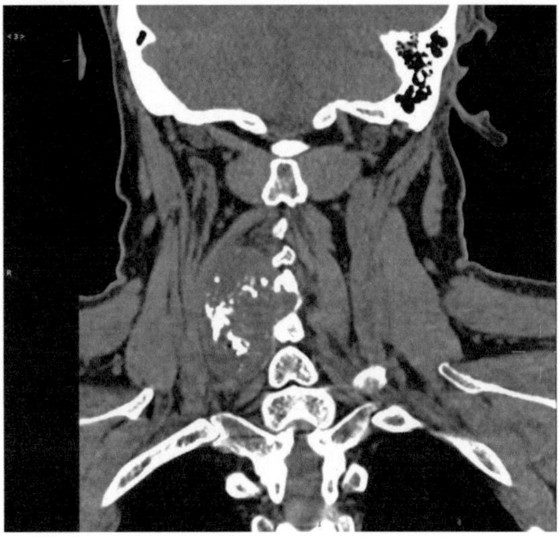

Fig. 5.7 Coronal CT image of the cervical spine in soft tissue window

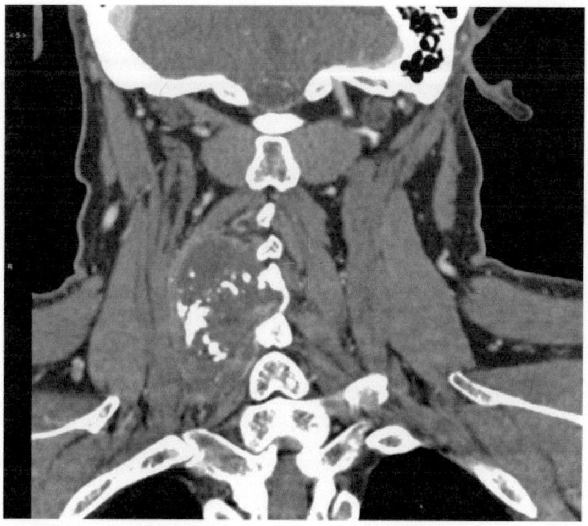

Fig. 5.8 Coronal post-contrast CT image of the cervical spine in soft tissue window

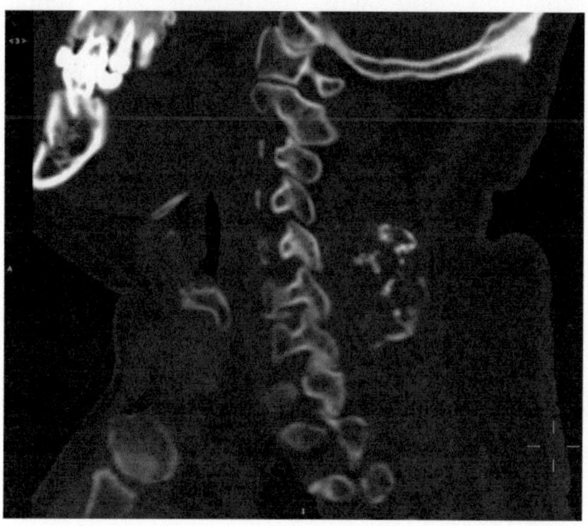

Fig. 5.9 Sagittal CT image of the cervical spine in bone window

5.3.3 MR Imaging (Figs. 5.10, 5.11, 5.12, and 5.13)

MRI of the cervical spine demonstrated bone destruction around spinous process of C5 with lobulated soft tissue mass extending to the cortex with low T1 and high T2 signal. There are scattered irregular patch low signal with adjacent bone and soft tissue edema. There is avid peripheral enhancement.

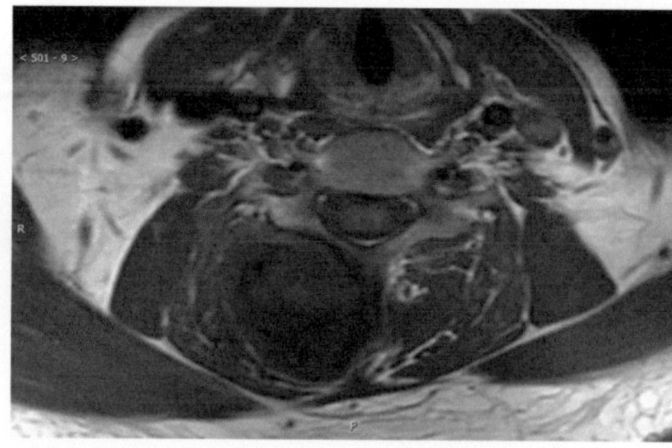

Fig. 5.10 Axial T1-weighted MR image of the cervical spine

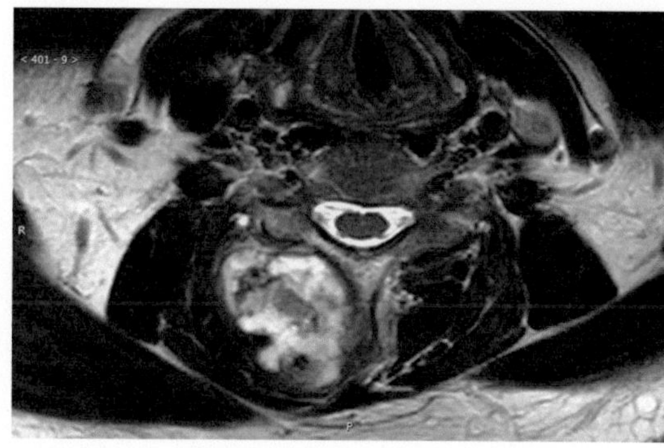

Fig. 5.11 Axial T2-weighted MR image of the cervical spine

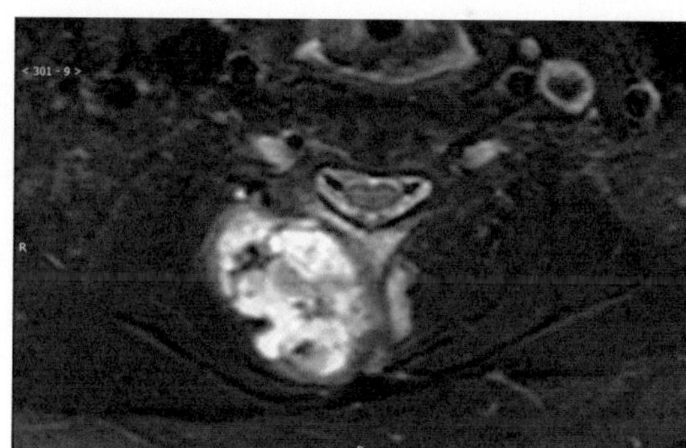

Fig. 5.12 Axial fat-suppressed T2-weighted MR image of the cervical spine

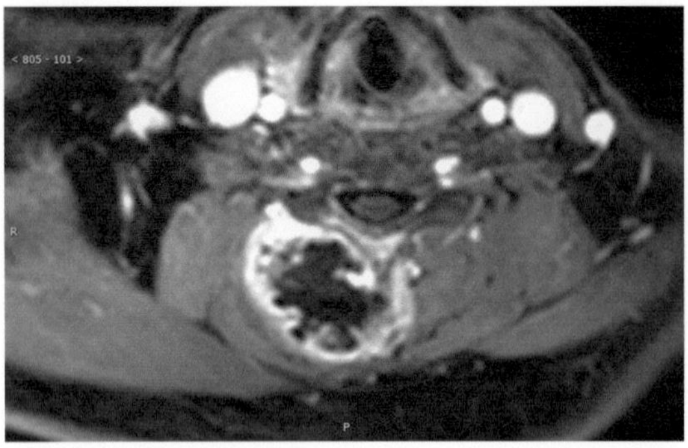

Fig. 5.13 Axial post-contrast fat-suppressed T1-weighted MR image of the cervical spine

5.4 Description and Discussion from Residents

The cervical spine radiographs demonstrated focal expansion around spinous processes from C5 to C7 with irregular shape and heterogeneous densities. CT images show bone destruction of C5 spinous process and right lateral lamina with irregular soft mass with irregular margin and internal multiple irregular high densities, likely of chondroid calcifications. There was avid peripheral enhancement and no enhancement internally, most suggestive of chondrogenic tumor. The mass showed low T1 signal and predominant high signal on T2 and fat-suppressed T2-weighted MR images, suggestive of chondroid matrix and avid peripheral enhancement also very suggestive of chondrogenic tumor. Given internal calcifications, our top consideration is low-grade chondrosarcoma. The differential diagnosis includes other chondrogenic tumor, such as chondromyxoid fibroma and chondroblastoma.

5.5 Analysis and Comments from Professor Cheng Xiao-Guang

The cervical spine radiographs showed irregular high density mass around posterior C5 and C6 vertebral bodies. It is very hard to differentiate the origin and type of the lesion based on radiograph alone. CT images showed the lesion originated around the spinous process of C5 with soft tissue mass on the right and compress on the adjacent lamina. The density of the soft tissue mass is lower than the muscle with internal multiple calcifications with peripheral and septal enhancement. The mass showed low T1 and high T2 signal indicating high water content of the lesion with internal low signal calcifications and septations and with peripheral and septal enhancement, very typical of chondrosarcoma. For some older patients, there is potential malignant transformation of preexisting osteochondroma. However, there is no clear sign of osteochondroma in this case.

5.6 Diagnosis

Chondrosarcoma grade 1, focal region can't exclude grade 2.

Suggested Reading

Gietzen L, Pokorski P. Chondrosarcoma of the cervical spine. JAAPA. 2017;30(12):23–5.

Pennington Z, Ehresman J, Pittman PD, et al. Chondrosarcoma of the spine: a narrative review. Spine J. 2021;21(12):2078–96.

Solitary Plasmacytoma of Bone: Case 6

6

6.1 Medical History

Patient is a 55-year-old male. He experienced back pain about 1 month ago and was seen at the local hospital, and the CT scan of the thoracic spine showed no clear abnormality. He had no treatment and was without relief of symptoms. Later, he experienced neck pain, with numbness, decreased muscle tone, and decreased sensory function in the lower extremities.

6.2 Physical Examination

Not recorded in the hospital system.

6.3 Imaging Findings

6.3.1 CT Imaging (Figs. 6.1, 6.2, 6.3, 6.4, 6.5, 6.6, and 6.7)

CT images of the thoracic spine demonstrated compression deformity of T2. There were lytic bone destruction of the vertebral body and posterior elements with soft tissue mass with cortical break and narrow of the central canal.

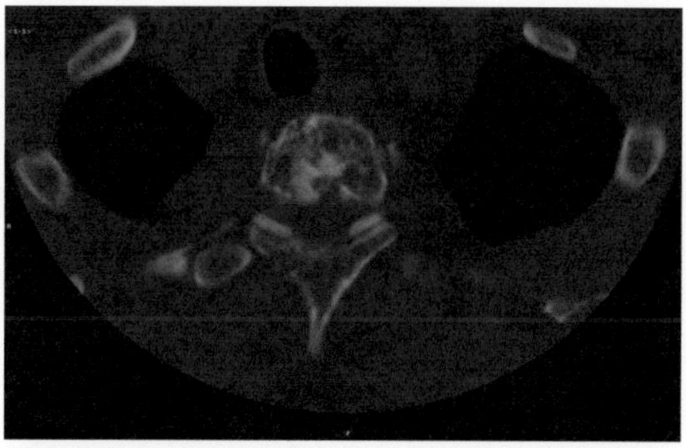

Fig. 6.1 Axial CT image of the thoracic spine in bone window (superior T2 level)

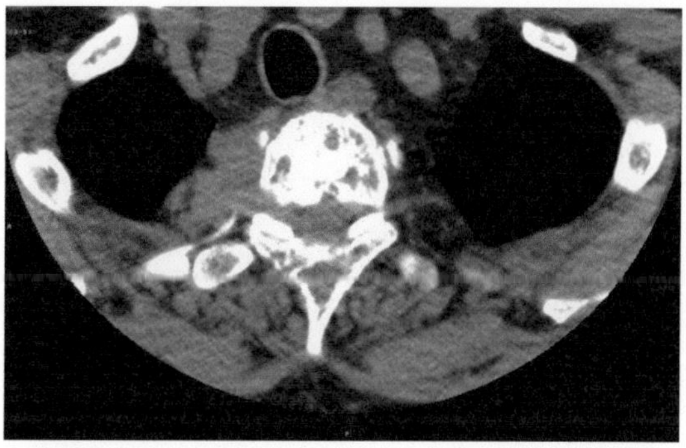

Fig. 6.2 Axial CT image of the thoracic spine in soft tissue window (superior T2 level)

X. Cheng et al., *Imaging of Bone Tumors in Axial Bones*,
https://doi.org/10.1007/978-981-95-2262-0_6

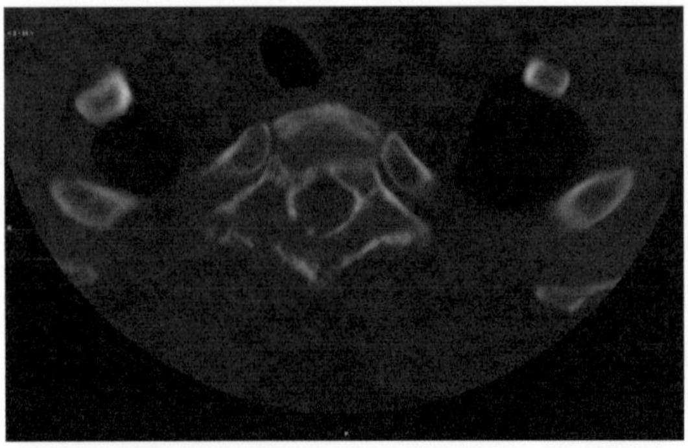

Fig. 6.3 Axial CT image of the thoracic spine in bone window (inferior T2 level)

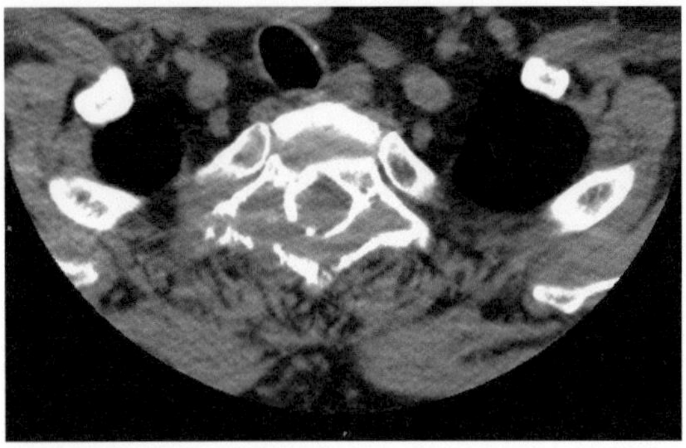

Fig. 6.4 Axial CT image of the thoracic spine in soft tissue window (inferior T2 level)

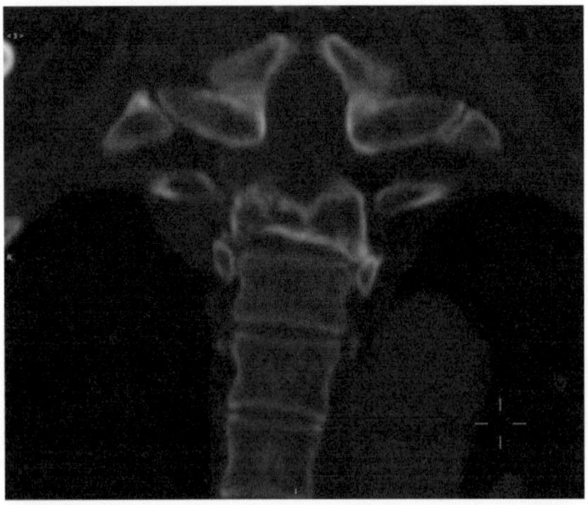

Fig. 6.5 Coronal CT image of the thoracic spine in bone window

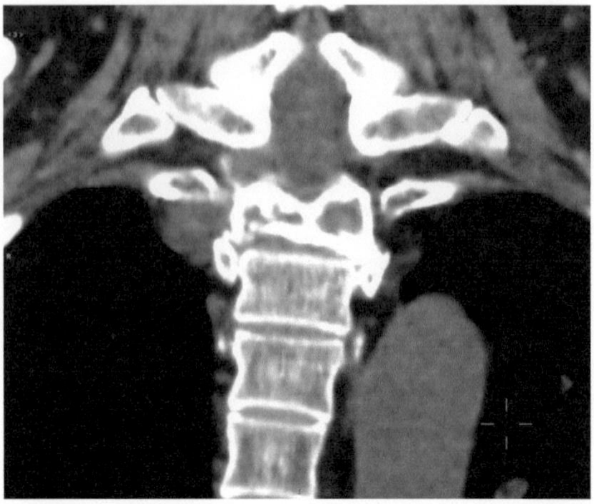

Fig. 6.6 Coronal CT image of the thoracic spine in soft tissue window

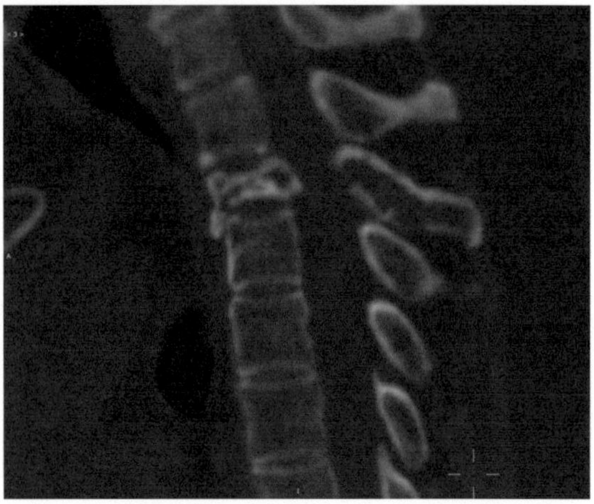

Fig. 6.7 Sagittal CT image of the thoracic spine in bone window

6.3.2 MR Imaging (Figs. 6.8, 6.9, 6.10, and 6.11)

MRI of the thoracic spine demonstrated compression deformity of T2 vertebral body with heterogeneous signals. There is adjacent soft tissue mass. High signal noted around the vertebral body and posterior elements on fat-suppressed T2-weighted sequence and small patchy high signal in the corresponding spinal cord.

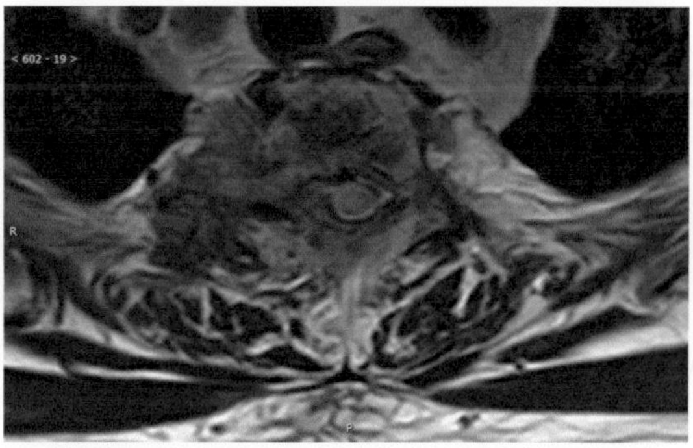

Fig. 6.8 Axial T2-weighted MR image of the thoracic spine

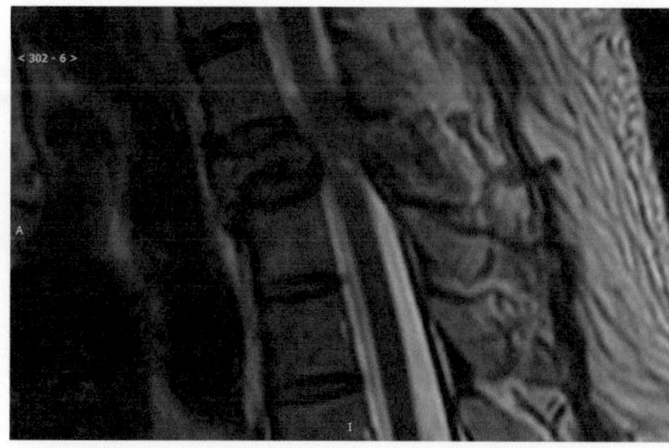

Fig. 6.10 Sagittal T2-weighted MR image of the thoracic spine

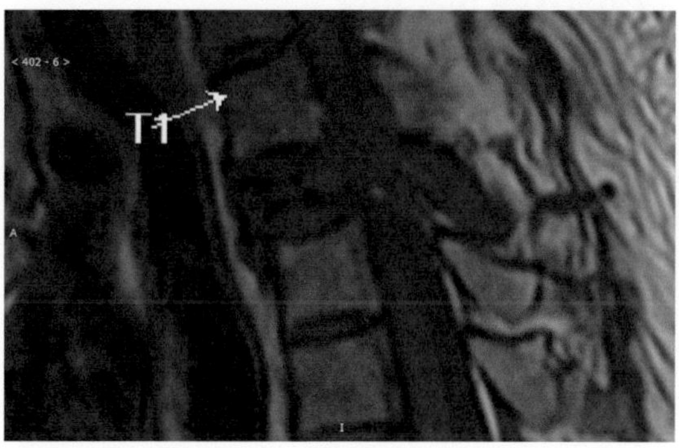

Fig. 6.9 Sagittal T1-weighted MR image of the thoracic spine

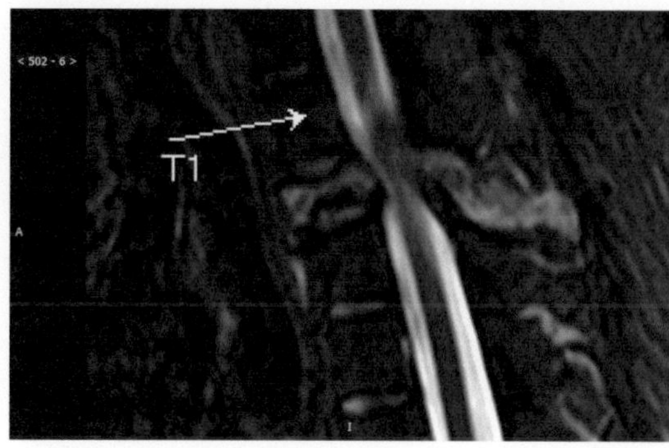

Fig. 6.11 Sagittal fat-suppressed T2-weighted MR image of the thoracic spine

6.4 Description and Discussion from Residents

CT images demonstrated lytic bone destruction of the T2 vertebral body and posterior elements with heterogeneous densities and focal ill defined margin with peripheral mild sclerosis and soft tissue mass. There was compression deformity of the T2 vertebral body on the sagittal images. The soft tissue mass was likely from the tumor growth or from compression, hard to differentiate based on imaging alone. Compression again was noted on the MR images with relative iso-intense signal on T1-weighted and T2-weighted sequences of the vertebral body and posterior elements. Fat-suppressed T2-weighted images showed high signal of the lesion, with narrowing of the spinal canal and change in the spinal cord. Non-contrast MR images are useful for depicting the spinal cord and nerve compressive changes, not helpful at narrowing down the differential diagnosis regarding the pathology of the lesion. With single vertebral body lytic bone destruction, our consideration includes plasmacytoma and giant cell tumor of the bone. Patient is older; we favor plasmacytoma. Differential diagnosis includes eosinophilic granuloma and chondroblastoma. However, usually these entities involve patients of much younger age and with more apparent reactive changes, not consistent with the current case, and thus, can be excluded.

6.5 Analysis and Comments from Professor Cheng Xiao-Guang

Spinal CT showed bone destruction of T2 vertebral body and posterior elements. MR images demonstrated the lesion with discontinuous cortex, indicating an aggressive process. The lesion was isolated to one vertebral segment and involved both the vertebral body and posterior elements extensively, not consistent with giant cell tumor of bone; my top consideration is aggressive hematologic disease. Given the patient's age, my first consideration is plasmacytoma or multiple myeloma. Plasmacytoma and multiple myeloma have similar processes in different stages. Differential diagnosis includes aggressive hemangioma; further evaluation with contrast-enhanced CT/MRI can be helpful.

6.6 Diagnosis

Solitary plasmacytoma of bone.

Suggested Reading

Ariyaratne S, Jenko N, Iyengar KP, et al. Primary osseous malignancies of the spine. Diagnostics (Basel). 2023;13(10):1801.

Major NM, Helms CA, Richardson WJ. The "mini brain": plasmacytoma in a vertebral body on MR imaging. AJR Am J Roentgenol. 2000;175(1):261–3.

7 Schwannoma: Case 7

7.1 Medical History

Patient is a 37-year-old male. He suffered from back pain without clear causes with left leg numbness after long distance walking about 2 weeks ago.

7.2 Physical Examination

Large area of numbness in the left leg.

7.3 Imaging Findings

7.3.1 CT Imaging (Figs. 7.1, 7.2, 7.3, 7.4, and 7.5)

CT images of the thoracic spine demonstrated lytic bone destruction around T3 vertebral body, right pedicle, bilateral lamina, and transverse process with peripheral sclerosis. There is enlargement of the right neuroforamen with soft tissue mass extending out from the neuroforamen and compression of the spinal cord. Mild enhancement of the soft tissue mass was noted.

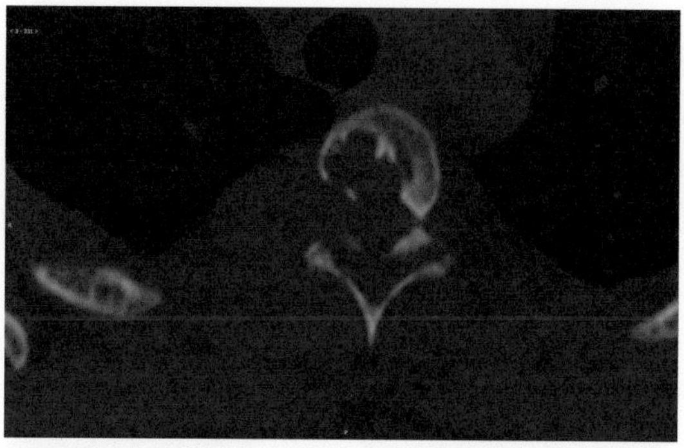

Fig. 7.1 Axial CT image of the thoracic spine in bone window (T3 level)

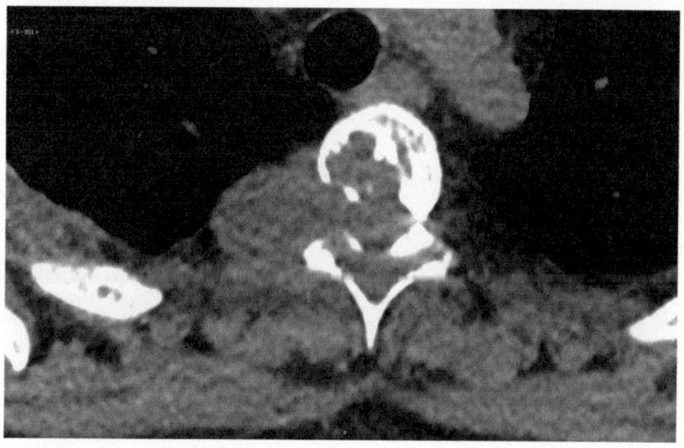

Fig. 7.2 Axial CT image of the thoracic spine in soft tissue window (T3 level)

X. Cheng et al., *Imaging of Bone Tumors in Axial Bones*,
https://doi.org/10.1007/978-981-95-2262-0_7

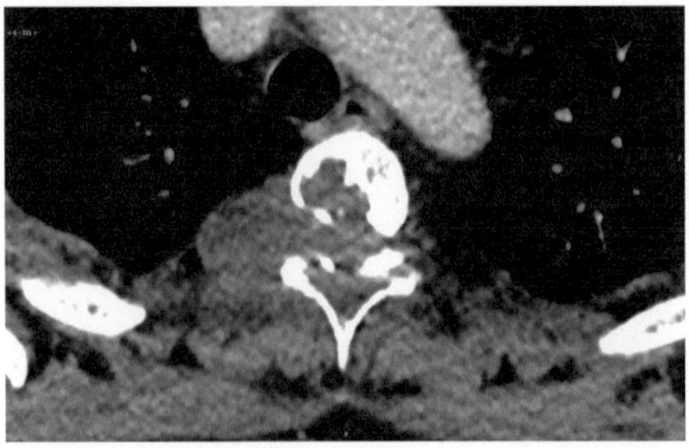

Fig. 7.3 Axial post-contrast CT image of the thoracic spine in soft tissue window (T3 level)

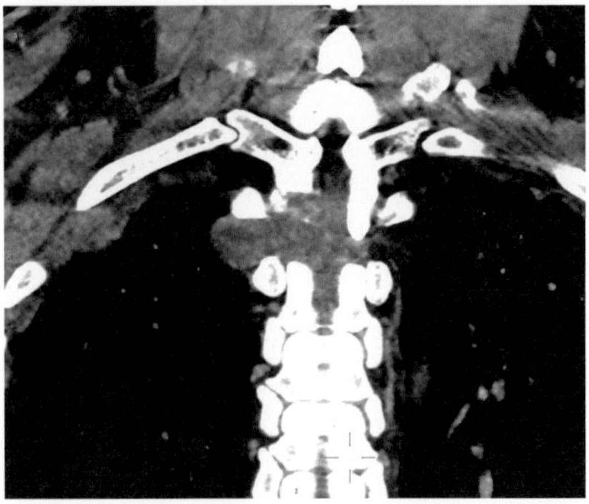

Fig. 7.4 Coronal post-contrast CT image of the thoracic spine in soft tissue window

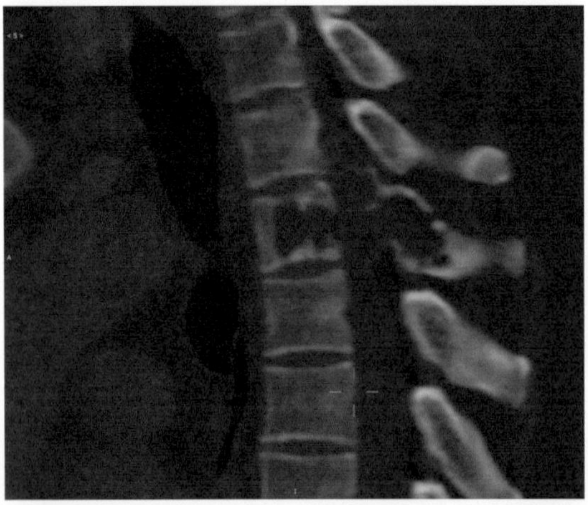

Fig. 7.5 Sagittal CT image of the thoracic spine in bone window

7.3.2 MR Imaging (Figs. 7.6, 7.7, 7.8, 7.9, 7.10, 7.11, 7.12, 7.13, and 7.14)

MRI of the thoracic spine demonstrated dumbbell-shaped soft tissue mass around the neuroforamen of T3–4 on the right. The lesion demonstrated isointense T1, heterogeneous slightly high T2 signals with destruction of the right T3 vertebral body, right pedicle, bilateral lamina, and transverse process with compression of the spinal cord at the level. Avid enhancement was noted.

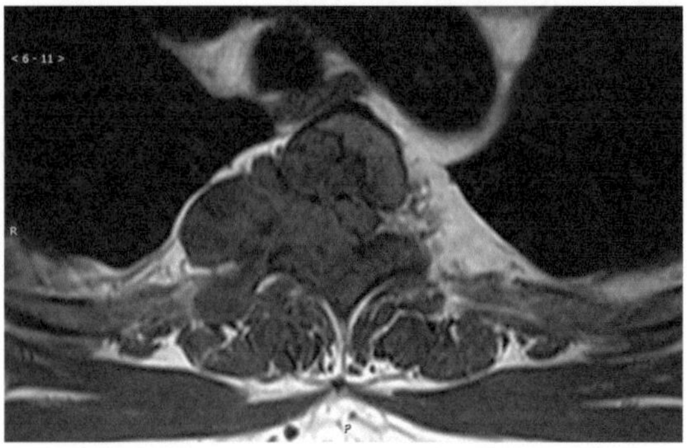

Fig. 7.6 Axial T1-weighted MR image of the thoracic spine (T3 level)

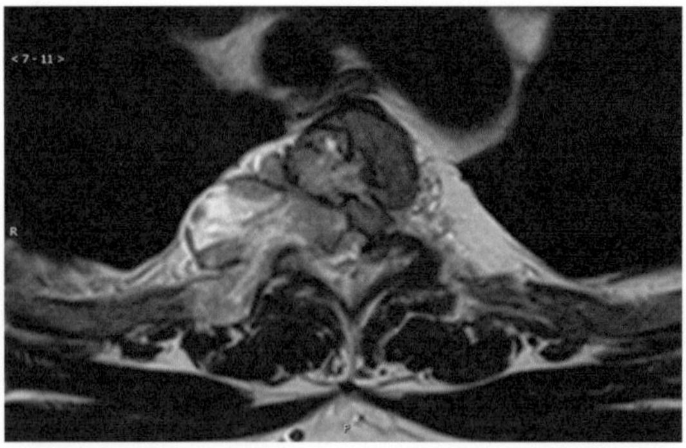

Fig. 7.7 Axial T2-weighted MR image of the thoracic spine (T3 level)

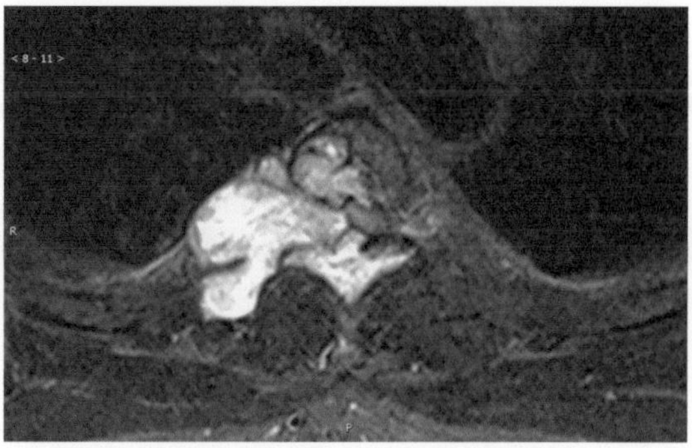

Fig. 7.8 Axial fat-suppressed T2-weighted MR image of the thoracic spine (T3 level)

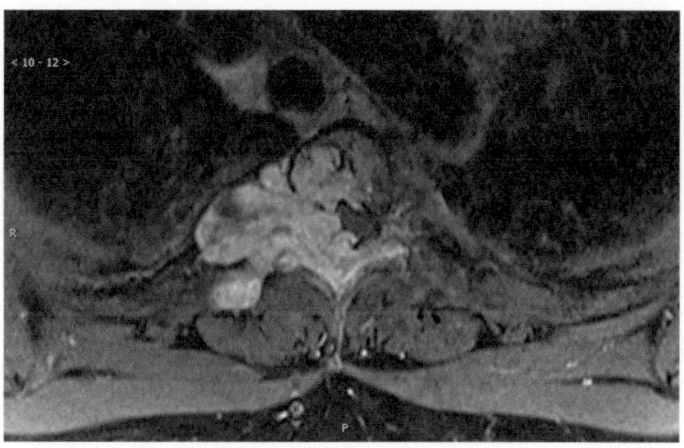

Fig. 7.9 Axial post-contrast fat-suppressed T1-weighted MR image of the thoracic spine (T3 level)

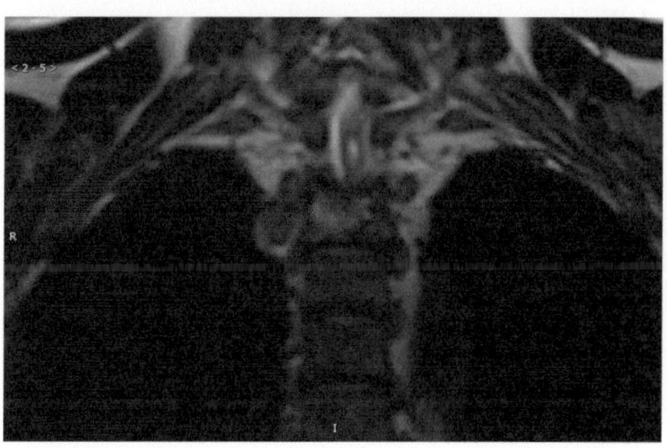

Fig. 7.10 Coronal T2-weighted MR image of the thoracic spine

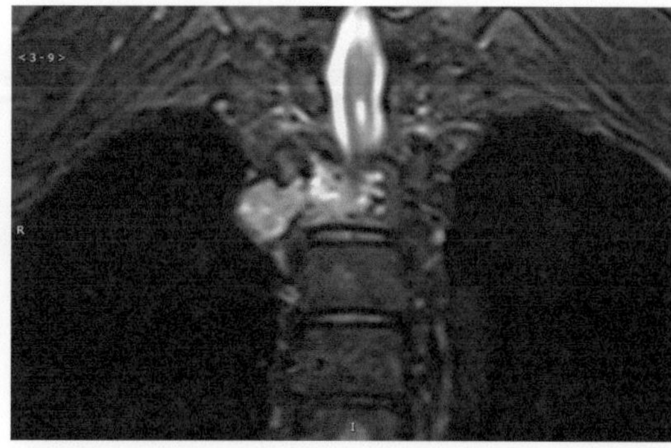

Fig. 7.11 Coronal fat-suppressed T2-weighted MR image of the thoracic spine

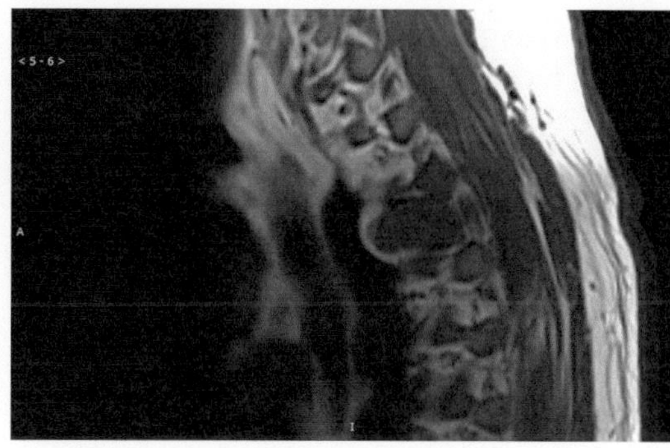

Fig. 7.12 Sagittal T1-weighted MR image of the thoracic spine

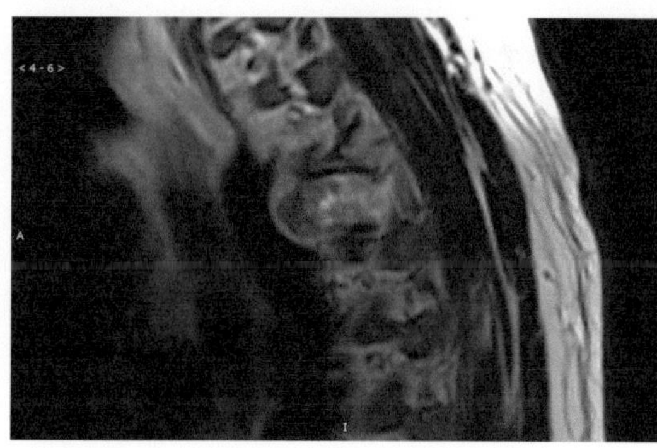

Fig. 7.13 Sagittal T2-weighted MR image of the thoracic spine

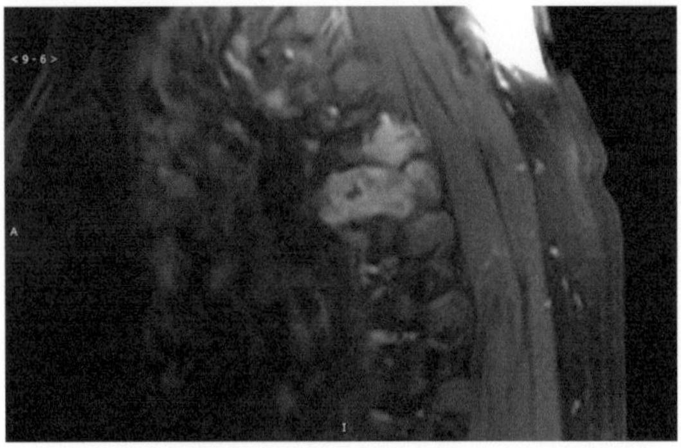

Fig. 7.14 Sagittal post-contrast fat-suppressed T1-weighted MR image of the thoracic spine

7.4 Description and Discussion from Residents

CT images demonstrated lytic destruction of the T3 vertebral body and posterior elements, with lobulated morphology and bony crests with peripheral sclerosis and soft tissue mass on the right. The sagittal images showed the center of the lesion is around the right neuroforamen with invasion to both anterior and posterior cortices. Homogenous densities noted on the non-contrast scan without calcification or ossification. There was irregular margin of the lesion posteriorly, indicating some aggressiveness. The above findings pointed to a peripheral nerve sheath tumor originated from the neuroforamen with epidural tumor in the differential diagnosis, such as metastatic lesion or lymphoma. With no significant enhancement, we can exclude metastatic lesion.

MRI images demonstrated the mass centered around the right neuroforamen of T3–4 with obvious enlargement and mass effect in the central canal and extension both anteriorly and posteriorly affecting the vertebral body and posterior elements. Heterogeneous signal noted of the lesion with some high T2 signal indicating fluid. Avid enhancement was noted, which can exclude lymphoma. We need to include bone tumor, such as giant cell tumor of bone. However, with bone tumor, there can be para-vertebral soft tissue mass but usually without enlargement of the neuroforamen and usually with osseous expansile changes, not consistent with the current case. Overall, we favor peripheral nerve sheath tumor with some invasiveness and epidural neoplasm in the differential diagnosis.

7.5 Analysis and Comments from Professor Cheng Xiao-Guang

The CT images showed bone destruction of the T3 vertebral body and posterior elements with soft tissue mass around the right neuroforamen. We need to focus on the center of the lesion and the relationship with the neuroforamen. The right neuroforamen was significantly enlarged; the top consideration is peripheral nerve sheath tumor. The MR images showed the extent of the disease more precisely and clearly depicted the origin of the lesion from the neuroforamen with invasion to the adjacent osseous structures, with malignant neurogenic neoplasm of our top consideration. Plasmacytoma and lymphoma are in the differential diagnosis; however, involvement of the neuroforamen is rare with these entities.

7.6 Diagnosis

Schwannoma.

Suggested Reading

Wang YQ, Hu JX, Yang SM, et al. Intraosseous schwannoma of the mobile spine: a report of twenty cases. Eur Spine J. 2018;27(12):3092–104.

Zadeh FS, Azhideh A, Mantilla JG, et al. Imaging features of intraosseous schwannoma: a case series and review of the literature. Diagnostics (Basel). 2023;13(9):1610.

8 Hobnail Hemangioma of Bone: Case 8

8.1 Medical History

Patient is a 26-year-old male. He started to experience increasing back pain without clear causes about 11 months ago. Abnormalities around T4 vertebral body and left 4th and 5th ribs were discovered about 7 months ago and followed with biopsy.

8.2 Physical Examination

Point tenderness around transverse process of T4 and left posterior 4th and 5th ribs without palpable mass.

8.3 Imaging Findings

8.3.1 CT Imaging (Figs. 8.1, 8.2, 8.3, 8.4, 8.5, 8.6, 8.7, and 8.8)

CT images of the thoracic spine demonstrated multiple areas of osseous changes involving the left T4 vertebral body, left pedicle, lamina, and left posterior 4th rib. There were increased bone densities with focal disruption of the cortex and soft tissue mass. Avid enhancement noted.

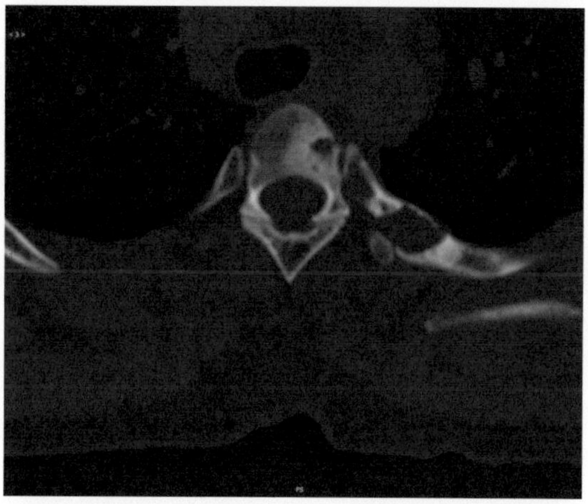

Fig. 8.1 Axial CT image of the thoracic spine in bone window (superior T4 level)

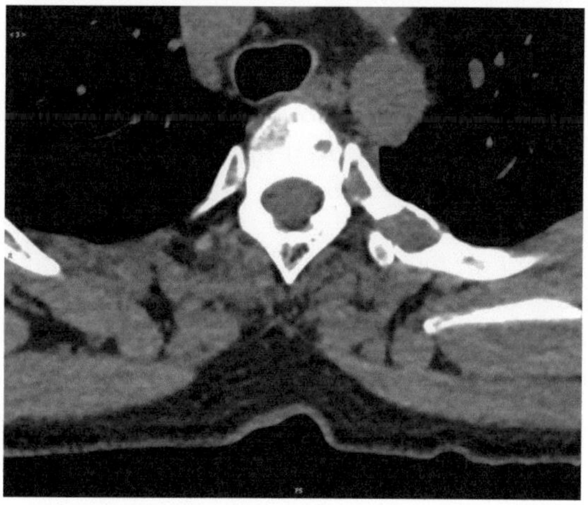

Fig. 8.2 Axial CT image of the thoracic spine in soft tissue window (superior T4 level)

X. Cheng et al., *Imaging of Bone Tumors in Axial Bones*,
https://doi.org/10.1007/978-981-95-2262-0_8

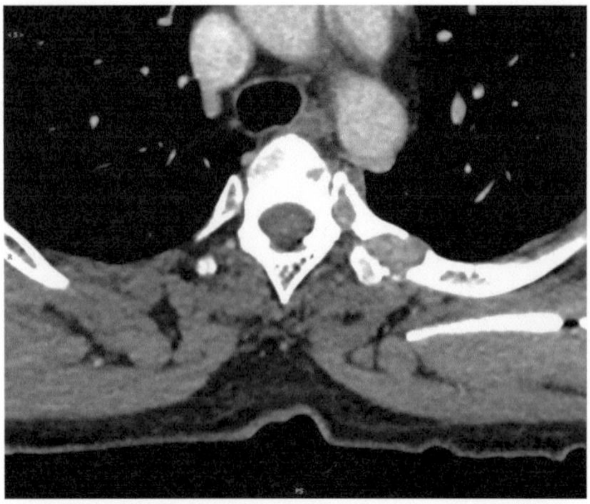

Fig. 8.3 Axial post-contrast CT image of the thoracic spine in soft tissue window (superior T4 level)

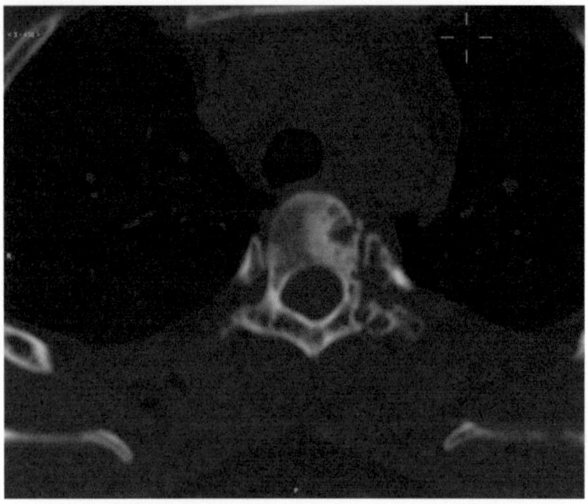

Fig. 8.4 Axial CT image of the thoracic spine in bone window (inferior T4 level)

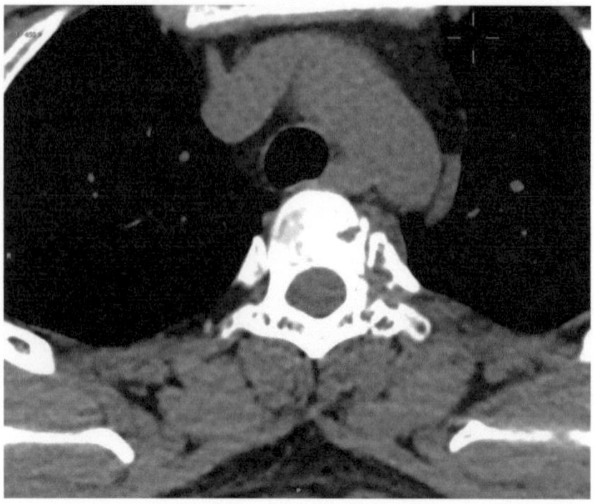

Fig. 8.5 Axial CT image of the thoracic spine in soft tissue window (inferior T4 level)

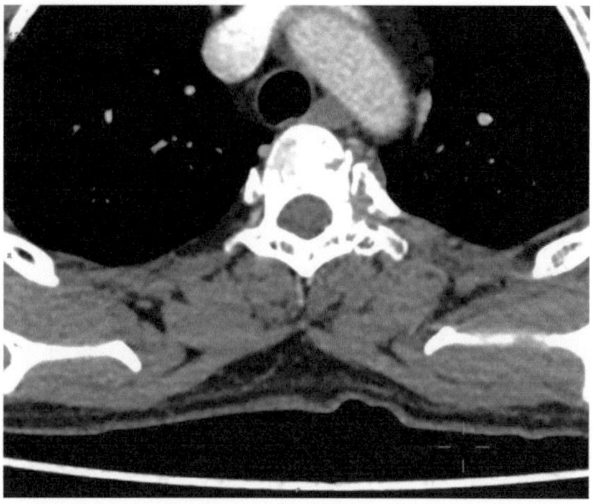

Fig. 8.6 Axial post-contrast CT image of the thoracic spine in soft tissue window (inferior T4 level)

8.3.2 MR Imaging (Figs. 8.9, 8.10, 8.11, and 8.12)

MRI of the thoracic spine demonstrated multiple areas of bone destruction involving left T4 vertebral body, left pedicle, lamina and transverse process, and left posterior 4th rib. The lesions demonstrated isointense T1, high T2, and heterogeneous high T2 signal on fat-suppressed sequences. There was focal soft tissue mass disrupting the cortex and avid heterogeneous enhancement.

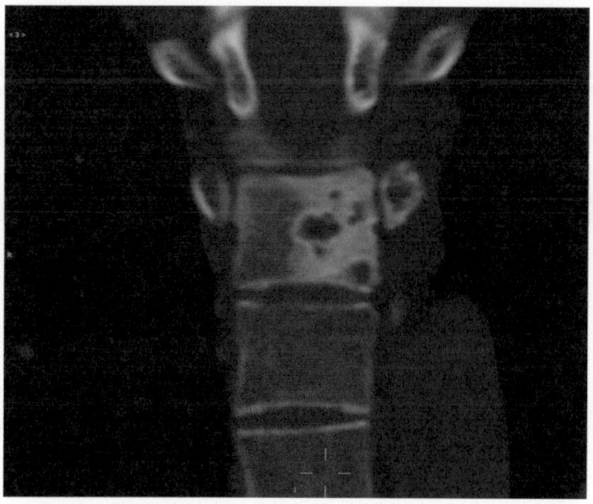

Fig. 8.7 Coronal CT image of the thoracic spine in bone window

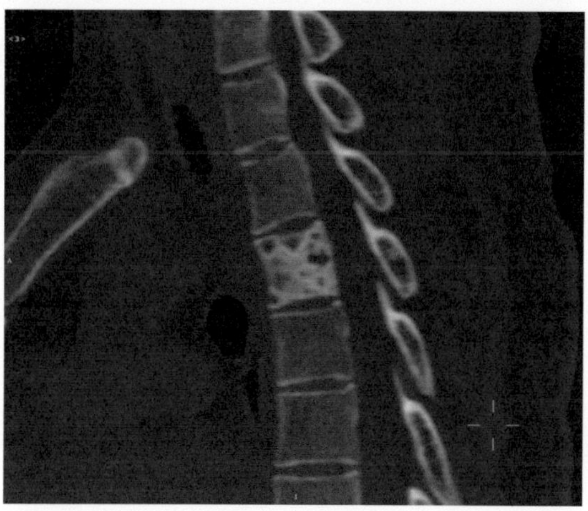

Fig. 8.8 Sagittal CT image of the thoracic spine in bone window

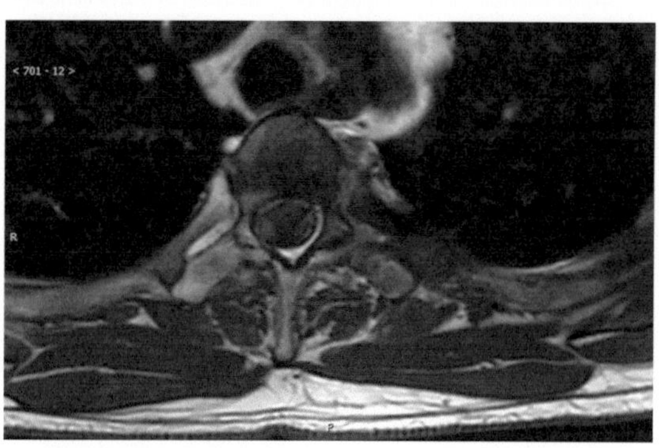

Fig. 8.9 Axial T1-weighted MR image of the thoracic spine

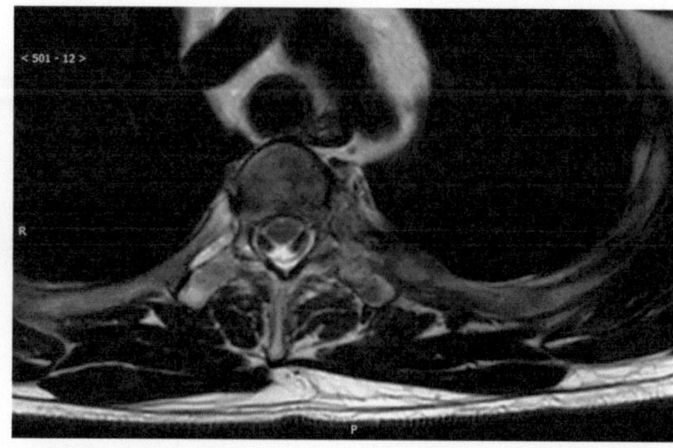

Fig. 8.10 Axial T2-weighted MR image of the thoracic spine

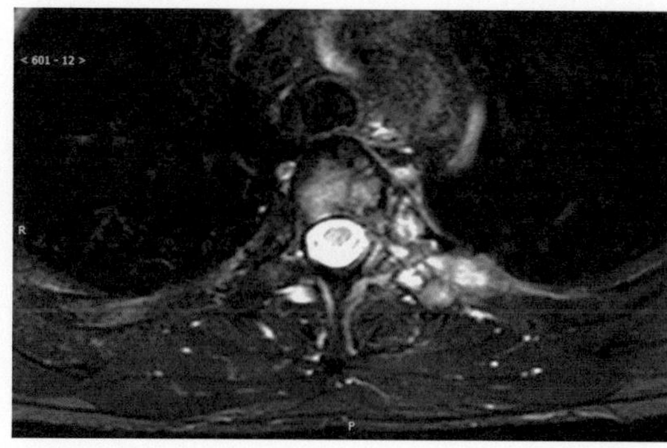

Fig. 8.11 Axial fat-suppressed T2-weighted MR image of the thoracic spine

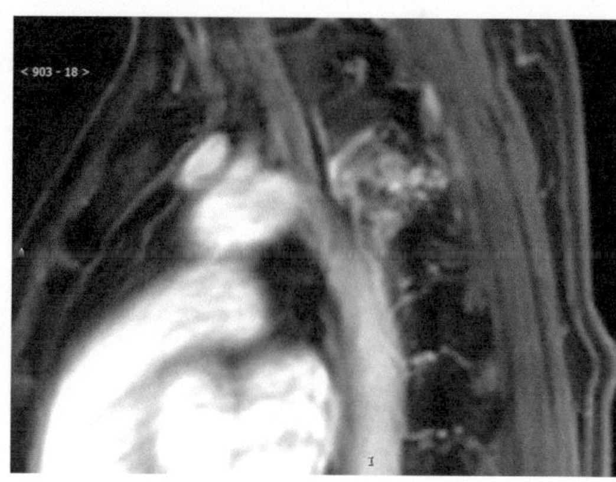

Fig. 8.12 Sagittal post-contrast fat-suppressed T1-weighted MR image of the thoracic spine

8.4 Description and Discussion from Residents

Patient is a young male. CT images demonstrated multiple areas of bone destruction involving left T4 vertebral body, posterior elements, and left posterior 4th rib. There was focal reactive sclerosis with mild enhancement and no involvement of the costovertebral joints. Multiple areas of bone destruction with reactive sclerosis involving multiple bones in a young male patient are unlikely to be neoplasm. We consider low virulent infection or eosinophilic granuloma (Langerhans cell histiocytosis). MR images demonstrated heterogeneous high T2 signal on fat-suppressed T2-weighted images with mild surrounding edema with avid heterogeneous enhancement. Given this type of "destroy and repair at the same time, multifocal, peri-lesion edema and avid enhancement" imaging pattern, we favor eosinophilic granuloma with low virulent infection and tuberculosis in the differential diagnosis. However, no sequestrum was noted of the current case. In addition, there were many solid components with the lesion, raising the possibility of vascular tumor, such as hemangioendothelioma.

8.5 Analysis and Comments from Professor Cheng Xiao-Guang

Patient is a young male. CT images demonstrated multiple areas of bone destruction involving left T4 vertebral body, posterior elements, left posterior 4th rib with focal sclerosis, and preserved costovertebral joints and facet joints. Enhancement was present. With the above findings, eosinophilic granuloma is a consideration. MR images showed clear high T2 signal on fat-suppressed sequences within the lesion with multifocal appearances, most suggestive of vascular tumor, such as hemangioendothelioma. However, that is usually seen around the long bones in the extremities, rare in the spine. Joint spaces are clearly preserved in this case, so infectious causes are not considered.

8.6 Diagnosis

Hobnail hemangioma (also known as targetoid hemosiderotic hemangioma) of bone.

Suggested Reading

Haseli S, Mansoori B, Shafiei M, et al. A review of posteromedial lesions of the chest wall: what should a chest radiologist know? Diagnostics (Basel). 2022;12(2):301.

Kato K, Teferi N, Challa M, et al. Vertebral hemangiomas: a review on diagnosis and management. J Orthop Surg Res. 2024;19(1):310.

Wang B, Zhang L, Yang S. Atypical radiographic features of aggressive vertebral hemangiomas. J Bone Joint Surg Am. 2019;101(11):979–86.

9 Giant Cell Tumor of Bone: Case 9

9.1 Medical History

Patient is a 53-year-old female. She started to experience back pain without clear causes about 8 months ago and worsening. She was seen at an outside institution and suggested "pulmonary mass."

9.2 Physical Examination

There is a protuberance around the spinous process of T6 on the left with a palpable bony protuberance with point tenderness and increased skin temperature in the region.

9.3 Imaging Findings

9.3.1 Radiograph (Figs. 9.1 and 9.2)

Radiographs of the thoracic spine show semicircle soft tissue mass around the left lateral T5 to T7 with smooth border and relatively homogeneous density. No abnormality noted of the adjacent vertebral body and intervertebral disc space.

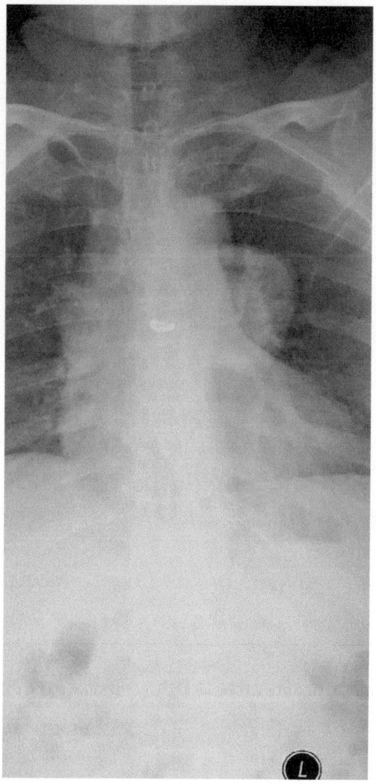

Fig. 9.1 Frontal view of the thoracic spine

X. Cheng et al., *Imaging of Bone Tumors in Axial Bones*,
https://doi.org/10.1007/978-981-95-2262-0_9

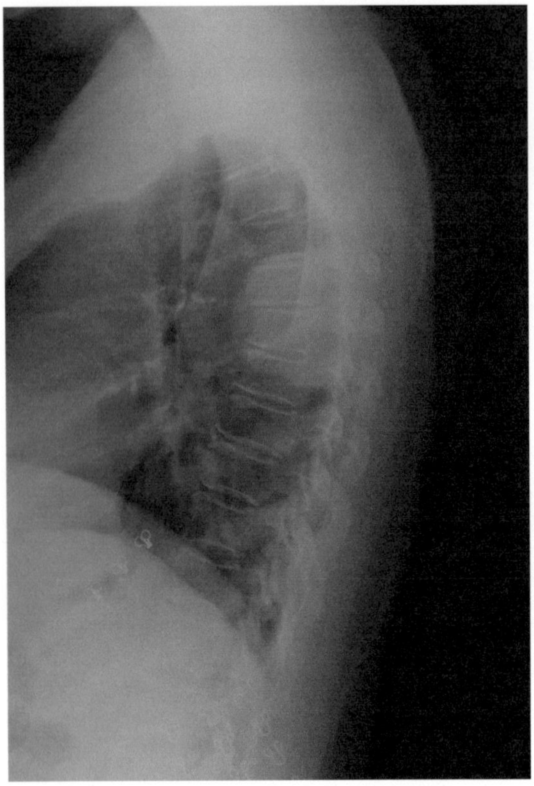

Fig. 9.2 Lateral view of the thoracic spine

9.3.2 CT Imaging (Figs. 9.3, 9.4, 9.5, 9.6, and 9.7)

CT images of the thoracic spine demonstrated partial bone destruction around the left 6th rib and left T6 posterior elements and some of the vertebral body with soft tissue mass of transverse diameter of 5.5 cm. There was noncontinuous peripheral bony shell. The soft tissue mass shows low and intermediate density with heterogeneous avid enhancement.

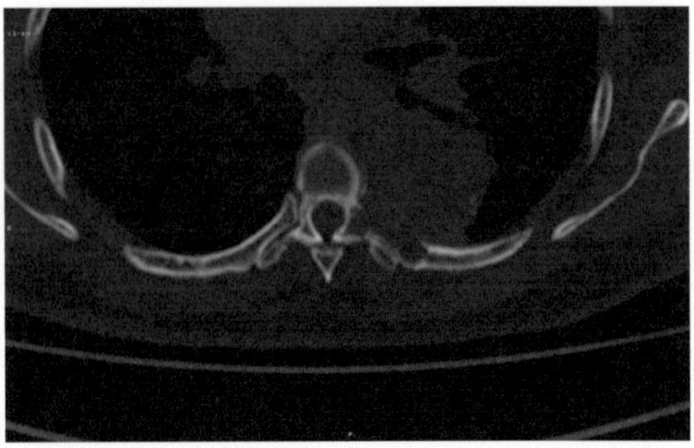

Fig. 9.3 Axial CT image of the thoracic spine in bone window

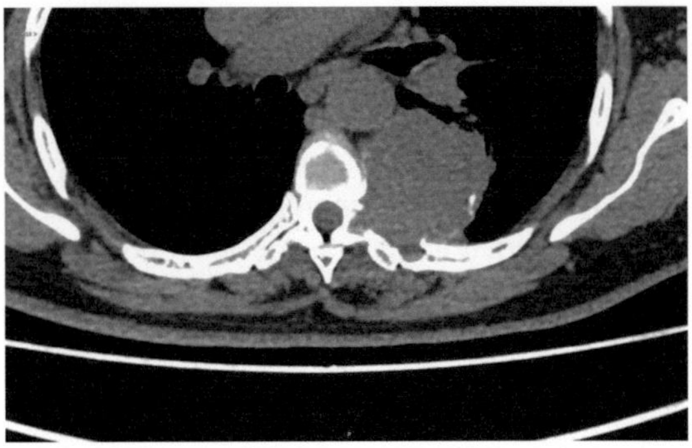

Fig. 9.4 Axial CT image of the thoracic spine in soft tissue window

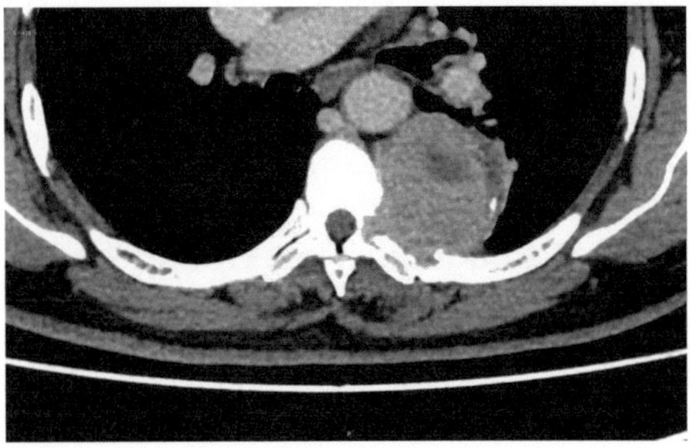

Fig. 9.5 Axial post-contrast CT image of the thoracic in soft tissue window

9.3.3 MR Imaging (Figs. 9.8, 9.9, 9.10, and 9.11)

MRI of the thoracic spine demonstrated bone destruction around the left posterior 6th rib with soft tissue mass and extends to the thoracic cavity, involving the costovertebral junction and posterior element of T6 on the left. There was heterogeneous signal within the lesion, with majority of the lesion demonstrated relatively low T2 signal and heterogeneous enhancement.

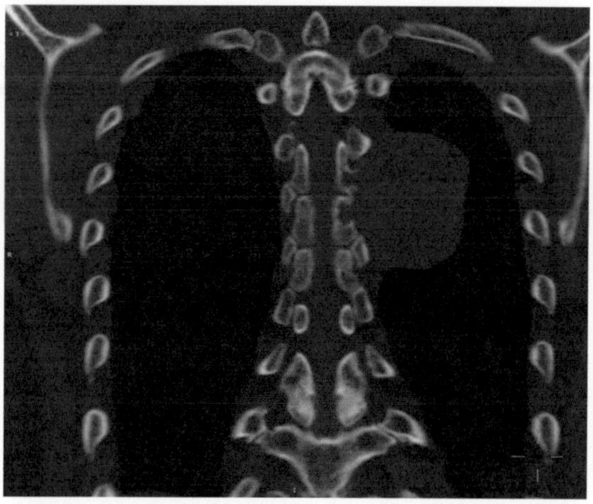

Fig. 9.6 Coronal CT image of the thoracic spine in bone window

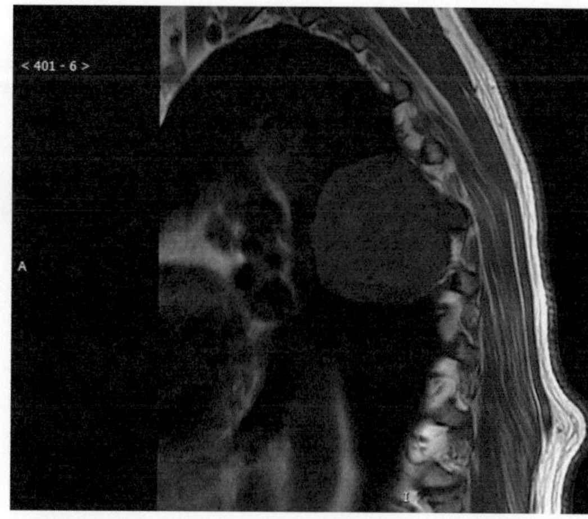

Fig. 9.9 Sagittal T1-weighted MR image of the thoracic spine

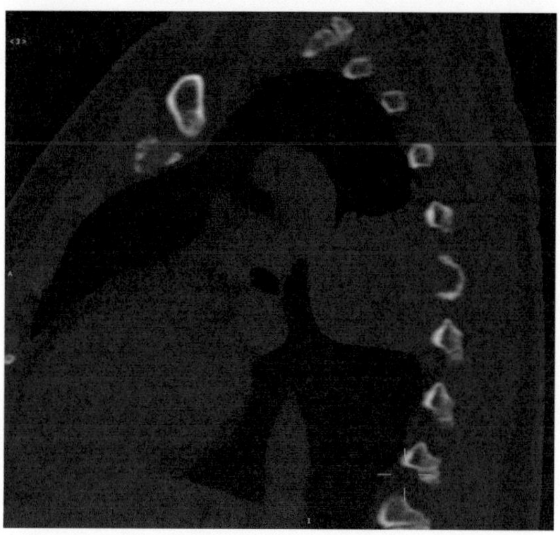

Fig. 9.7 Sagittal CT image of the thoracic spine in bone window

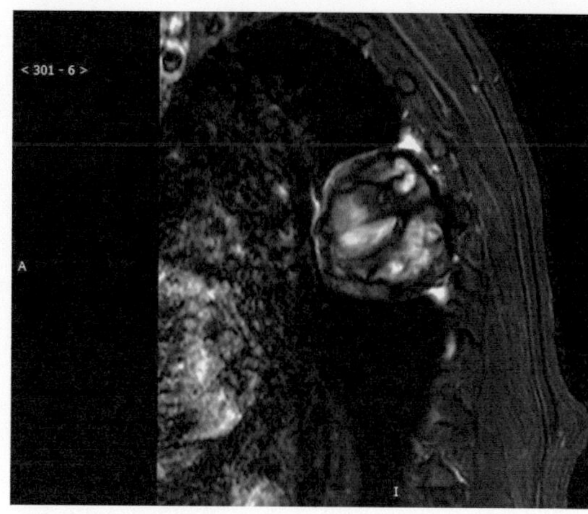

Fig. 9.10 Sagittal fat-suppressed T2-weighted MR image of the thoracic spine

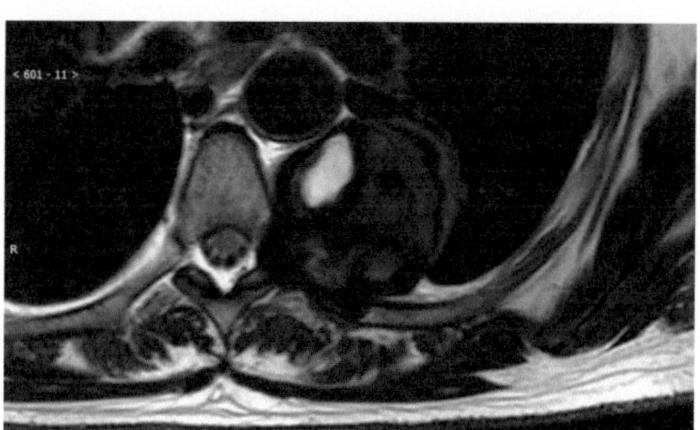

Fig. 9.8 Axial T2-weighted MR image of the thoracic spine

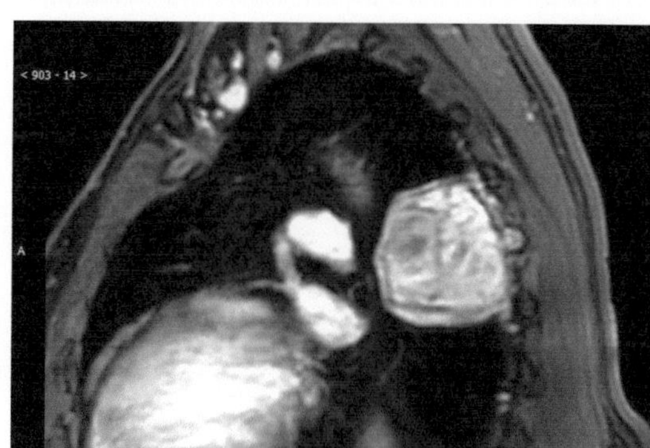

Fig. 9.11 Sagittal post-contrast fat-suppressed T1-weighted MR image of the thoracic spine

9.4 Description and Discussion from Residents

The patient is a middle-aged female. The radiographs showed a large soft tissue mass around left T6 vertebral body with clear and sharp margin and intact adjacent vertebral body and intervertebral disc space, suggesting mass from the posterior mediastinum. CT images demonstrated soft tissue mass on the left of T6 vertebral body with heterogeneous density, focal low density, and peripheral bony shell. There was bone destruction noted at adjacent rib and facet joint with compression of the pulmonary tissue. Avid enhancement was present with area of non-enhancing necrosis internally. There was sharp margin between the mass and adjacent pulmonary tissue with bone destruction, indicating extrapulmonary origin; top consideration is neoplasm from the posterior mediastinum which usually is neurogenic. However, there was no enlargement of the intervertebral foramen. Our next consideration is the neoplasm from the pleura, such as pleural mesothelioma. But with mesothelioma, the shape is usually flat, not consistent with the current case. Our other consideration includes osseous neoplasm. MR images showed heterogeneous T2 signal inside the soft tissue mass and focal high signal on the T1-weighted sequences, suggesting hemorrhage. Given the above findings, our top consideration is peripheral nerve sheath tumor with hemorrhage and paraganglioma, solitary fibrous tumor from the pleura, and pleural mesothelioma in the differential diagnosis.

9.5 Analysis and Comments from Professor Cheng Xiao-Guang

Radiographs of the thoracic spine demonstrated a large soft tissue mass to the left of the thoracic spine with preserved intervertebral spaces. CT images showed likely calcified shell at the periphery of the mass, indicating slow growth. Given the location of the mass, top consideration is neurogenic neoplasm. Attention needs to focus on the change of intervertebral foramen. There was no enlargement of the foramen of this case. Bone destruction of rib, T6 vertebral body, and posterior elements noted on the bone window CT images, especially of the rib, and osseous neoplasm can't be entirely excluded, such as chondrosarcoma.

9.6 Diagnosis

Giant cell tumor of bone.

Suggested Reading

Goldbach AR, Kumaran M, Donuru A, et al. The spectrum of rib neoplasms in adults: a practical approach and multimodal imaging review. AJR Am J Roentgenol. 2020;215(1):165–77.

Haseli S, Mansoori B, Shafiei M, et al. A review of posteromedial lesions of the chest wall: what should a chest radiologist know? Diagnostics (Basel). 2022;12(2):301.

Sakanoue I, Hamakawa H, Onishi E, et al. Giant cell tumor of the rib with direct invasion into the thoracic spine. Gen Thorac Cardiovasc Surg. 2017;65(5):293–6.

10 Hemangioma of Bone: Case 10

10.1 Medical History

Patient is a 50-year-old female. She was found to have a mass at left back at medical evaluation about 5 months ago with mild pain, slightly more at night. She had biopsy afterward.

10.2 Physical Examination

Suspicious mass with point tenderness at left mid-back area.

10.3 Imaging Findings

10.3.1 Radiograph (Figs. 10.1 and 10.2)

Radiographs of ribs show focal heterogeneous high-density mass around the T6 costovertebral joint.

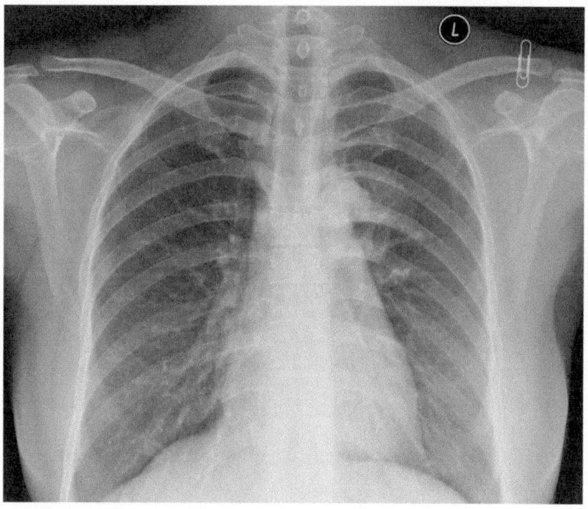

Fig. 10.1 Frontal view of the bilateral ribs

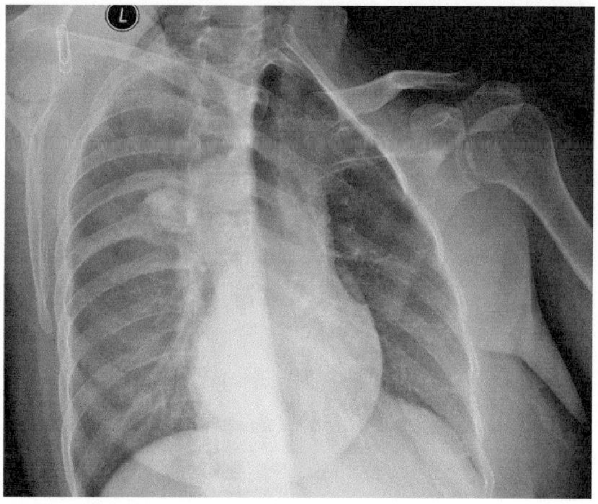

Fig. 10.2 Oblique view of the left rib

10.3.2 CT Imaging (Figs. 10.3, 10.4, 10.5, 10.6, 10.7, and 10.8)

CT images of the thoracic spine and rib demonstrated irregular bony density mass around the 6th costovertebral junction, measuring 3.4 cm × 2.7 cm × 2.4 cm (transverse, anterior

X. Cheng et al., *Imaging of Bone Tumors in Axial Bones*,
https://doi.org/10.1007/978-981-95-2262-0_10

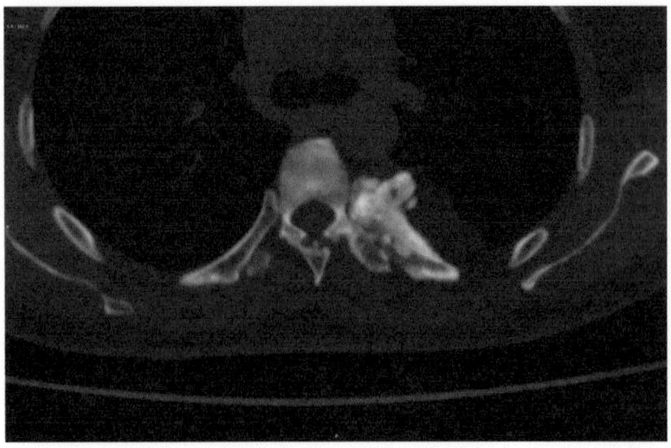

Fig. 10.3 Axial CT image of the thoracic spine in bone window (T6 level)

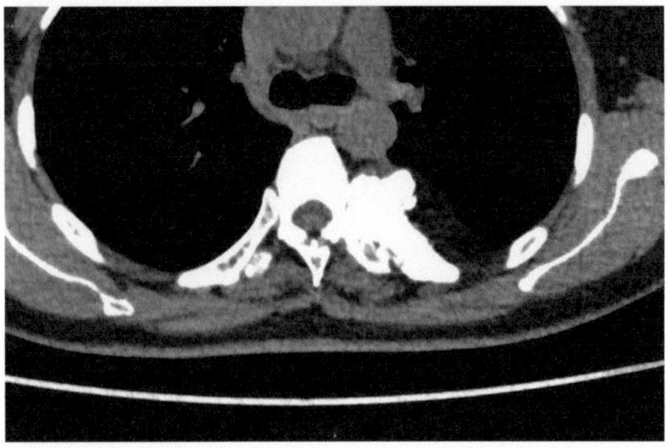

Fig. 10.4 Axial CT image of the thoracic spine in soft tissue window (T6 level)

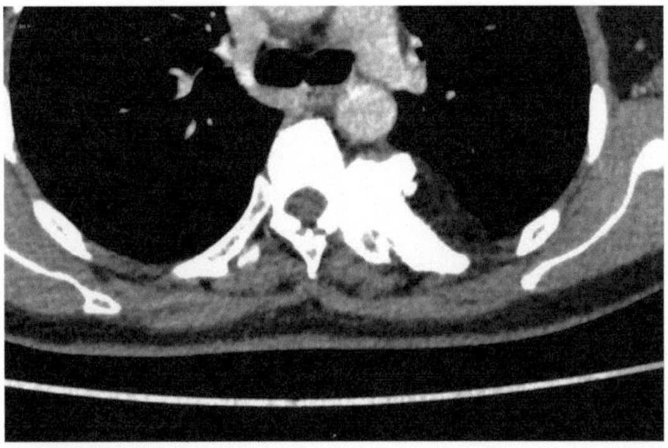

Fig. 10.5 Axial post-contrast CT image of the thoracic in soft tissue window (T6 level)

to posterior, cranial to caudal), with clear margin and internal heterogeneous density and focal periosteal reaction with anterior soft tissue mass. There was also increased density of the T5-T7 vertebral bodies and left posterior 7th rib.

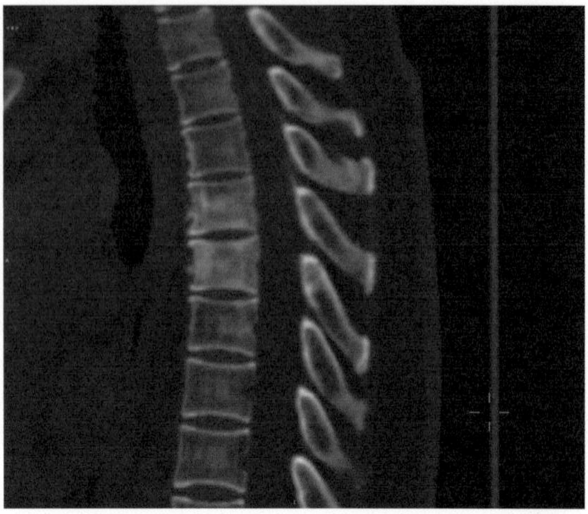

Fig. 10.6 Sagittal CT image of the thoracic spine in bone window

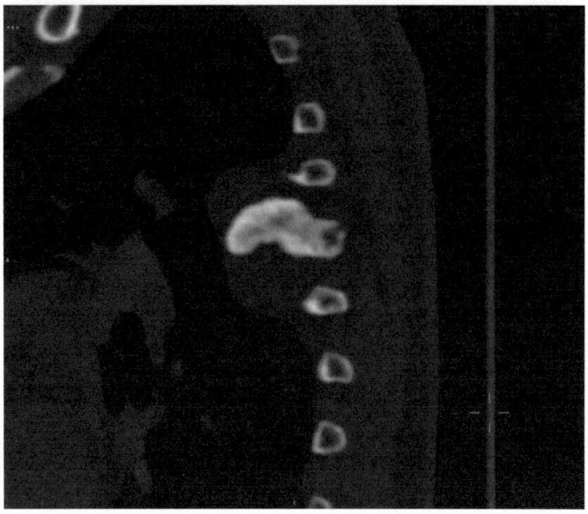

Fig. 10.7 Sagittal CT image of the left 6th rib in bone window

10.3.3 MR Imaging (Figs. 10.9, 10.10, 10.11, 10.12, 10.13, and 10.14)

MRI of the thoracic spine demonstrated irregular shape of the posterior 6th rib head with cauliflower-like protuberance and internal heterogeneous signal with peripheral wrapped flaky high T1WI, high T2WI, and heterogeneous slightly low T2 signal on fat-suppressed sequences with heterogeneous enhancement. Some of these could be post-biopsy changes. There were focal high T2 signals in the T4–T6 vertebral bodies on the fat-suppressed sequences.

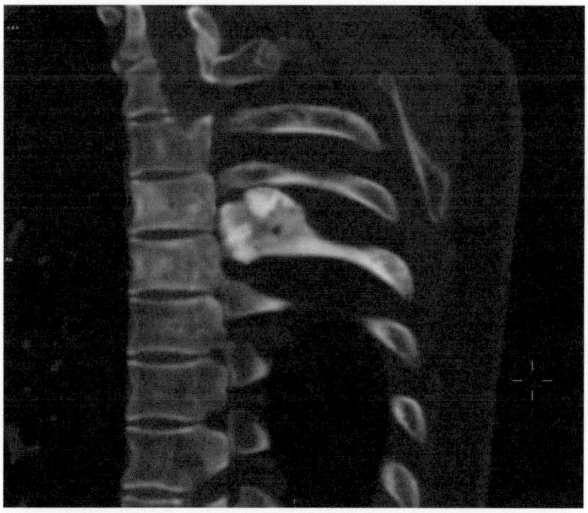

Fig. 10.8 Coronal CT image of the left 6th rib in bone window

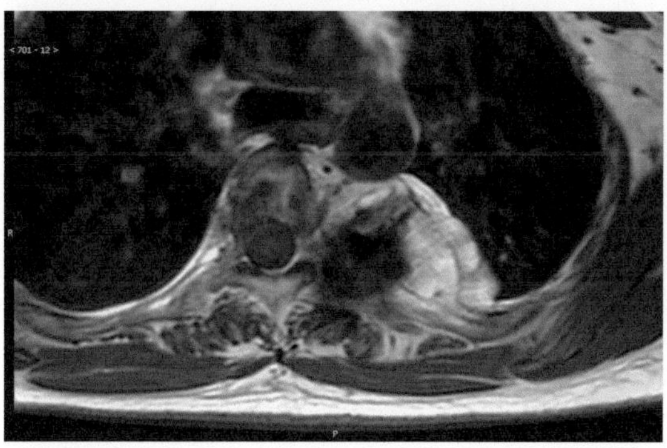

Fig. 10.9 Axial T1-weighted MR image of the thoracic spine

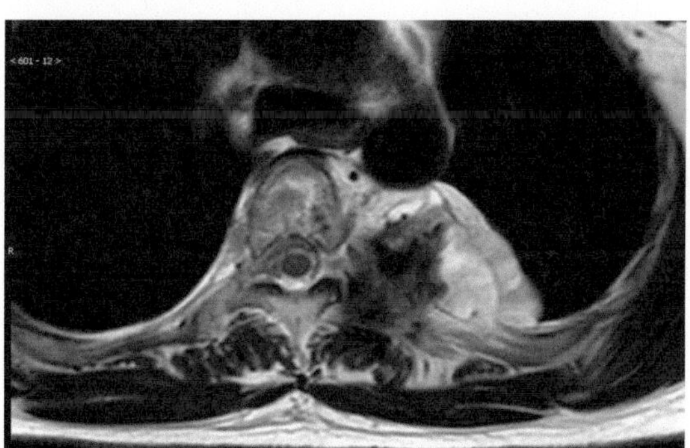

Fig. 10.10 Axial T2-weighted MR image of the thoracic spine

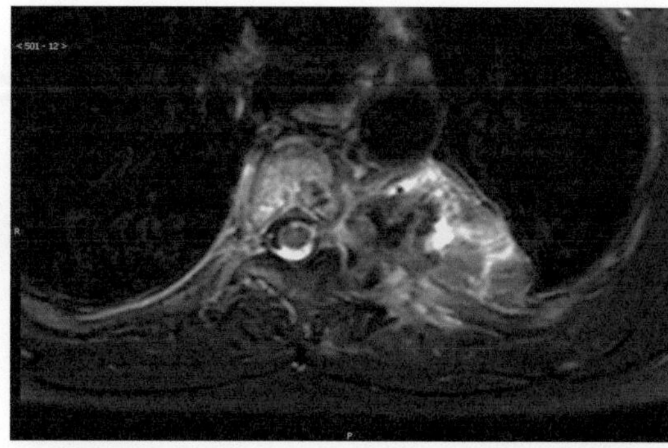

Fig. 10.11 Axial fat-suppressed T2-weighted MR image of the thoracic spine

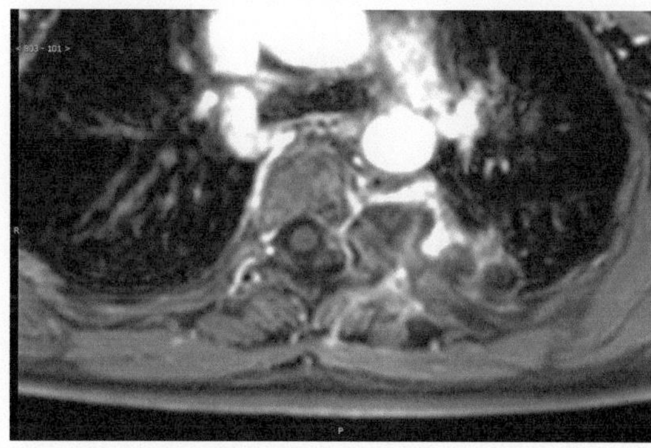

Fig. 10.12 Axial post-contrast fat-suppressed T1-weighted MR image of the thoracic spine

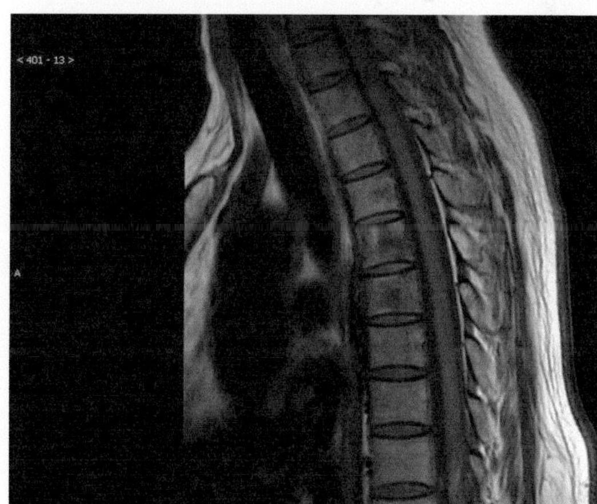

Fig. 10.13 Sagittal T1-weighted MR image of the thoracic spine

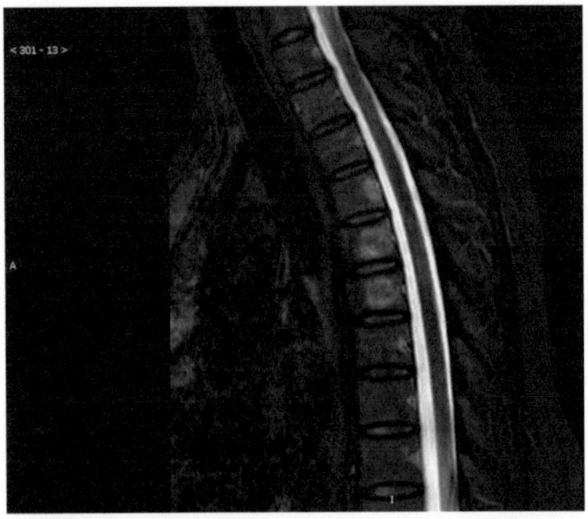

Fig. 10.14 Sagittal fat-suppressed T2-weighted MR image of the thoracic spine

10.4 Description and Discussion from Residents

There were expansile changes around the left T5 and T6 costovertebral junction with increased internal density on radiographs. CT images showed cauliflower-like protuberance at the left posterior 6th rib with internal heterogeneous density and non-smooth margin. There was extensive involvement with focal periosteal reaction. The track from biopsy was noted. There was adjacent soft tissue mass with internal fat density. Focal flaky or septate enhancement noted. The adjacent vertebral bodies demonstrated irregular increased bone density, involving the posterior elements and without narrowing of the central canal and preservation of the costovertebral joint space. Patient is a middle-aged female with multifocal lesions, significant sclerosis, soft tissue mass, and most suggestive of aggressive bone tumor, such as multifocal osteosarcoma, with osteoblastoma, osteoid osteoma in the differential diagnosis. Majority of the lesion showed heterogeneous low signal on MR images. High T1, high T2 signal with focal low T2 signal on the fat-suppressed sequences seen in the adjacent soft tissue, indicating fat component in the lesion. Majority of the lesion showed no obvious enhancement with focal avid enhancement of the surrounding soft tissue and intra-vertebral body lesion. The findings on MR images supported the findings on CT images.

10.5 Analysis and Comments from Professor Cheng Xiao-Guang

Radiographs demonstrated bony density around the left 6th rib head. CT images show the origin of the lesion around the left 6th rib head with obvious sclerosis and fat density noted in the adjacent soft tissue mass. MR images also demonstrated fat components within the lesion. Heterogeneous enhancement noted on the CT images with focal enhancement along the septation and no enhancement of the fatty components. There was increased density of the adjacent vertebral bodies but with preserved shape, which might indicate multifocal lesions, but reactive changes can't be excluded. Bone marrow edema seen of the adjacent vertebral bodies on MR images, not of typical bone destruction. Fatty components within the lesion do not support diagnose of osteosarcoma and osteosarcoma with fatty changes is very rare. The lesion was found at medical evaluation without symptoms and with plenty of mature fat cells; my top consideration is benign process, such as hemangioma. The imaging findings of this case is rather complex; diagnosis needs to be made based on combining pathology findings.

10.6 Diagnosis

Hemangioma of bone.

Suggested Reading

Haseli S, Mansoori B, Shafiei M, et al. A review of posteromedial lesions of the chest wall: what should a chest radiologist know? Diagnostics (Basel). 2022;12(2):301.

Kato K, Teferi N, Challa M, et al. Vertebral hemangiomas: a review on diagnosis and management. J Orthop Surg Res. 2024;19(1):310.

Wang B, Zhang L, Yang S. Atypical radiographic features of aggressive vertebral hemangiomas. J Bone Joint Surg Am. 2019;101(11):979–86.

Langerhans Cell Histiocytosis: Case 11

11

11.1 Medical History

Patient is a 49-year-old male. He suffered from focal swelling and back pain without clear causes about 2 months ago, with stringy feel around the junction of the chest and abdomen and powerless in the left lower extremity.

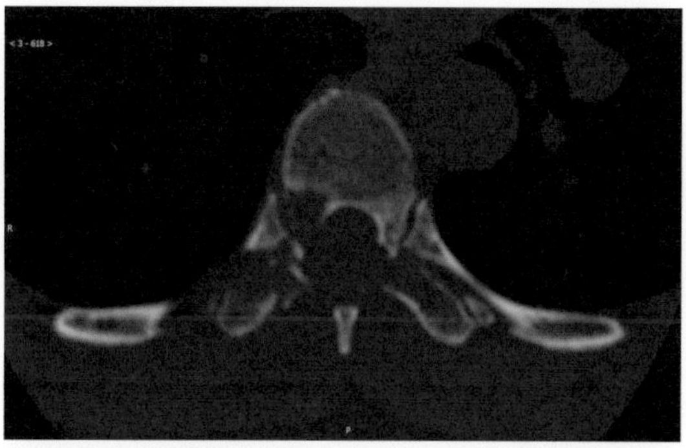

Fig. 11.1 Axial CT image of the thoracic spine in bone window (T7 level)

11.2 Physical Examination

No abnormality.

11.3 Imaging Findings

11.3.1 CT Imaging (Figs. 11.1, 11.2, 11.3, 11.4, 11.5, 11.6, 11.7, 11.8, and 11.9)

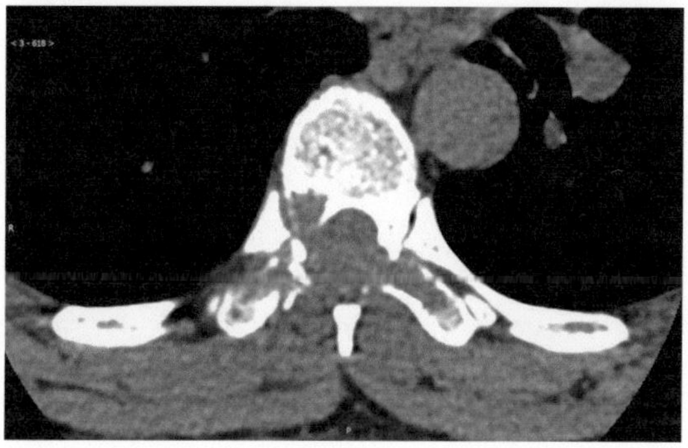

Fig. 11.2 Axial CT image of the thoracic spine in soft tissue window (T7 level)

CT images of the thoracic spine demonstrated relatively well-defined lytic bone destruction of the posterior elements of T7 and right posterior vertebral body with relative homogeneous density and moderate enhancement. There was some residual bone crest and no peripheral sclerosis with focal discontinued cortex with compression to the spinal canal.

X. Cheng et al., *Imaging of Bone Tumors in Axial Bones*,
https://doi.org/10.1007/978-981-95-2262-0_11

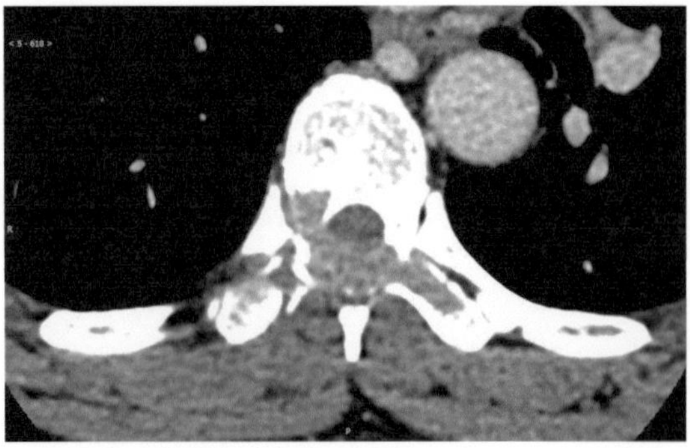

Fig. 11.3 Axial post-contrast CT image of the thoracic spine in soft tissue window (T7 level)

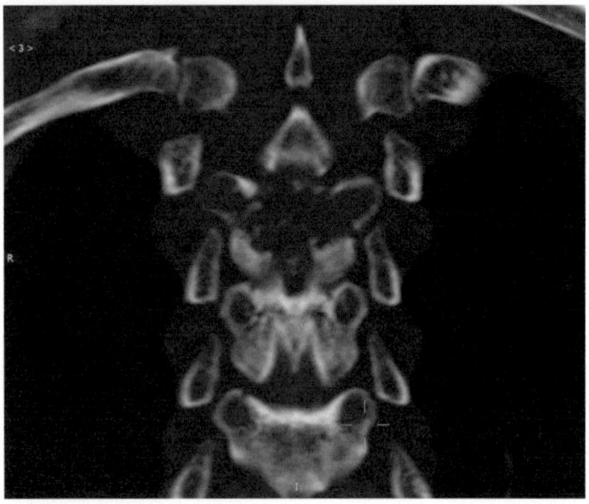

Fig. 11.4 Coronal CT image of the thoracic spine in bone window

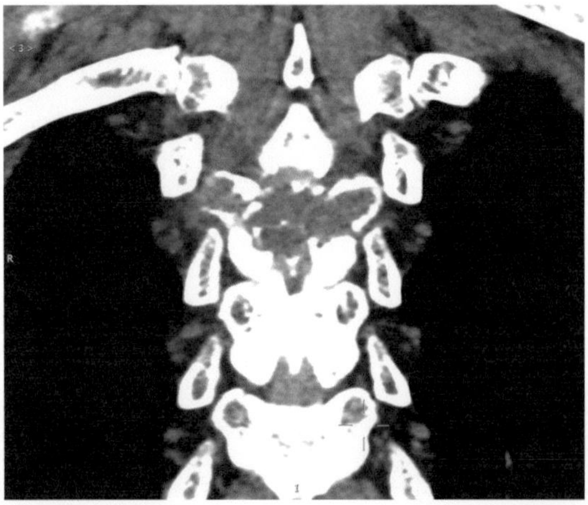

Fig. 11.5 Coronal CT image of the thoracic spine in soft tissue window

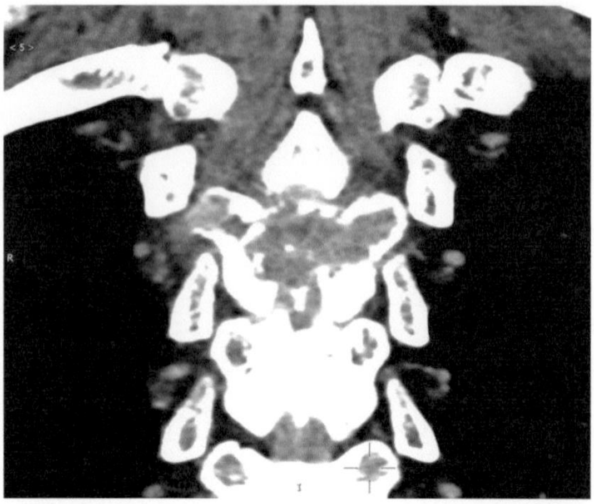

Fig. 11.6 Coronal post-contrast CT image of the thoracic spine in soft tissue window

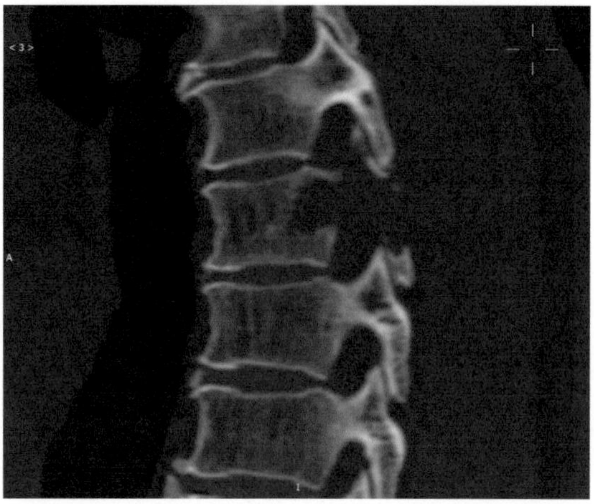

Fig. 11.7 Sagittal CT image of the thoracic spine in bone window

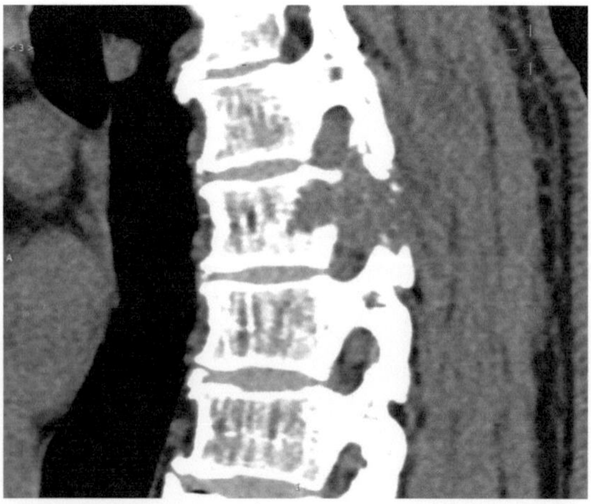

Fig. 11.8 Sagittal CT image of the thoracic spine in soft tissue window

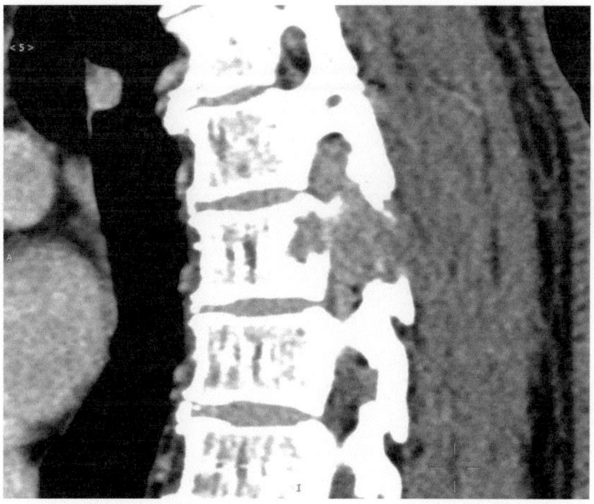

Fig. 11.9 Sagittal post-contrast CT image of the thoracic spine in soft tissue window

11.4 Description and Discussion from Residents

Vertebral body right posterior part, bilateral transverse process, pedicle, and lamina and spinous process of T7 had bone destruction with homogeneous density, clear margin, and focal residual trabeculae. There was extensive bone destruction but mostly confined within the bone, without soft tissue mass protrusion, suggesting benign nature of the lesion. The patient is older; metastatic lesion is a possibility. However, with metastatic disease, with extensive bone destruction usually with relatively large soft tissue mass, not consistent with the current case. Additionally, the pattern bone destruction seen in of this case is similar to plasmacytoma. However, there was no avid enhancement with just heterogeneous enhancement, not consistent with plasmacytoma/multiple myeloma. Overall, the imaging features not supporting aggressive lesion, we favor non-aggressive lesion.

11.5 Analysis and Comments from Professor Cheng Xiao-Guang

The patient is a middle-aged male. There was bone destruction of the T7 vertebral body, bilateral transverse process, pedicle, and lamina and spinous process of multifocal lesions. There was no internal calcification with clear margin and focal cortex disruption without soft tissue protrusion and mild enhancement. Given multicentric feature of the lesion, indicating aggressive lesion, such as metastatic lesion or multiple myeloma.

11.6 Diagnosis

Langerhans cell histiocytosis.

Suggested Reading

Huang W, Yang X, Cao D. Eosinophilic granuloma of spine in adults: a report of 30 cases and outcome. Acta Neurochir (Wien). 2010;152(7):1129–37.

Rodallec MH, Feydy A, Larousserie F, et al. Diagnostic imaging of solitary tumors of the spine: what to do and say. Radiographics. 2008;28(4):1019–41.

Vidal JA, Murphey MD. Primary tumors of the osseous spine. Magn Reson Imaging Clin N Am. 2007;15(2):239–55. vii

12 Paget Disease of Bone: Case 12

12.1 Medical History

Patient is a 49-year-old female. She started to suffer from back pain about 7 months ago and worsened in the last 1 month.

12.2 Physical Examination

Point tenderness and percussion tenderness around the spinous process of T12 with restricted motion of thoracolumbar spine.

12.3 Imaging Findings

12.3.1 Radiograph (Figs. 12.1 and 12.2)

Radiographs of the thoracolumbar spine show increased bone density of the T12 vertebral body and posterior elements with compression deformity. Bone proliferative changes noted in the adjacent vertebral bodies.

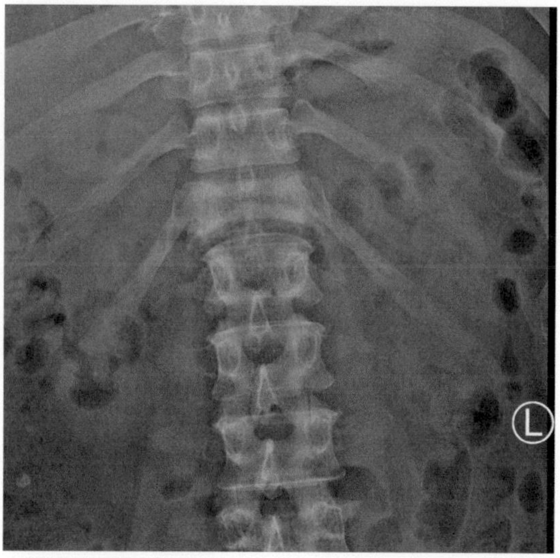

Fig. 12.1 Frontal view of the thoracolumbar spine

12.3.2 CT Imaging (Figs. 12.3, 12.4, 12.5, 12.6, and 12.7)

CT images of the thoracolumbar spine demonstrated compression deformity of T12 vertebral body with thickening of the cortex and coarsen-

X. Cheng et al., *Imaging of Bone Tumors in Axial Bones*,
https://doi.org/10.1007/978-981-95-2262-0_12

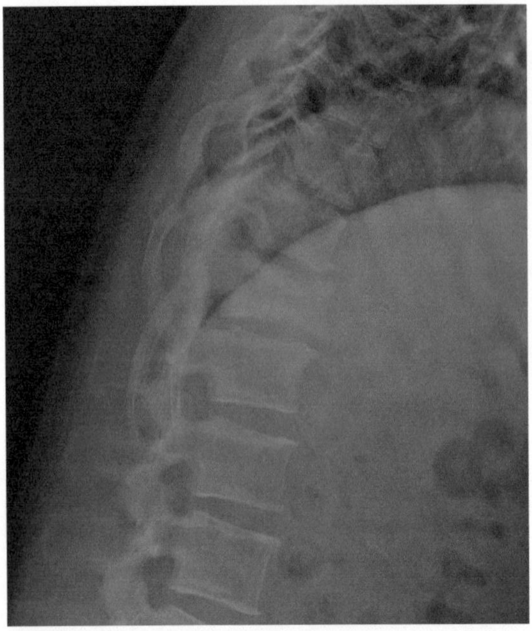

Fig. 12.2 Lateral view of the thoracolumbar spine

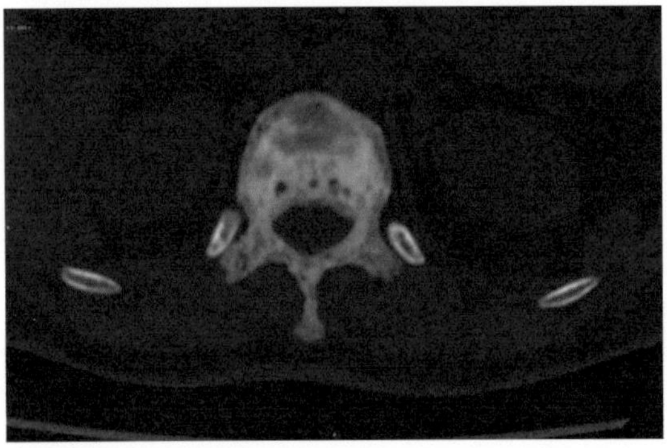

Fig. 12.3 Axial CT image of the thoracolumbar spine in bone window (T12 level)

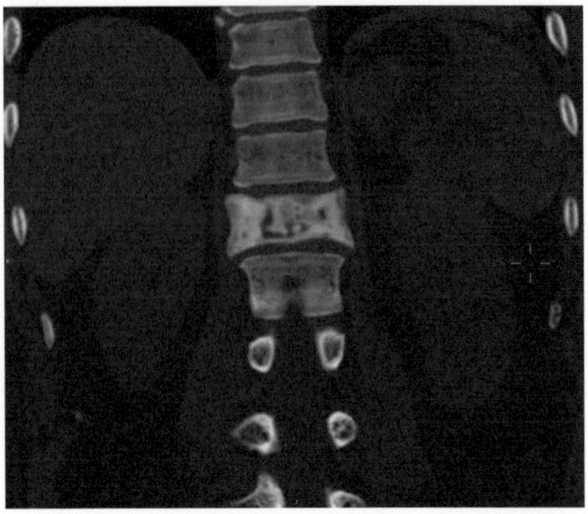

Fig. 12.4 Coronal CT image of the thoracolumbar spine in bone window

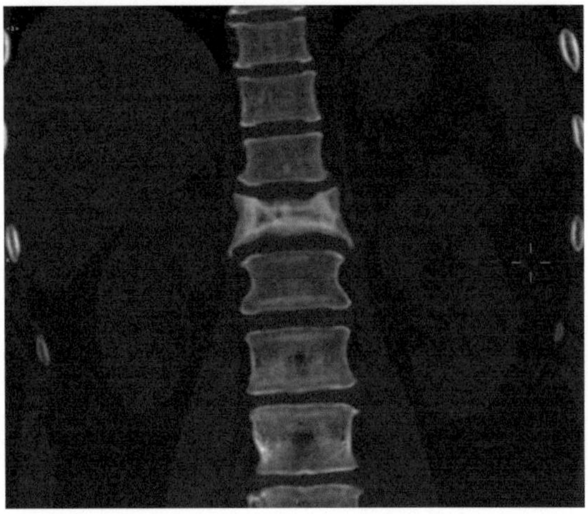

Fig. 12.5 Coronal CT image of the thoracolumbar spine in bone window

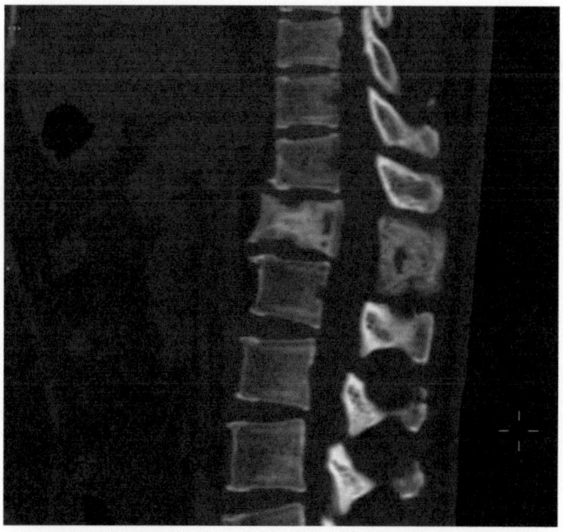

Fig. 12.6 Sagittal CT image of the thoracolumbar spine in bone window

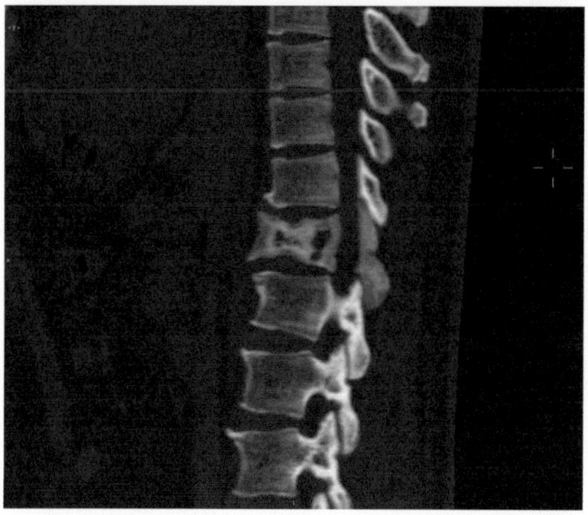

Fig. 12.7 Sagittal CT image of the thoracolumbar spine in bone window

ing of trabeculae and internal multiple linear low-density regions. Bone proliferative changes noted in the adjacent vertebral bodies.

12.4 Description and Discussion from Residents

The radiographs show enlargement, flattening of T12 vertebral body with peripheral sclerosis. The CT images demonstrated enlargement of the T12 vertebral body and posterior elements with increased densities and indistinct boundary between the cortex and cancellous bone (typical "picture frame" pattern) with thickened trabeculae and internal low-density region. There was biconcave appearance of the vertebral body with preserved intervertebral space. Other vertebral bodies demonstrated linear high densities along the endplates. Given above findings, our top consideration is Paget disease of bone with fibrous dysplasia as differential diagnosis.

12.5 Analysis and Comments from Professor Cheng Xiao-Guang

The radiographs show compression deformity of T12 vertebral body with increased densities of the vertebral body and posterior elements—typical "picture frame" sign. Some adjacent vertebral bodies demonstrated linear radiodensities along the endplates. CT images show enlargement and increased densities of the T12 vertebral body and posterior elements, consistent with abnormal bone remodeling. Given above findings, my top consideration is osteitis deformans (Paget disease of bone). This is more common in European countries and rare in China. Paget disease of bone has the following characteristics: bone deformity, such as enlargement of the vertebral body, "picture frame" sign, bowing of the tibia or femur; osteitis as coarsened trabeculae, clinically presenting with pain and elevated alkaline phosphatase with good results when treating with bisphosphonates.

12.6 Diagnosis

Paget disease of bone.

Suggested Reading

Dell'Atti C, Cassar-Pullicino VN, Lalam RK. The spine in Paget's disease. Skeletal Radiol. 2007;36(7):609–26.

Morales H. MR imaging findings of Paget's disease of the spine. Clin Neuroradiol. 2015;25(3):225–32.

Saifuddin A, Hassan A. Paget's disease of the spine: unusual features and complications. Clin Radiol. 2003;58(2):102–11.

13 Giant Cell Tumor of Bone: Case 13

13.1 Medical History

Patient is a 34-year-old male. He started to suffer from back pain about 4 months ago without clear causes. The pain is dull without radiation and intermittent and worsen after activity, improved with rest. He had biopsy afterward.

13.2 Physical Examination

Point tenderness around the spinous process in the thoracolumbar spine without radiation.

13.3 Imaging Findings

13.3.1 Radiograph (Figs. 13.1 and 13.2)

Radiographs of the thoracolumbar spine show expansile bone destruction of L1 vertebral body with compression deformity and secondary focal kyphosis.

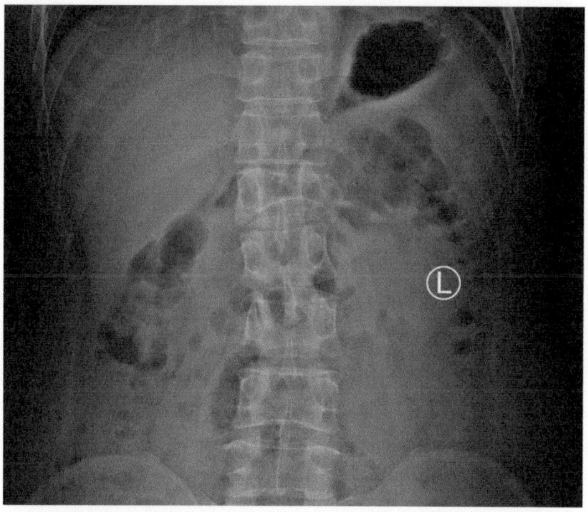

Fig. 13.1 Frontal view of the thoracolumbar spine

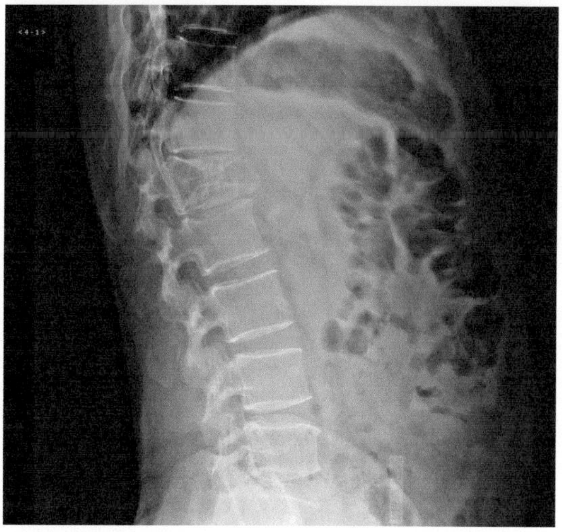

Fig. 13.2 Lateral view of the thoracolumbar spine

X. Cheng et al., *Imaging of Bone Tumors in Axial Bones*,
https://doi.org/10.1007/978-981-95-2262-0_13

13.3.2 CT Imaging (Figs. 13.3, 13.4, 13.5, 13.6, 13.7, 13.8, 13.9, 13.10, and 13.11)

CT images of the lumbar spine demonstrated expansile bone destruction of L1 vertebral body with compression deformity and involving bilateral pedicles with internal ridges. The lesion was with thin shell with posterior soft tissue mass protruding toward the spinal canal with homogenous avid enhancement.

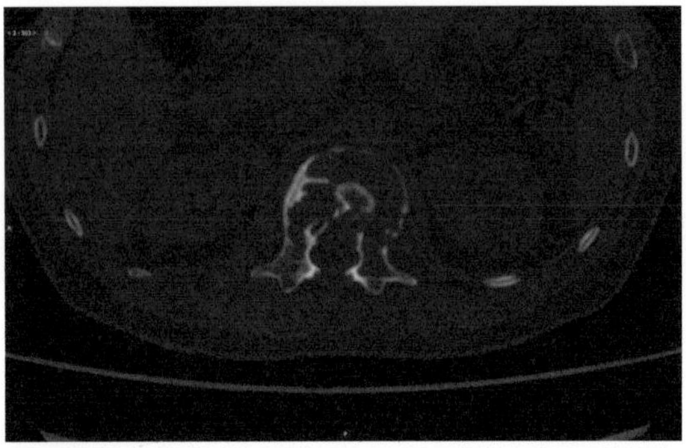

Fig. 13.3 Axial CT image of the lumbar spine in bone window

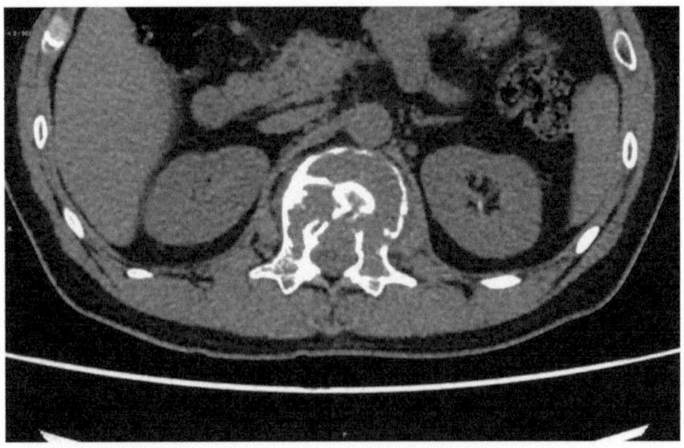

Fig. 13.4 Axial CT image of the lumbar spine in soft tissue window

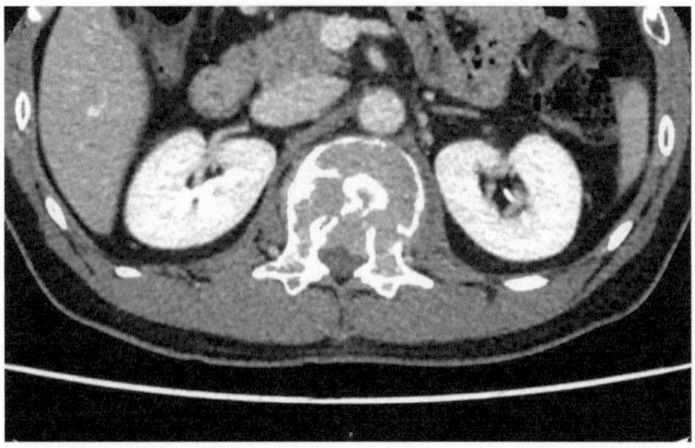

Fig. 13.5 Axial post-contrast CT image of the lumbar spine in soft tissue window

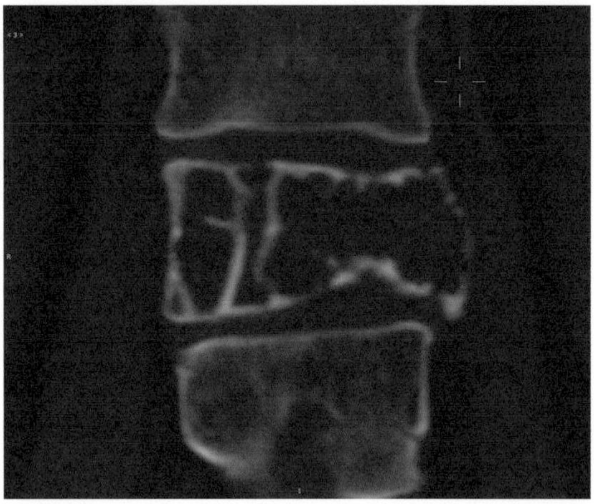

Fig. 13.6 Coronal CT image of the lumbar spine in bone window

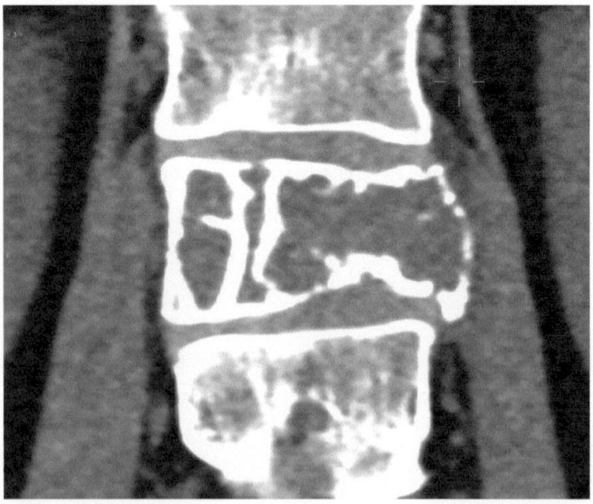

Fig. 13.7 Coronal CT image of the lumbar spine in soft tissue window

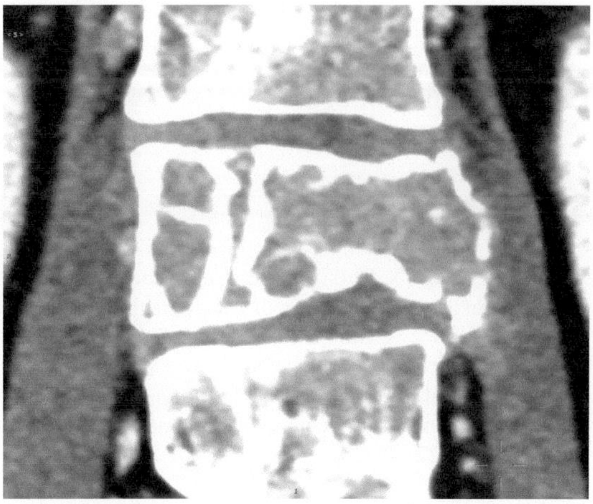

Fig. 13.8 Coronal post-contrast CT image of the lumbar spine in soft tissue window

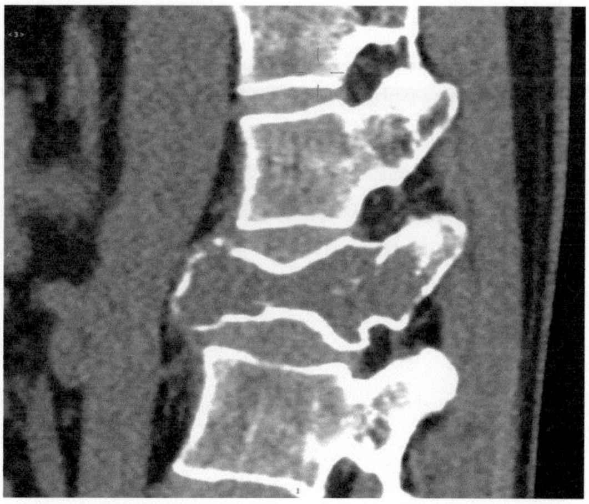

Fig. 13.10 Sagittal CT image of the lumbar spine in soft tissue window

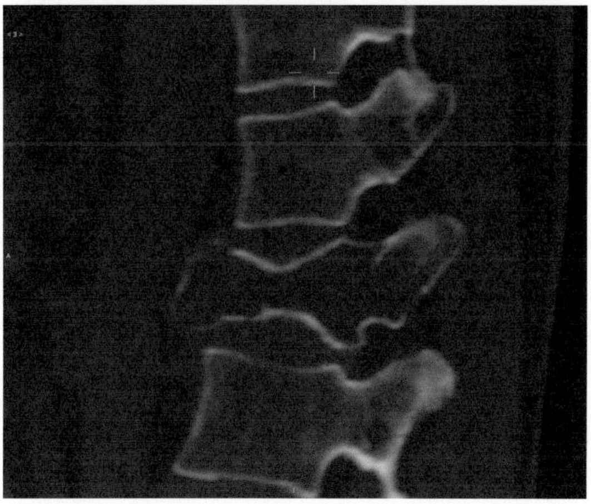

Fig. 13.9 Sagittal CT image of the lumbar spine in bone window

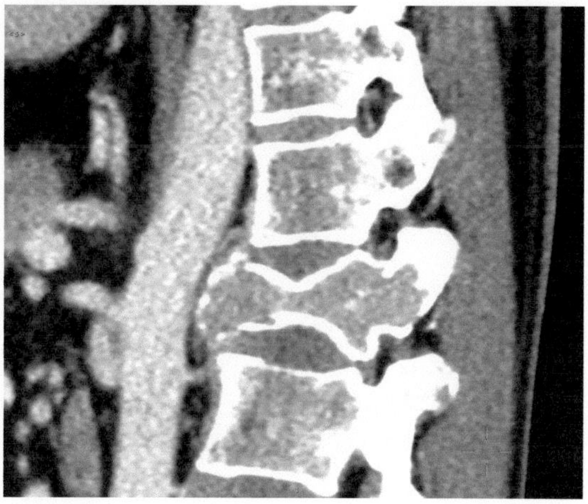

Fig. 13.11 Sagittal post-contrast CT image of the lumbar spine in soft tissue window

13.4 Description and Discussion from Residents

Lateral view of radiograph showed L1 vertebral body expansile bone destruction with biconcave deformity of pathologic fracture. CT images showed L1 expansile vertebral body destruction, involving the posterior elements with internal trabeculations, with thinned cortex with focal disruption. The solid portion of the lesion showed CT value of 46 HU before the contrast with avid enhancement, of CT value of 120 HU. There was mild expansion with peripheral sclerosis, indicating benign process, such as vascular tumors, with plasmacytoma, eosinophilic granuloma and giant cell tumor of bone in the differential diagnosis. If there was obvious T2 signal on MR images, then supporting hemangioma.

13.5 Analysis and Comments from Professor Cheng Xiao-Guang

Radiographs showed collapse of the L1 vertebral body with internal lytic bone destruction and protruding of the anterior cortex, indicating neoplastic process. CT images showed bone destruction of L1 vertebral body and posterior elements with homogeneous enhancement. However, the degree of enhancement is not as avid as giant cell tumor of bone. There were multiple ridges in the lesion, brain sulcus like, could be "mini brain" sign, characteristics of solitary plasmacytoma. MR images would be helpful at diagnose.

13.6 Diagnosis

Giant cell tumor of bone.

Suggested Reading

Bukata SV, Blay JY, Rutkowski P, et al. Denosumab treatment for giant cell tumor of the spine including the sacrum. Spine (Phila Pa 1976). 2021;46(5):277–84.

Leggett AR, Berg AR, Hullinger H, et al. Diagnosis and treatment of lumbar giant cell tumor of the spine: update on current management strategies. Diagnostics (Basel). 2022;12(4):857.

Extraskeletal Myxoid Chondrosarcoma of Bone: Case 14

14

14.1 Medical History

Patient is a 45-year-old female. She started to experience back pain after activities about 5 months ago, more in the night, and migrating and not relieved by rest. She had biopsy about 2 weeks ago and was presented with pain around the anterior left thigh.

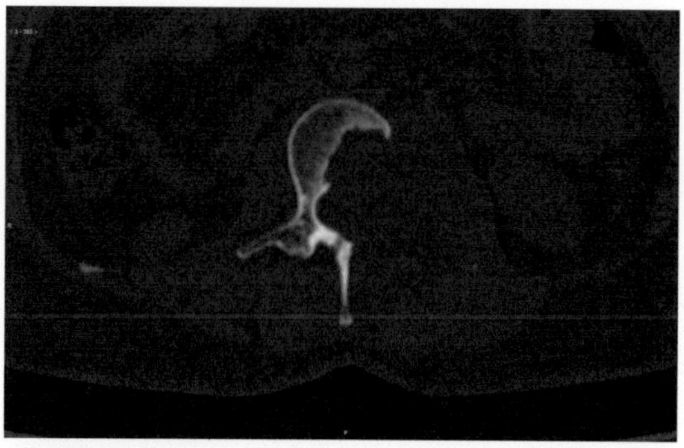

Fig. 14.1 Axial CT image of the lumbar spine in bone window (superior L2 level)

14.2 Physical Examination

No abnormalities at the back. Left lower extremity muscle strength at IV with numbness at the anterior left thigh.

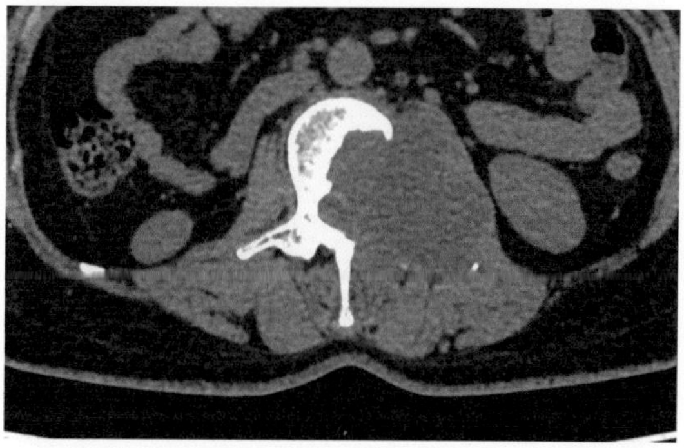

Fig. 14.2 Axial CT image of the lumbar spine in soft tissue window (superior L2 level)

14.3 Imaging Findings

14.3.1 CT Imaging (Figs. 14.1, 14.2, 14.3, 14.4, 14.5, 14.6, 14.7, and 14.8)

CT images of the lumbar spine demonstrated lytic bone destruction of the L2 vertebral body and left posterior elements with large soft tissue mass. The lesion showed a clear margin with peripheral sclerosis and invaded the central canal with narrowing. Avid peripheral enhancement noted of the soft tissue mass and no enhancement at the center of the lesion.

X. Cheng et al., *Imaging of Bone Tumors in Axial Bones*,
https://doi.org/10.1007/978-981-95-2262-0_14

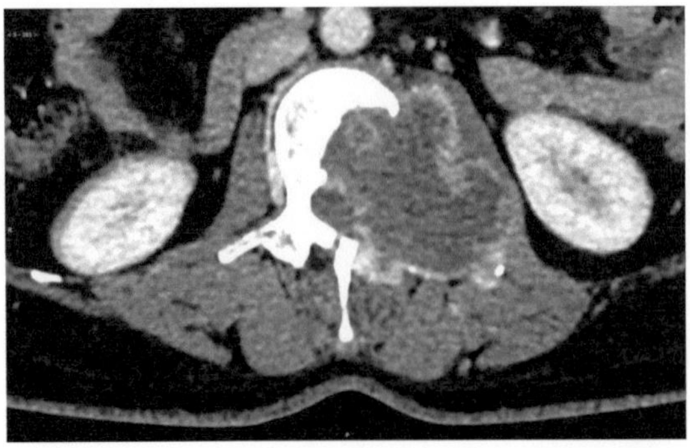

Fig. 14.3 Axial post-contrast CT image of the lumbar spine in soft tissue window (superior L2 level)

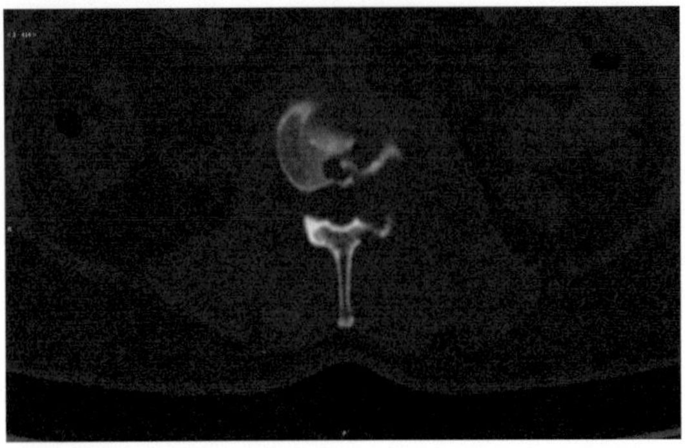

Fig. 14.4 Axial CT image of the lumbar spine in bone window (inferior L2 level)

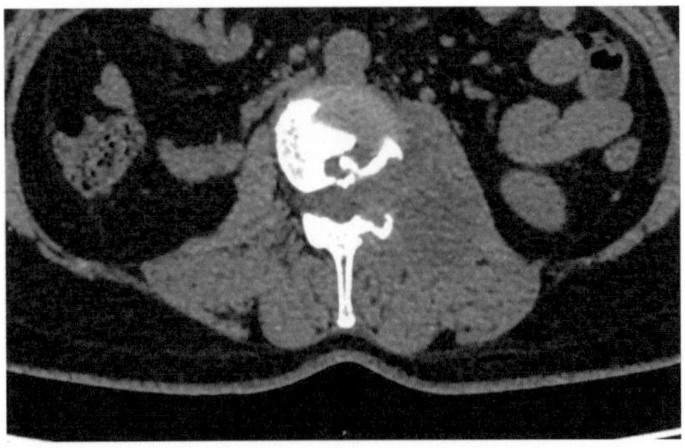

Fig. 14.5 Axial CT image of the lumbar spine in soft tissue window (inferior L2 level)

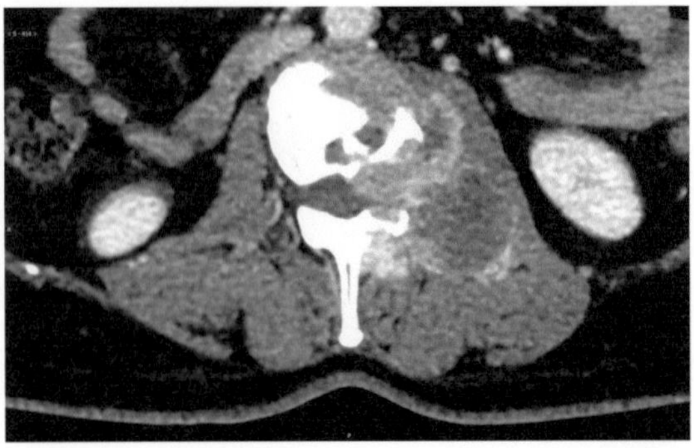

Fig. 14.6 Axial post-contrast CT image of the lumbar spine in soft tissue window (inferior L2 level)

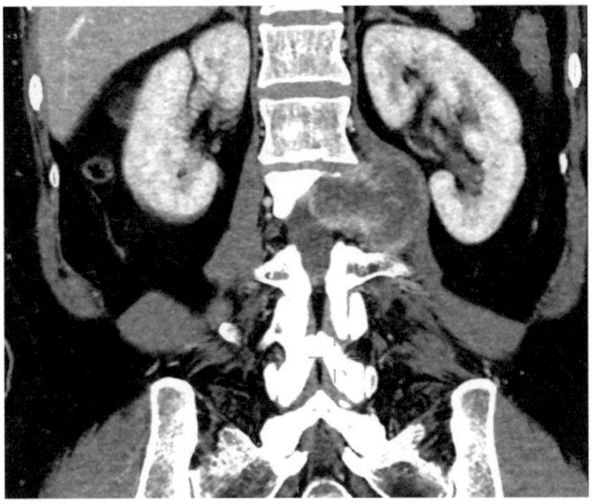

Fig. 14.7 Coronal post-contrast CT image of the lumbar spine in soft tissue window

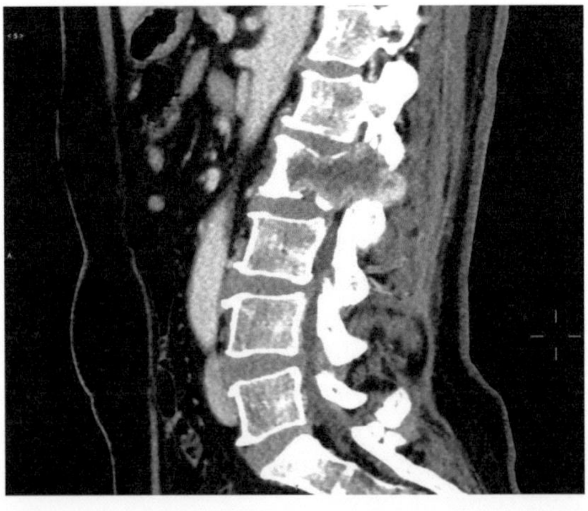

Fig. 14.8 Sagittal post-contrast CT image of the lumbar spine in soft tissue window

14.4 Description and Discussion from Residents

CT images demonstrated lytic bone destruction around the L2 vertebral body and left pedicle with peripheral sclerosis and large soft tissue mass without internal calcification with distinct margin and peripheral enhancement. Our consideration is low-grade aggressive neoplasm originated in the lumbar spine, such as small blue cell tumor. However, the age was not typical of it. We include giant cell tumor of bone (features not supportive of the diagnosis: large soft tissue mass and no peripheral bone shell), metastatic lesion (features not supportive of the diagnosis: relative young age of the patient and peripheral sclerosis), and chordoma and chondrosarcoma (features not supportive of the diagnosis: no internal calcifications) in the differential diagnosis. Additionally, there was relative low density internally of the lesion, similar to fluid densities and peripheral enhancement; spinal tuberculosis should also be included in the differential diagnosis.

14.5 Analysis and Comments from Professor Cheng Xiao-Guang

Patient is a middle-aged male. He suffered from lytic bone destruction of the L2 vertebral body and left posterior elements with mild expansion and clear margin. There was low density of the soft tissue mass with cystic central portion and no calcifications. Peripheral avid enhancement was noted. Given patient's age, expansile nature of the lesion, and focal avid enhancement, my top consideration is giant cell tumor of bone. Chondrosarcoma and neurogenic tumors are included in the differential diagnosis. Given no change in the intervertebral disc space, I would not consider spinal tuberculosis.

14.6 Diagnosis

Extraskeletal myxoid chondrosarcoma (*EWSR1-NR4A3* fusion) of bone.

Suggested Reading

Demicco EG, Wang WL, Madewell JE, et al. Osseous myxochondroid sarcoma: a detailed study of 5 cases of extraskeletal myxoid chondrosarcoma of the bone. Am J Surg Pathol. 2013;37(5):752–62.

Kapoor N, Shinagare AB, Jagannathan JP, et al. Clinical and radiologic features of extraskeletal myxoid chondrosarcoma including initial presentation, local recurrence, and metastases. Radiol Oncol. 2014;48(3):235–42.

15 Lymphoma of Bone: Case 15

15.1 Medical History

Patient is a 62-year-old male. He started to experience mild pain around the waist about 2 months ago without clear causes. The pain worsened in the past 1 month with night pain. An exophytic mass noted at the superior pole of the left kidney on his PET-CT scan images with increased uptake and considered as aggressive neoplasm, likely renal cell cancer. Lytic bone destruction of L2 vertebral body noted with pathologic fracture and large soft tissue mass with increased uptake, highly suggestive of metastatic lesion.

15.2 Physical Examination

Not recorded in the hospital system.

15.3 Imaging Findings

15.3.1 Radiograph (Fig. 15.1)

Radiograph of the lumbar spine showed focal depression along the superior L2 vertebral body with disruption of the cortex with focal decreased bone density.

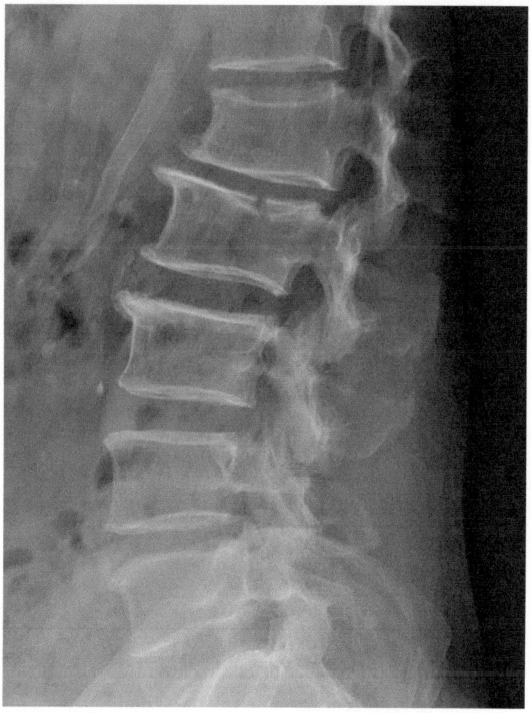

Fig. 15.1 Lateral view of the lumbar spine

15.3.2 CT Imaging (Figs. 15.2, 15.3, 15.4, 15.5, and 15.6)

CT images of the lumbar spine demonstrated bone destruction of the L2 vertebral body with pathologic fracture. There was complete destruc-

X. Cheng et al., *Imaging of Bone Tumors in Axial Bones*,
https://doi.org/10.1007/978-981-95-2262-0_15

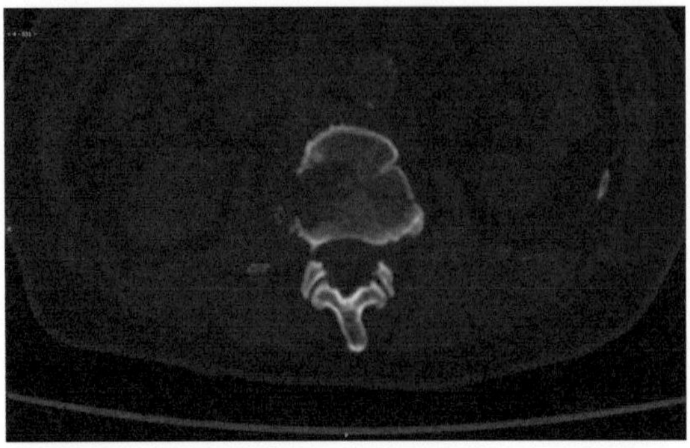

Fig. 15.2 Axial CT image of the lumbar spine in bone window (L2 level)

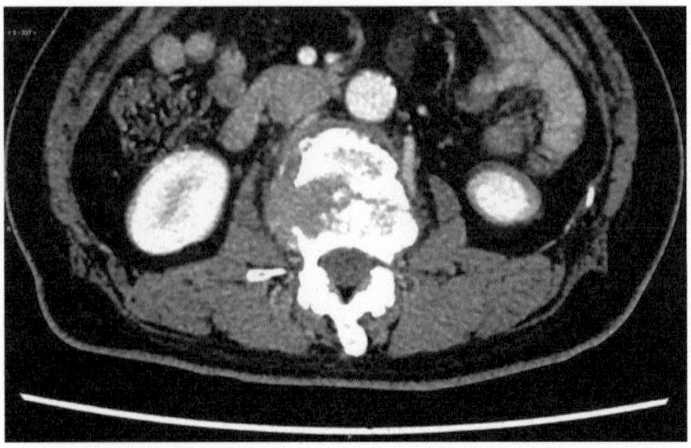

Fig. 15.4 Axial post-contrast CT image of the lumbar spine in soft tissue window (L2 level)

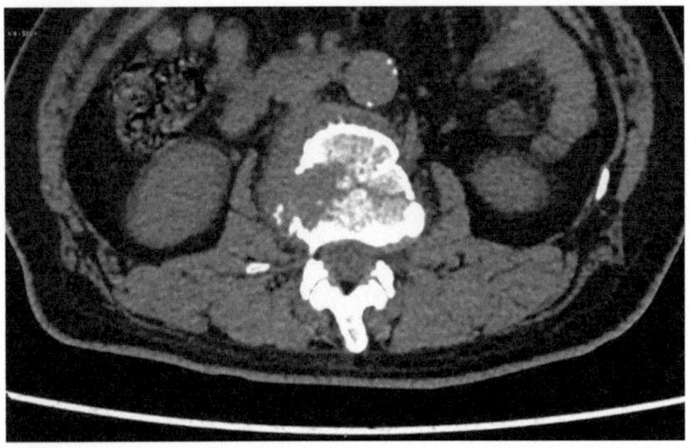

Fig. 15.3 Axial CT image of the lumbar spine in soft tissue window (L2 level)

tion of the cortex with formation of soft tissue mass and moderate enhancement.

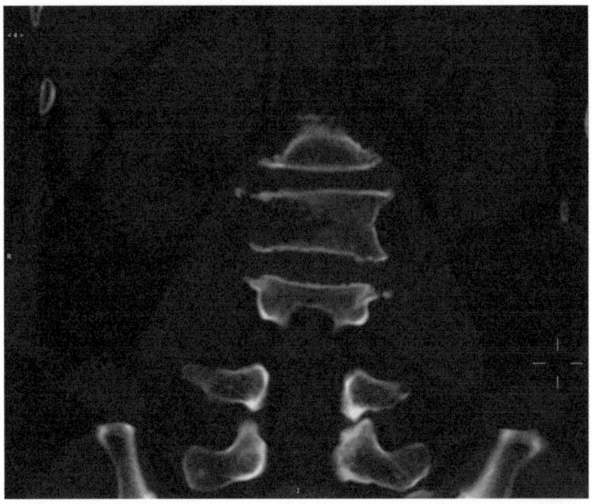

Fig. 15.5 Coronal CT image of the lumbar spine in bone window

15.3.3 MR Imaging (Figs. 15.7, 15.8, 15.9, 15.10, 15.11, 15.12, and 15.13)

MR images demonstrated bone destruction of L2 vertebral body with compression deformity and permeated cortex destruction and soft tissue mass with low T1 and heterogeneous high T2 signal. There was thickening of surrounding soft tissue with edema. The mass extending posteriorly with mass effect upon the spinal canal. The lesion demonstrated avid enhancement.

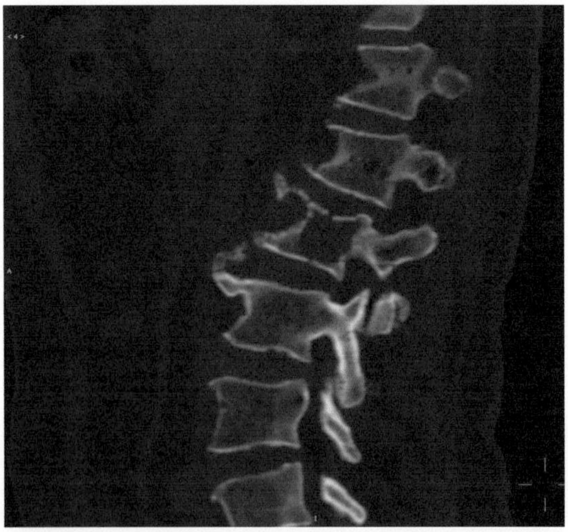

Fig. 15.6 Sagittal CT image of the lumbar spine in bone window

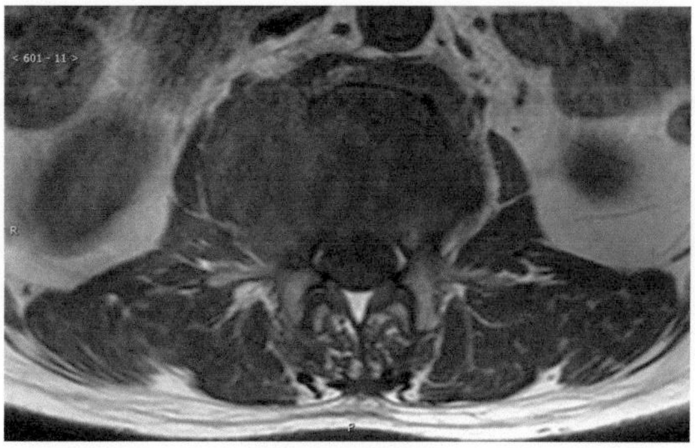

Fig. 15.7 Axial T1-weighted MR image of the lumbar spine (L2 level)

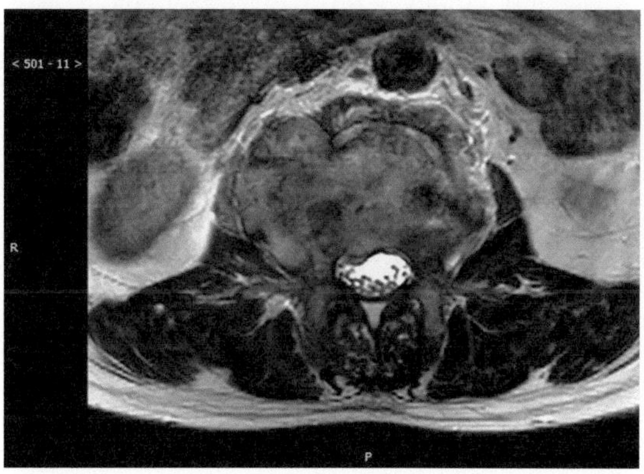

Fig. 15.8 Axial T2-weighted MR image of the lumbar spine (L2 level)

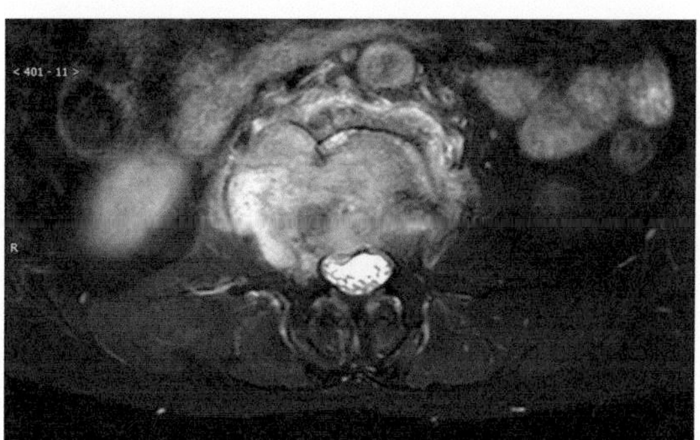

Fig. 15.9 Axial fat-suppressed T2-weighted MR image of the lumbar spine (L2 level)

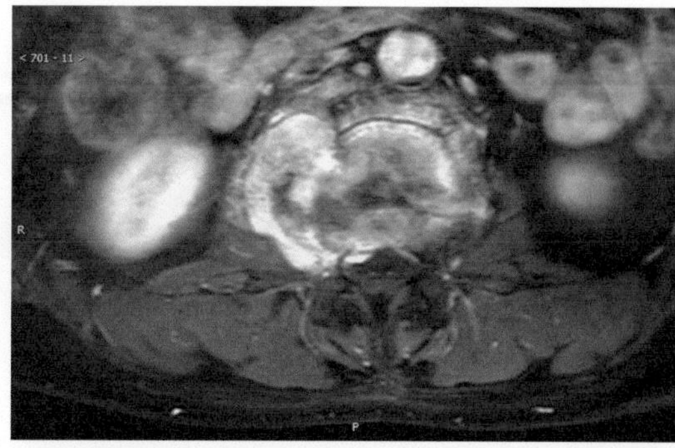

Fig. 15.10 Axial post-contrast fat-suppressed T1-weighted MR image of the lumbar spine (L2 level)

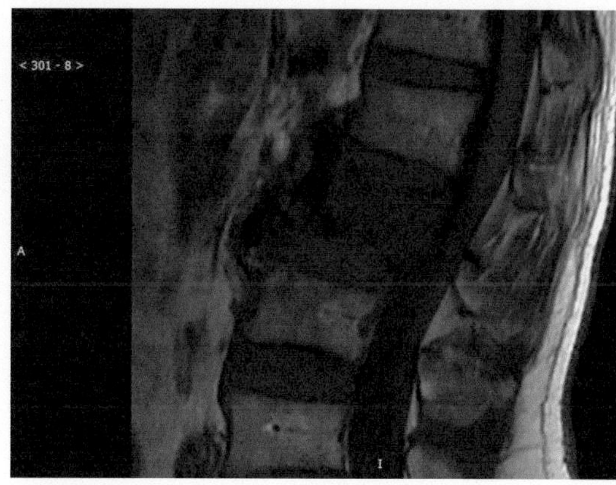

Fig. 15.11 Sagittal T1-weighted MR image of the lumbar spine

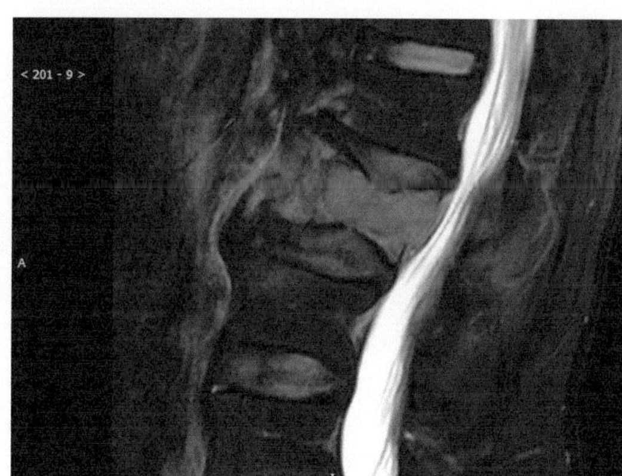

Fig. 15.12 Sagittal fat-suppressed T2-weighted MR image of the lumbar spine

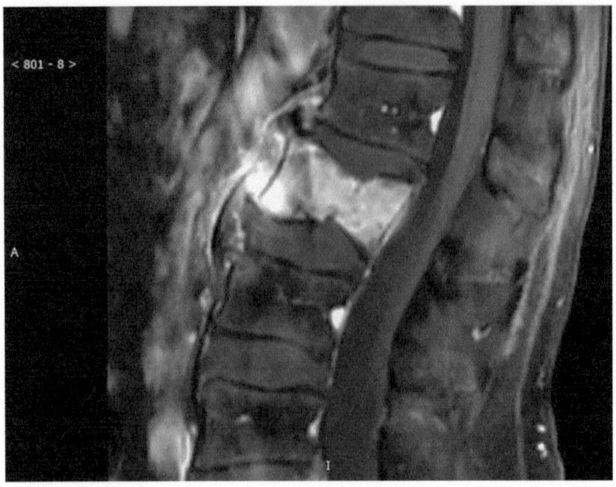

Fig. 15.13 Sagittal post-contrast fat-suppressed T1-weighted MR image of the lumbar spine

15.4 Description and Discussion from Residents

The patient is an older male. Radiograph showed collapse of the superior L2 vertebral body and focal cortical disruption with internal low bone density of the vertebral body. CT images showed isointense mass at the superior pole of the left kidney with avid enhancement and lytic bone destruction of the L2 vertebral body with indistinct margin and no peripheral sclerosis. There was disruption of the cortex along the right side of the vertebral body with soft tissue mass with mild to moderate enhancement. Combining the history, our top consideration is bone metastatic lesion. MR images showed larger extent of the lesion with heterogeneous signals and avid enhancement of L2 vertebral body lytic area, soft tissue mass and adjacent soft tissues, suggestive of significant vascular supply of the lesion. Combining all the imaging findings and history, our top consideration is bone metastatic disease with lymphoma as differential diagnosis.

15.5 Analysis and Comments from Professor Cheng Xiao-Guang

This case had lots of information from the history; however, we need to be aware it could provide false lead. The lateral view radiograph showed clear bone proliferative changes along the vertebral bodies with narrowing of the L1–2 intervertebral disc space and decreased bone density of the posterior L2 vertebral body with mild collapse of the superior endplate. CT images demonstrated vertical fracture of L2 vertebral body with bone destruction without peripheral sclerosis and paraspinal soft tissue changes with mild to moderate enhancement. Additionally, we need to pay attention to the kidney; without the diagnosis of renal cell cancer, we would not prioritize the diagnosis of metastatic lesion. There was isointense protrusion along the superior pole of the left kidney with avid enhancement. MR images showed the paraspinal soft tissue changes clearly with avid enhancement. However, CT is superior at demonstrating degree of soft tissue enhancement when compared to MRI, so we should base our consideration of enhancement more on CT post-contrast images. The kidneys showed no abnormalities on the MR images, likely unrelated to the changes in the spine. Overall, this was an aggressive neoplastic process involving the L2 vertebral body, given patient's age, metastatic lesion is in consideration. Lymphoma, plasmacytoma are other possibilities.

15.6 Diagnosis

Lymphoma (B-cell origin) of bone.

Suggested Reading

Krishnan A, Shirkhoda A, Tehranzadeh J, et al. Primary bone lymphoma: radiographic-MR imaging correlation. Radiographics. 2003;23(6):1371–83. discussion 1384–7

Murphey MD, Kransdorf MJ. Primary musculoskeletal lymphoma. Radiol Clin North Am. 2016;54(4):785–95.

16 Bone Metastases: Case 16

16.1 Medical History

Patient is a 66-year-old female. She started to experience pain around her waist when open a window about 2 months ago. She had a radiograph taken then and showed no abnormalities. She was treated with oral anti-inflammatory drugs with no relief and symptoms worsened that she could no longer walk. CT images showed pathological fracture in the lumbar spine. Biopsy had been performed.

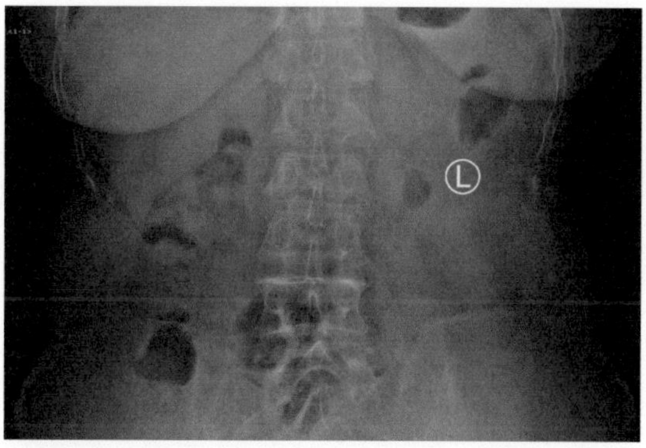

Fig. 16.1 Frontal view of the lumbar spine

16.2 Physical Examination

Scar noted from prior L2 vertebral body biopsy on the right.

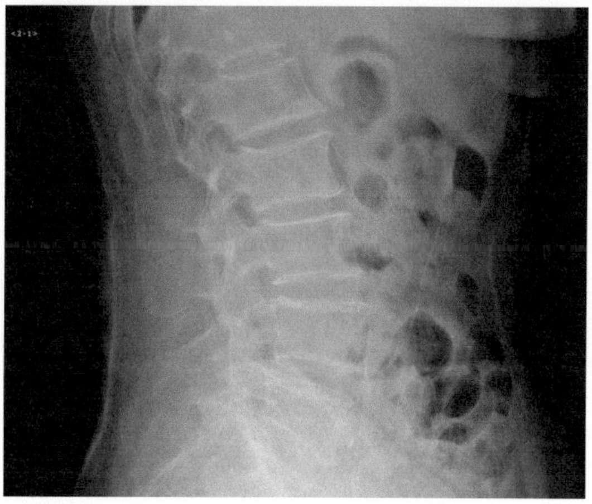

Fig. 16.2 Lateral view of the lumbar spine

16.3 Imaging Findings

16.3.1 Radiograph (Figs. 16.1 and 16.2)

Radiographs of the lumbar spine show degenerative changes in the lumbar spine with normal morphology of L2 vertebral body with mild decreased bone density and preserved intervertebral disc spaces.

X. Cheng et al., *Imaging of Bone Tumors in Axial Bones*,
https://doi.org/10.1007/978-981-95-2262-0_16

16.3.2 CT Imaging (Figs. 16.3, 16.4, 16.5, 16.6, 16.7, 16.8, and 16.9)

CT images of the lumbar spine demonstrated bone destruction of the L2 vertebral body on the right with disruption of the superior and inferior endplates. There was mild posterior expansion of the vertebral body, protruding to the spinal canal with narrowing of the spinal canal. There was relatively homogeneous density within the lesion with peripheral mild sclerosis with moderate enhancement.

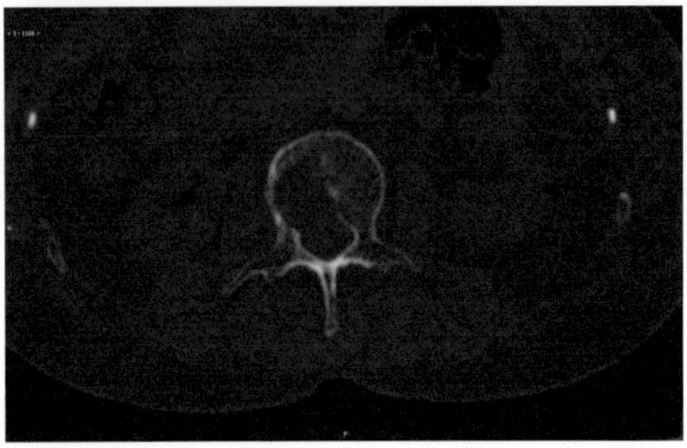

Fig. 16.3 Axial CT image of the lumbar spine in bone window

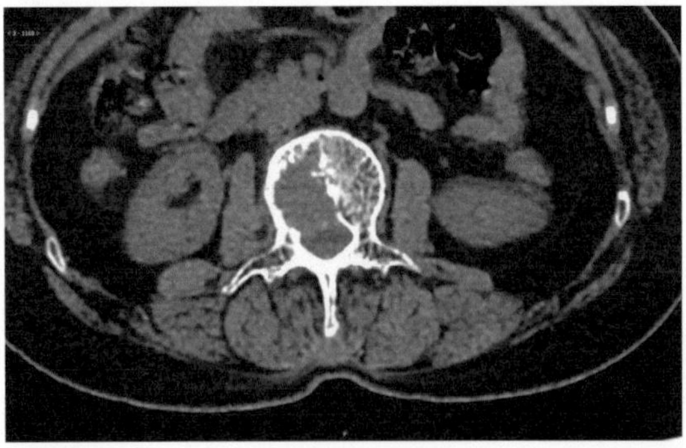

Fig. 16.4 Axial CT image of the lumbar spine in soft tissue window

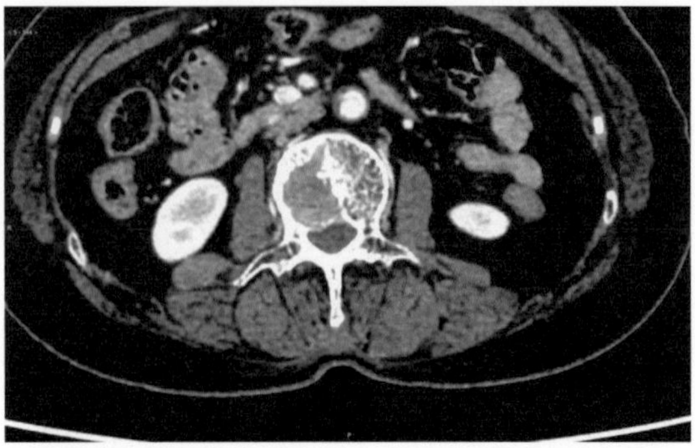

Fig. 16.5 Axial post-contrast CT image of the lumbar spine in soft tissue window

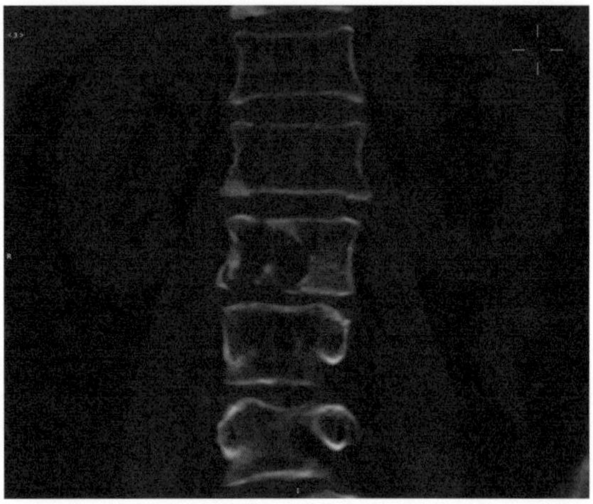

Fig. 16.6 Coronal CT image of the lumbar spine in bone window

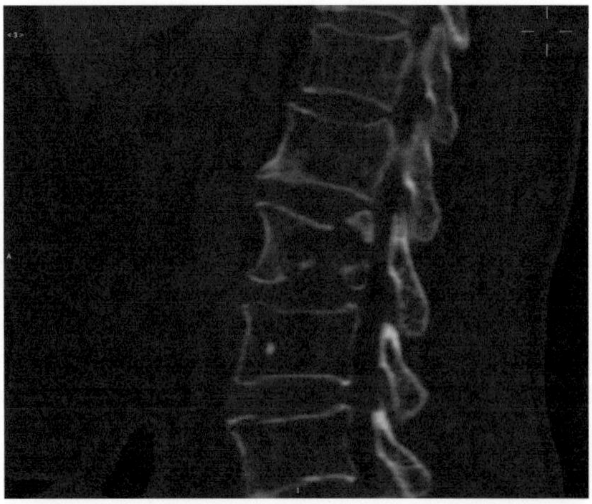

Fig. 16.7 Sagittal CT image of the lumbar spine in bone window

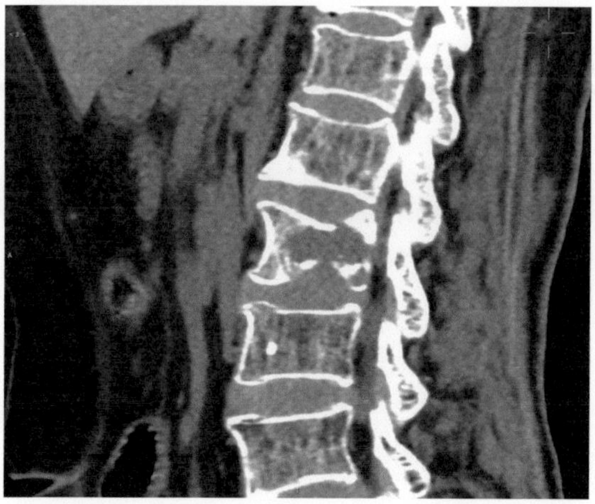

Fig. 16.8 Sagittal CT image of the lumbar spine in soft tissue window

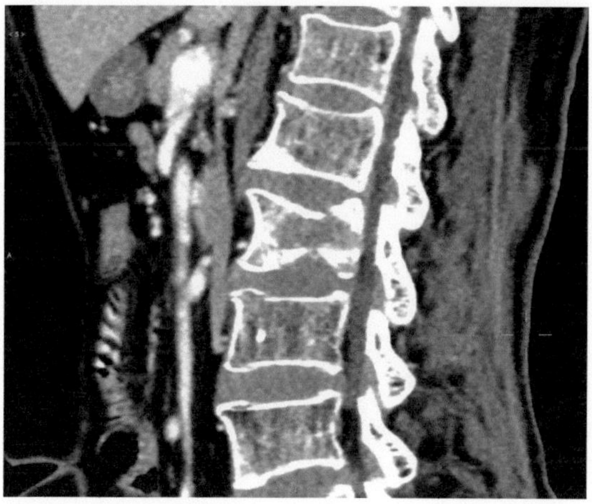

Fig. 16.9 Sagittal post-contrast CT image of the lumbar spine in soft tissue window

16.4 Description and Discussion from Residents

Lateral view radiograph of the lumbar spine showed suspected decreased bone density of L2 vertebral body. L2 vertebral body lytic bone destruction noted on CT images with peripheral mild sclerosis and posteriorly soft tissue mass protruding through the cortex with moderate enhancement. Given patient's age, metastatic disease is very likely. Differential diagnosis includes (1) solidary plasmacytoma, but this case lacks typical "mini brain" sign and (2) lymphoma, peripheral sclerosis of this case is not consistent with typical findings of lymphoma.

16.5 Analysis and Comments from Professor Cheng Xiao-Guang

The patient was an older female. Radiographs did not provide useful information for reaching the diagnosis. CT images showed bone destruction along the right L2 vertebral body with irregular margin and internal residual bone fragments and irregular high densities with pathologic fracture and moderate enhancement. No other abnormalities noted in the remaining osseous structures and abdominal organs. This was an aggressive lesion, given patient's age, my top consideration is metastatic lesion. Overall, this lesion lacks typical features of other aggressive pathologies.

16.6 Diagnosis

Bone metastases (primary site: lung or thyroid).

Suggested Reading

Costelloe CM, Lin PP, Chuang HH, et al. Bone metastases: mechanisms of the metastatic process, imaging and therapy. Semin Ultrasound CT MR. 2021;42(2):164–83.

O'Sullivan GJ, Carty FL, Cronin CG. Imaging of bone metastasis: an update. World J Radiol. 2015;7(8):202–11.

Poon D, Tang C, Vijayanathan S, et al. The use of MRI for the imaging of metastatic bone lesions. Q J Nucl Med Mol Imaging. 2023;67(4):271–9.

Langerhans Cell Histiocytosis: Case 17

17

17.1 Medical History

Patient is a 6-year-old boy. He started to experience mild swelling, erythema and increased temperature of the skin at the right forearm about 2 months ago without clear causes.

17.2 Physical Examination

Mild swelling of the proximal right forearm with point tenderness.

17.3 Imaging Findings

17.3.1 Radiograph (Figs. 17.1, 17.2, 17.3, and 17.4)

Radiographs of the right forearm show bone destruction of the right radial shaft with heterogeneous densities with continuous cortex and no periosteal reaction. Radiographs of lumbar spine show compression deformity of L2 vertebral body with preserved intervertebral disc spaces.

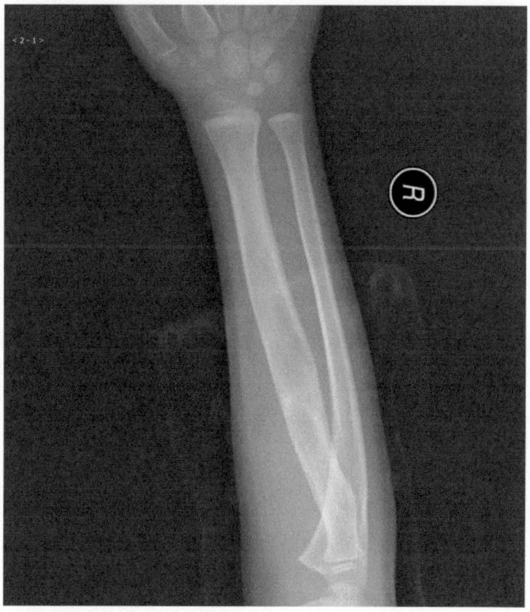

Fig. 17.1 Frontal view of the right forearm

17.3.2 CT Imaging (Figs. 17.5, 17.6, 17.7, 17.8, 17.9, and 17.10)

CT images demonstrated compression of L2 vertebral body with regional bone destruction, more on the left. No paraspinal soft tissue mass noted.

X. Cheng et al., *Imaging of Bone Tumors in Axial Bones*,
https://doi.org/10.1007/978-981-95-2262-0_17

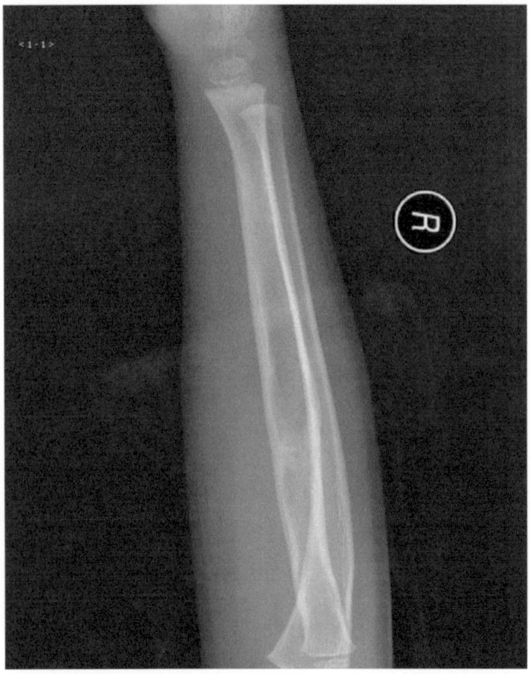

Fig. 17.2 Lateral view of the right forearm

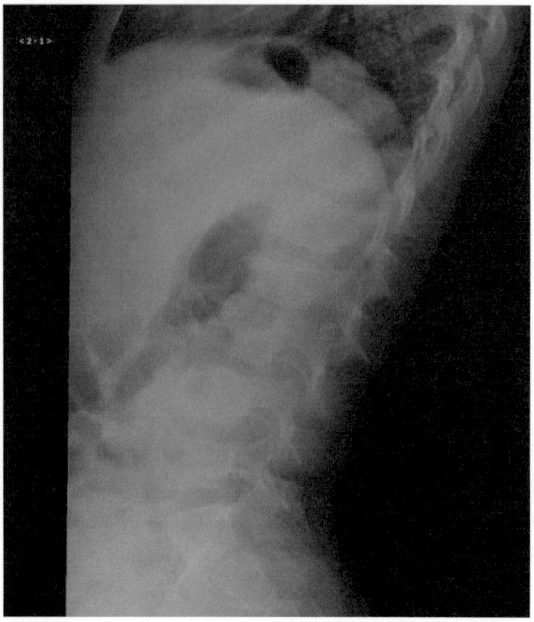

Fig. 17.4 Lateral view of the lumbar spine

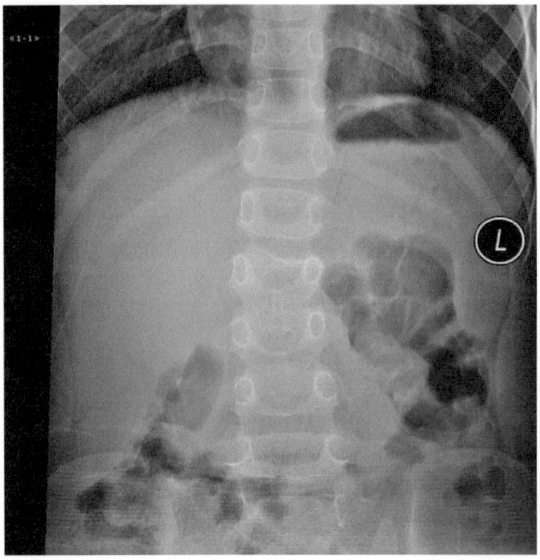

Fig. 17.3 Frontal view of the lumbar spine

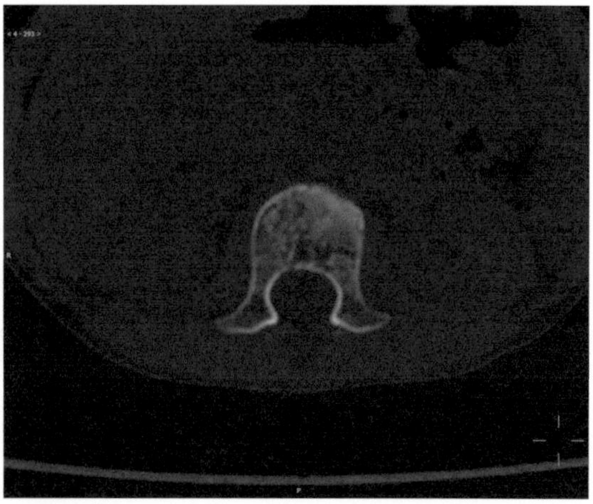

Fig. 17.5 Axial CT image of the lumbar spine in bone window (L2 level)

There was additional bone destruction of the right posterior superior iliac spine with focal cortical disruption and clear margin and heterogeneous enhancement.

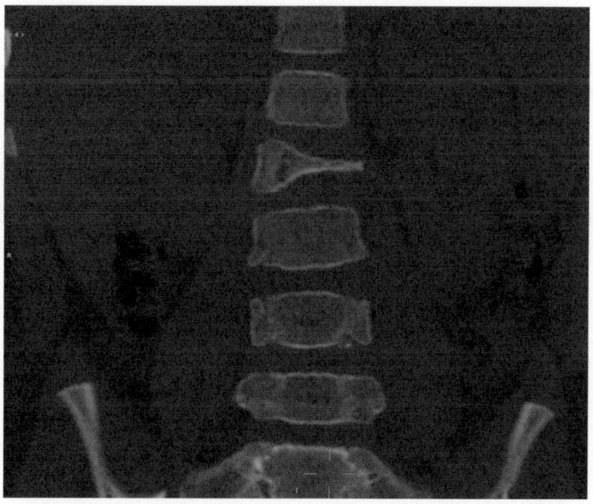

Fig. 17.6 Coronal CT image of the lumbar spine in bone window

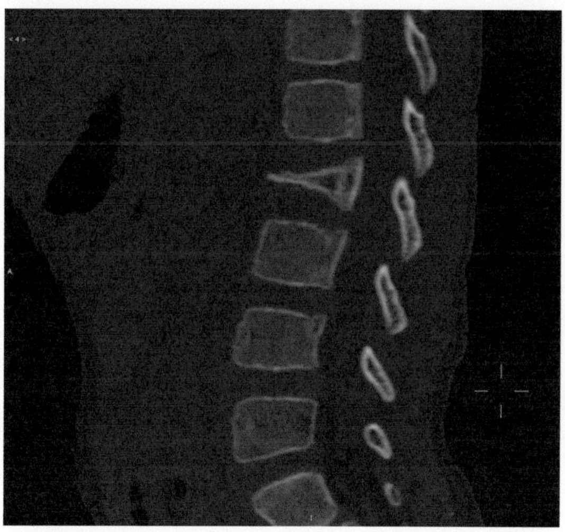

Fig. 17.7 Sagittal CT image of the lumbar spine in bone window

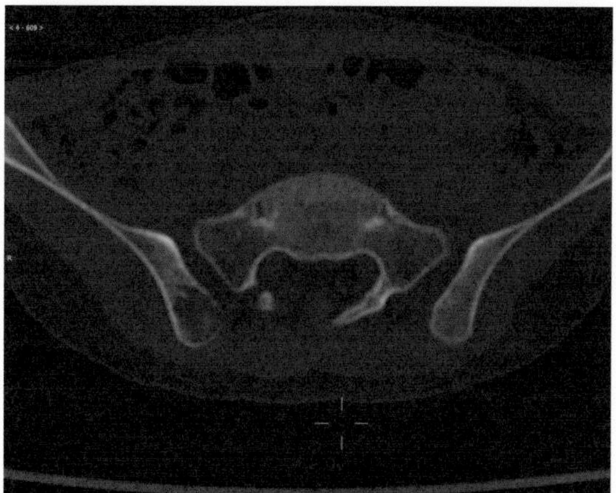

Fig. 17.8 Axial CT image of the iliac in bone window

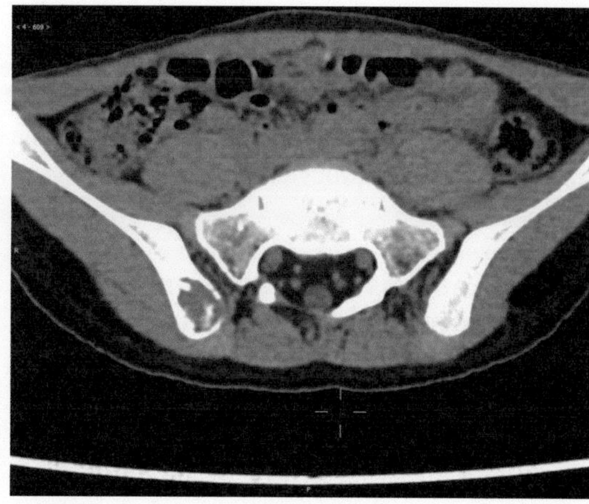

Fig. 17.9 Axial CT image of the iliac in soft tissue window

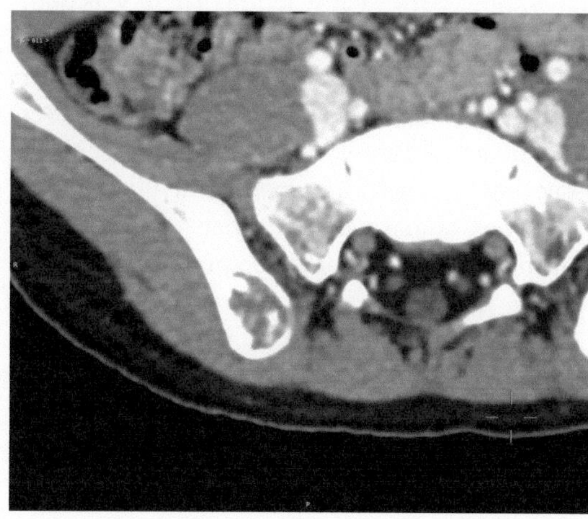

Fig. 17.10 Axial post-contrast CT image of the iliac in soft tissue window

17.4 Description and Discussion from Residents

There was mild expansile bone destruction along the radial shaft in a vertical fashion on the right forearm radiographs with indistinct margin and ground glass density changes within the lesion with preserved cortex and peripheral layered periosteal reaction. Lumbar spine radiographs showed focal vertebral body collapse and no narrowing of the intervertebral disc space. CT images showed apparent compression of L2 vertebral body with "plana" appearance with focal bone destruction and no paraspinal soft tissue mass and intact intervertebral spaces. There was additional bone destruction of the posterior superior iliac spine with internal high density and mild to moderate heterogeneous enhancement. Given patient's age and inflammatory symptoms, our top consideration is eosinophilic granuloma (Langerhans cell histiocytosis).

17.5 Analysis and Comments from Professor Cheng Xiao-Guang

Patient is a boy with lesions involving multiple bones. There was large area of expansile bone destruction around the mid right radial shaft on the radiographs with fracture noted at the proximal 1/3 of the shaft, likely of pathologic fracture and without periosteal reaction. There was additional compression deformity of L2 vertebral body. CT images showed compression of L2 vertebral body with increased density, typical "vertebral plana" deformity with normal adjacent soft tissue and preserved intervertebral disc spaces. There was additional lytic bone destruction at right posterior superior iliac spine with mild to moderate enhancement. Patient is a child with multiple bone involvements; my top consideration is eosinophilic granuloma, now known as Langerhans cell histiocytosis. When there are multiple sites of involvements, surgery is no longer considered, currently the main treatment is chemotherapy.

17.6 Diagnosis

Langerhans cell histiocytosis.

Suggested Reading

Angelini A, Mosele N, Gnassi A, et al. Vertebra plana: a narrative clinical and imaging overview among possible differential diagnoses. Diagnostics (Basel). 2023;13(8):1438.

Khung S, Budzik JF, Amzallag-Bellenger E, et al. Skeletal involvement in Langerhans cell histiocytosis. Insights Imaging. 2013;4(5):569–79.

Rajakulasingam R, Siddiqui M, Michelagnoli M, et al. Skeletal staging in Langerhans cell histiocytosis: a multimodality imaging review. Skeletal Radiol. 2021;50(6):1081–93.

18 Tenosynovial Giant Cell Tumor: Case 18

18.1 Medical History

Patient is a 42-year-old female. She started to experience back pain about 3 months ago without clear causes with numbness around the left gluteal region.

18.2 Physical Examination

Mild tenderness around left L2 to L3 region.

18.3 Imaging Findings

18.3.1 CT Imaging (Figs. 18.1, 18.2, 18.3, 18.4, 18.5, 18.6, and 18.7)

CT images of the lumbar spine demonstrated bone destruction around the facet joint on the left of L2–3 with thinning of the cortex and heterogeneous density internally. There was heterogeneous enhancement noted with focal avid enhancement.

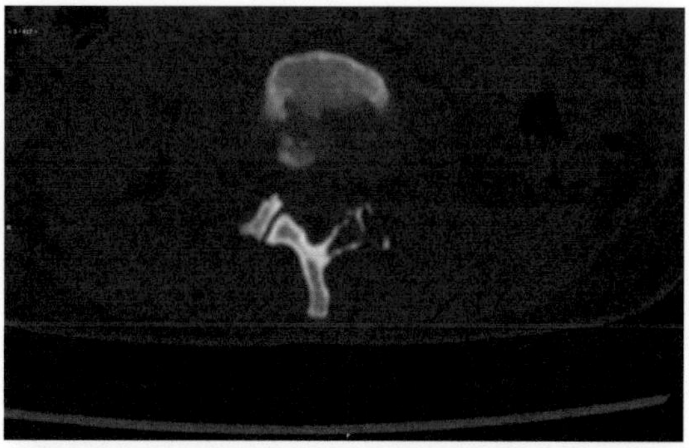

Fig. 18.1 Axial CT image of the lumbar spine in bone window

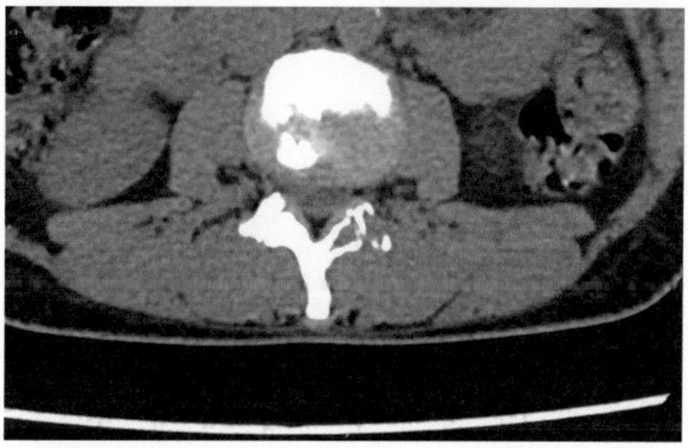

Fig. 18.2 Axial CT image of the lumbar spine in soft tissue window

X. Cheng et al., *Imaging of Bone Tumors in Axial Bones*,
https://doi.org/10.1007/978-981-95-2262-0_18

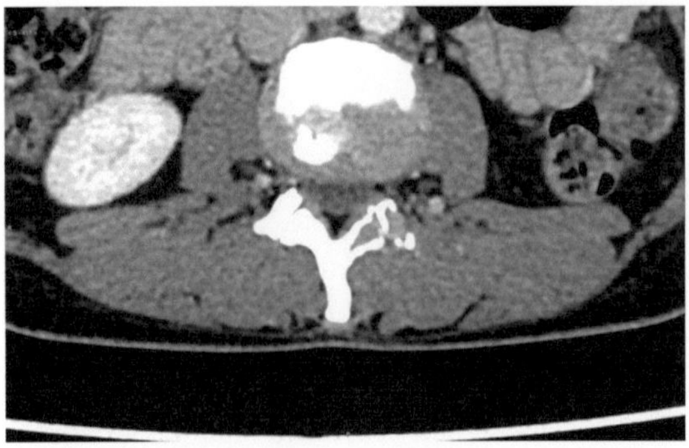

Fig. 18.3 Axial post-contrast CT image of the lumbar spine in soft tissue window

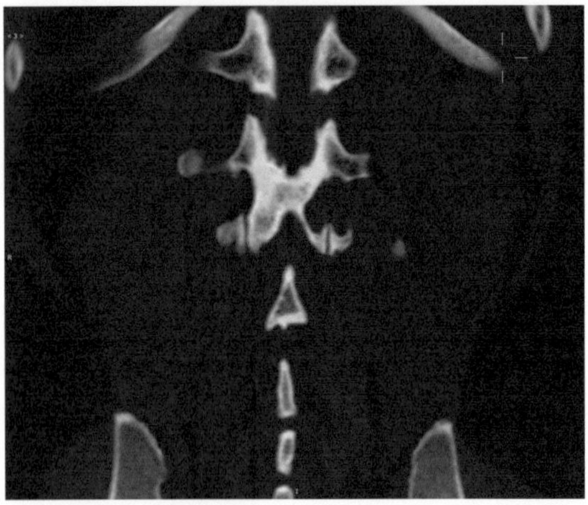

Fig. 18.4 Coronal CT image of the lumbar spine in bone window

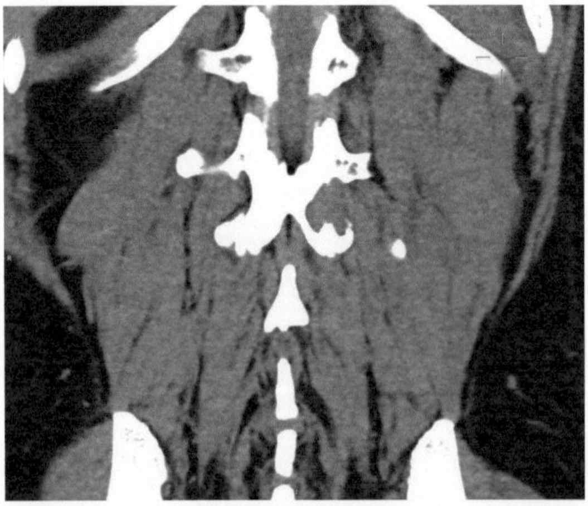

Fig. 18.5 Coronal CT image of the lumbar spine in soft tissue window

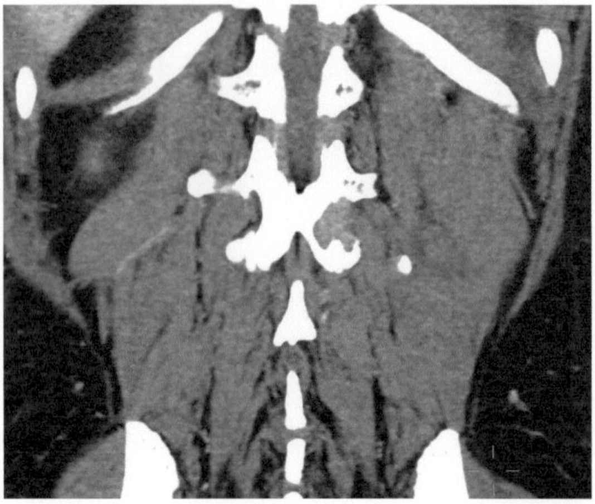

Fig. 18.6 Coronal post-contrast CT image of the lumbar spine in soft tissue window

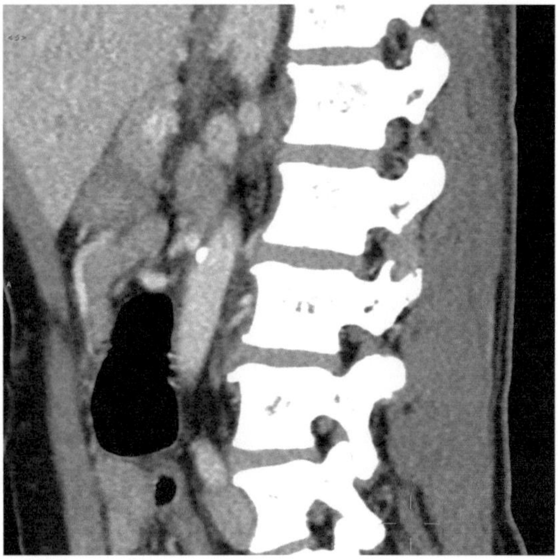

Fig. 18.7 Sagittal post-contrast CT image of the lumbar spine in soft tissue window

18.4 Description and Discussion from Residents

CT images of the lumbar spine demonstrated bone destruction around the facet joint on the left of L2–3 with thinning of the cortex and focal disruption and overall maintained morphology and preserved intervertebral disc spaces. Soft tissue density noted within the lesion without surrounding soft tissue mass. Avid enhancement noted. Given this pattern of involvement across the joint, our top consideration is tenosynovial giant cell tumor with tuberculosis and gout in the differential diagnosis.

18.5 Analysis and Comments from Professor Cheng Xiao-Guang

Patient is a middle-aged female. The lesion involved left facet joint of L2–3 with involvement of both superior and inferior articular process. Residents had described the lesion well on imaging. Facet joint is a synovial joint when lesion is involving across the joint without narrowing of the joint space; we can exclude tuberculosis. This was a lesion involving the synovial joint; my top consideration is pigmented villonodular synovitis (tenosynovial giant cell tumor). MRI usually is more sensitive at diagnosing this lesion. Gout is the differential diagnosis. Usually, we can see tophi as high densities on CT images, however, not a must.

18.6 Diagnosis

Tenosynovial giant cell tumor (diffuse type).

Suggested Reading

Anaya JEC, Coelho SRN, Taneja AK, et al. Differential diagnosis of facet joint disorders. Radiographics. 2021;41(2):543–58.

Zhang J, Li Y, Zhu Y, et al. FDG PET/CT in tenosynovial giant cell tumor of the lumbar facet joint. Clin Nucl Med. 2022;47(1):66–7.

Hemorrhage: Case 19

19

19.1 Medical History

Patient is a 64-year-old male. He suddenly started to experience severe right waist and gluteal pain after long time sitting about half a year ago and prevented him from standing up with relief after rest. This had become episodic, usually occurred after long time standing or walking and could be incited by coughing or sneezing and radiated to the right lower extremity. Patient took pain killer and ointment himself. He was also treated with pain killer, nerve nutritional medication, and acupuncture at the local community hospital without any relief.

19.2 Physical Examination

Muscle strength of bilateral lower extremity at V.

19.3 Imaging Findings

19.3.1 CT Imaging (Figs. 19.1, 19.2, 19.3, 19.4, 19.5, 19.6, and 19.7)

CT images of the lumbar spine demonstrated bone destruction along the right facet joint of L3–4 with internal high-density soft tissue nodule and no enhancement. There was mass effect upon the dura at the corresponding level with narrowing of the spinal canal.

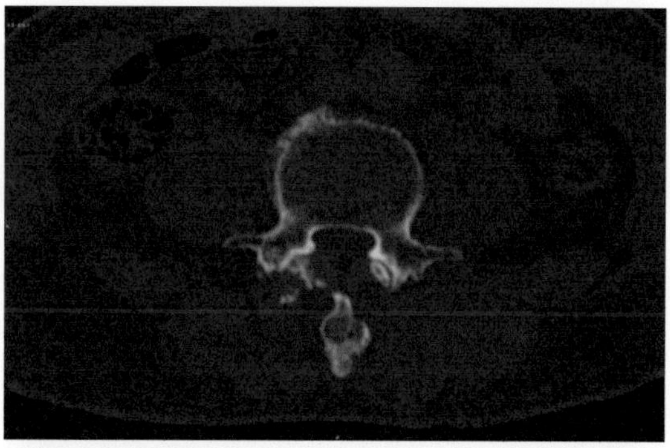

Fig. 19.1 Axial CT image of the lumbar spine in bone window (L3–4)

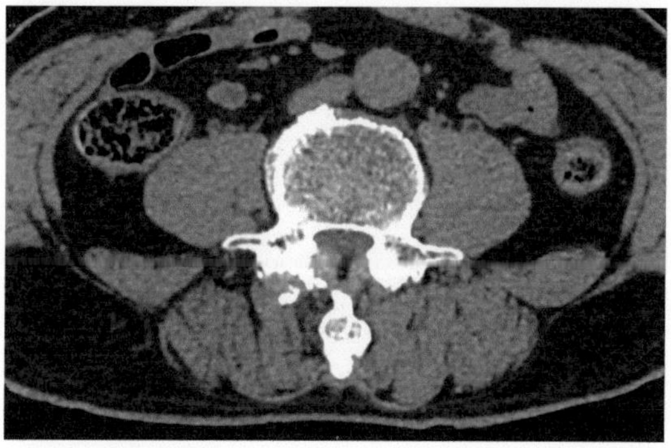

Fig. 19.2 Axial CT image of the lumbar spine in soft tissue window (L3–4)

X. Cheng et al., *Imaging of Bone Tumors in Axial Bones*,
https://doi.org/10.1007/978-981-95-2262-0_19

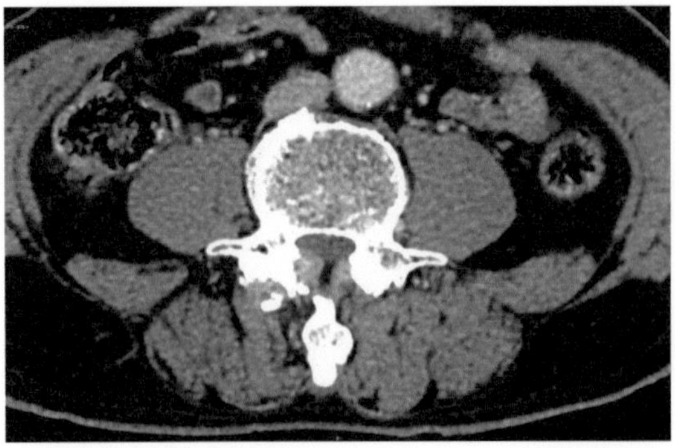

Fig. 19.3 Axial post-contrast CT image of the lumbar spine in soft tissue window (L3–4)

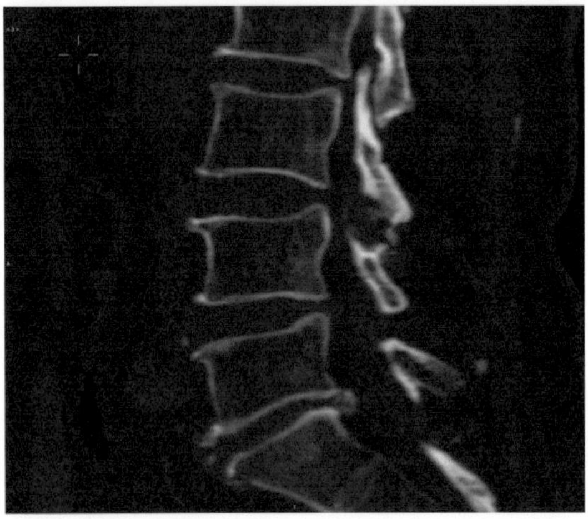

Fig. 19.4 Sagittal CT image of the lumbar spine in bone window

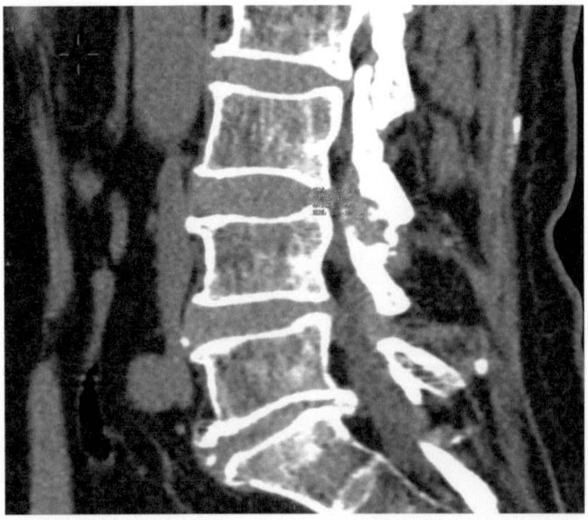

Fig. 19.5 Sagittal CT image of the lumbar spine in soft tissue window

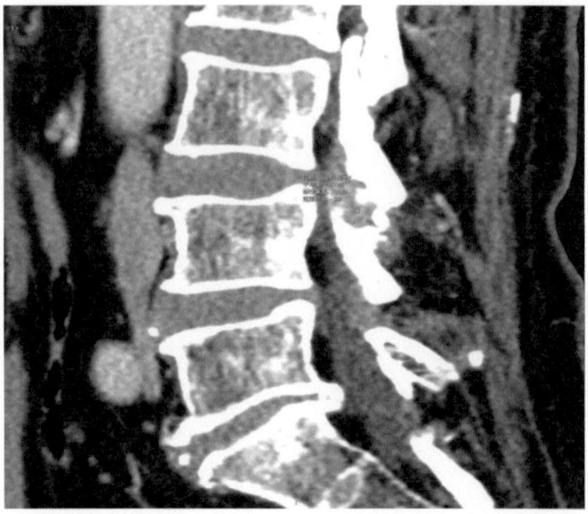

Fig. 19.6 Sagittal post-contrast CT image of the lumbar spine in soft tissue window

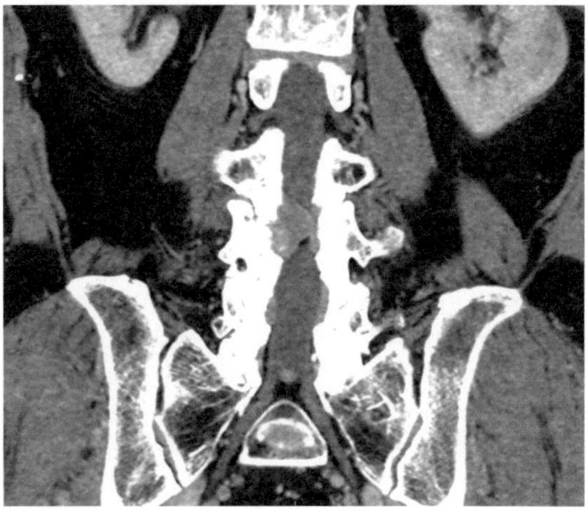

Fig. 19.7 Coronal CT image of the lumbar spine in soft tissue window

19.3.2 MR Imaging (Figs. 19.8, 19.9, 19.10, and 19.11)

MRI of the lumbar spine demonstrated bone destruction along the right facet joint of L3–4 with high T1 and low T2 signal with soft tissue mass extruding into the central canal causing compression of the cord. Heterogeneous enhancement was noted.

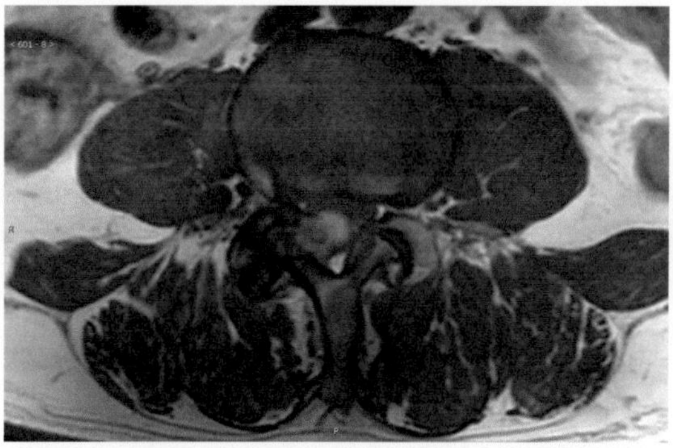

Fig. 19.8 Axial T1-weighted MR image of the lumbar spine (L3–4)

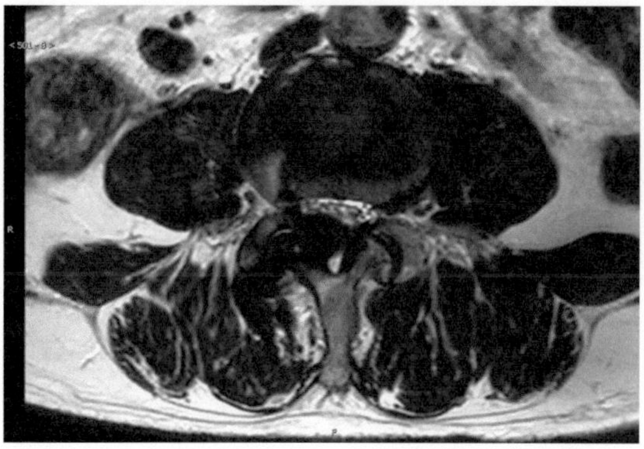

Fig. 19.9 Axial T2-weighted MR image of the lumbar spine (L3–4)

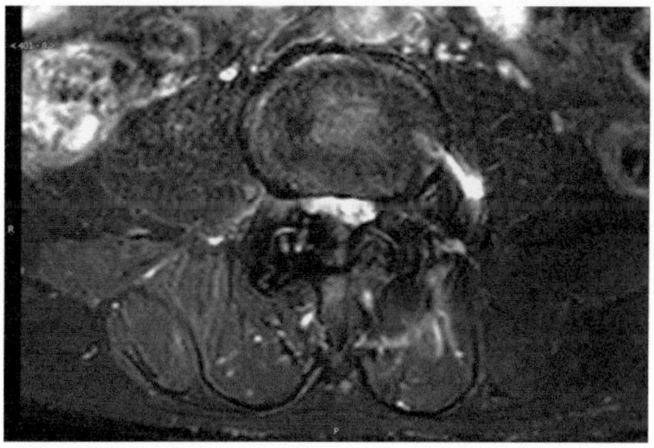

Fig. 19.10 Axial fat-suppressed T2-weighted MR image of the lumbar spine (L3–4)

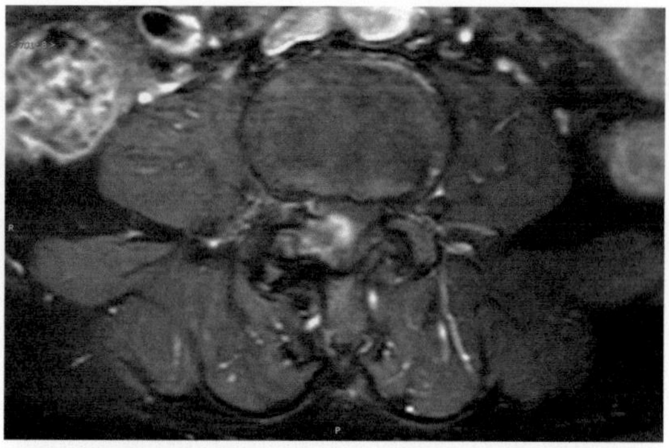

Fig. 19.11 Axial post-contrast fat-suppressed T1-weighted MR image of the lumbar spine (L3–4)

19.4 Description and Discussion from Residents

CT images demonstrated bone destruction around the right facet joint of L3–4 with surrounding nodular high densities (CT value measured at 114HU) and extruding into the central canal with compression on the dura. No enhancement was noted. We favor arthropathy, with increased density noted, raising the possibility of gout. The lesion demonstrated high T1 and low T2 signal with mass extruding to the central canal and heterogeneous enhancement, raising the possibilities of pigmented villonodular synovitis (PVNS). However, given patient's age, presentation, and CT findings, we put gout as our top consideration.

19.5 Analysis and Comments from Professor Cheng Xiao-Guang

CT images showed bone destruction of right facet joint at L3–4 with destruction involving the joint and superior and inferior articular processes and soft tissue mass of slightly high density extruding to the spinal canal. Top consideration is gout. However, with pigmented villonodular synovitis, there also could be high-density area on non-contrast CT images. MR images showed internal high T1, low T2 signal. High T1 signal usually represents fat or hemorrhage. While with tophi and PVNS, it should be low signal. With clinical experience, the lesion involved the joint, given that we consider gout and PVNS first, but not consistent with the MRI signal changes. Further evaluation with uric acid level and pathology biopsy are needed.

19.6 Diagnosis

Focal hemorrhage with surrounding fibrosis and ossification.

Suggested Reading

Anaya JEC, Coelho SRN, Taneja AK, et al. Differential diagnosis of facet joint disorders. Radiographics. 2021;41(2):543–58.

Nishida K, Iguchi T, Kurihara A, et al. Symptomatic hematoma of lumbar facet joint: joint apoplexy of the spine? Spine (Phila Pa 1976). 2003;28(11):E206–8.

20 Gout: Case 20

20.1 Medical History

Patient is a 39-year-old male. He started to experience bilateral lower extremities numbness with weakness about 2 months ago without clear causes. Sometimes, this was accompanied by burning sensation at the perineal area.

20.2 Physical Examination

Muscle strength of bilateral lower extremities at III. Decreased of both shallow and deep sensations.

20.3 Imaging Findings

20.3.1 CT Imaging (Figs. 20.1, 20.2, 20.3, 20.4, 20.5, and 20.6)

CT images of the lumbar spine demonstrated bone destruction along the bilateral L4–5 facet joints with high-density soft tissue masses with clear margin and relative homogeneous density of about 194 HU.

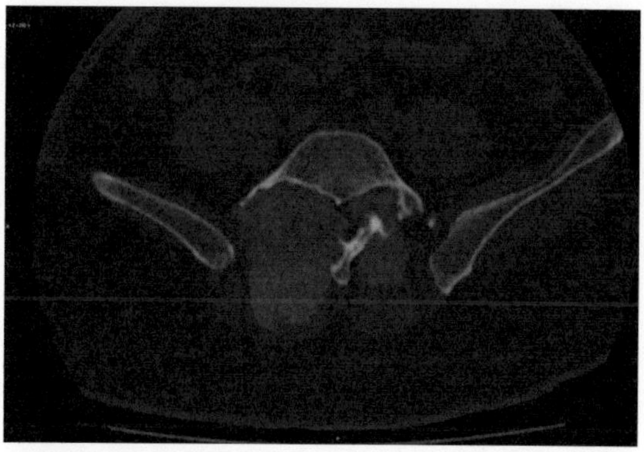

Fig. 20.1 Axial CT image of the lumbar spine in bone window (L4–5)

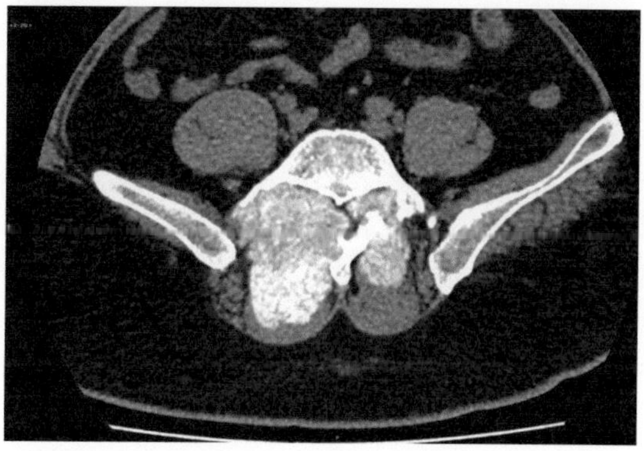

Fig. 20.2 Axial CT image of the lumbar spine in soft tissue window (L4–5)

X. Cheng et al., *Imaging of Bone Tumors in Axial Bones*,
https://doi.org/10.1007/978-981-95-2262-0_20

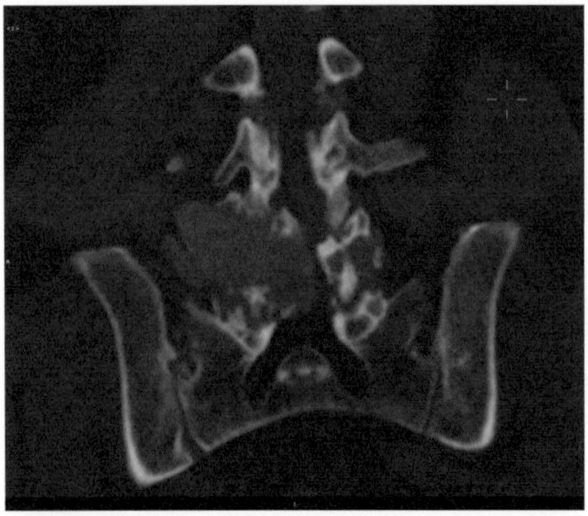

Fig. 20.3 Coronal CT image of the lumbar spine in bone window (L4–5)

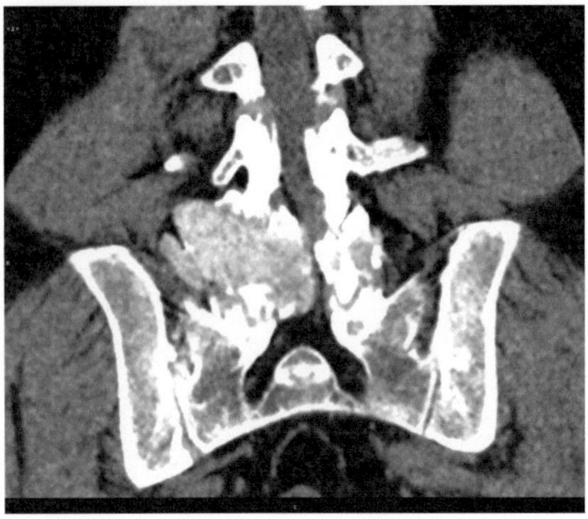

Fig. 20.4 Coronal CT image of the lumbar spine in soft tissue window

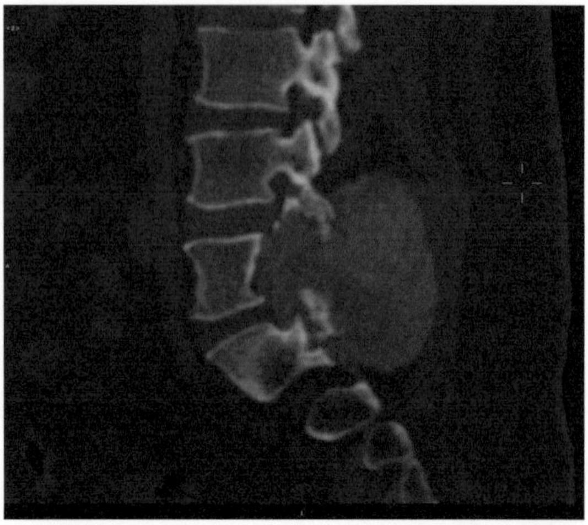

Fig. 20.5 Sagittal CT image of the lumbar spine in bone window

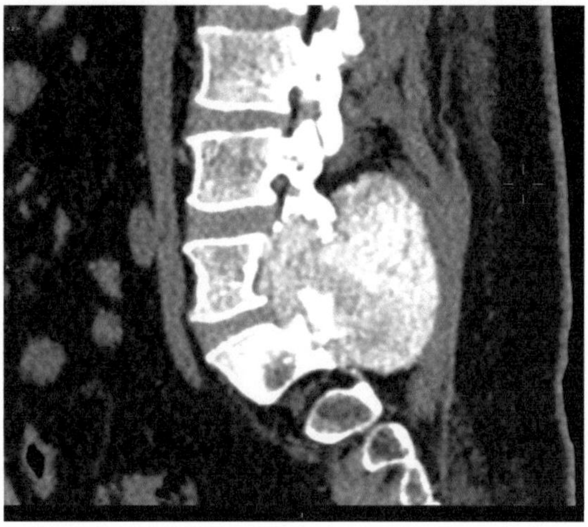

Fig. 20.6 Sagittal CT image of the lumbar spine in soft tissue window

20.3.2 MR Imaging (Figs. 20.7, 20.8, 20.9, and 20.10)

MRI of the lumbar spine demonstrated bone destruction along the bilateral facet joints of L4–5 with surrounding globular soft tissue masses with isointense T1 signal and slightly low T2 signal. With involving the bilateral pedicles, laminae, and right vertebral body, the bone destruction appeared as absorption changes from external compression. There was narrowing of the central canal at L5-S1 level. The lesion extended posterior and invading the bilateral erector spinae muscles.

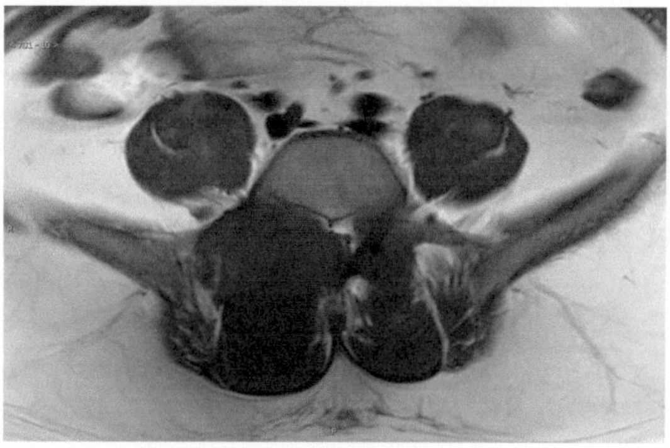

Fig. 20.7 Axial T1-weighted MR image of the lumbar spine (L4–5)

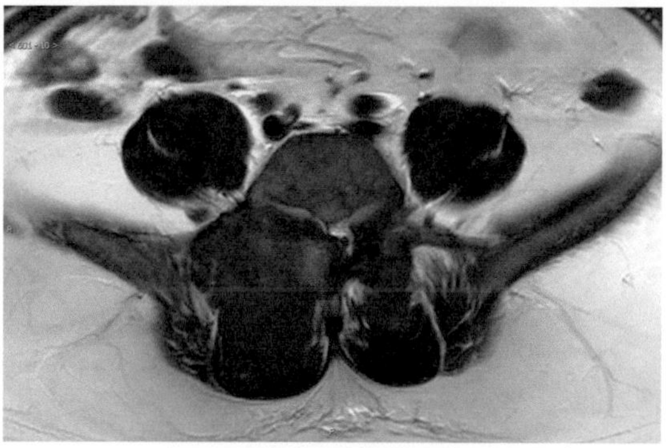

Fig. 20.8 Axial T2-weighted MR image of the lumbar spine (L4–5)

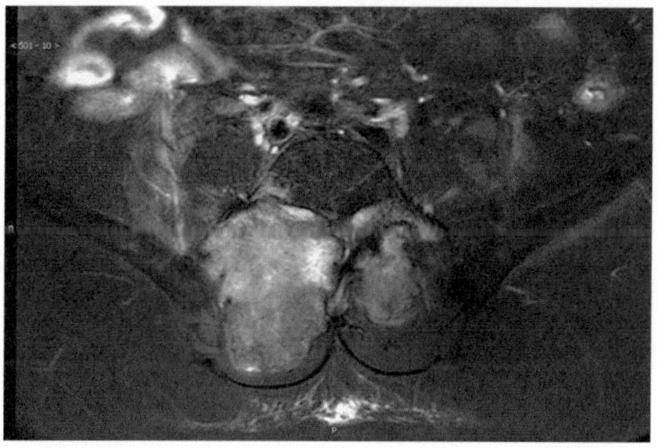

Fig. 20.9 Axial fat-suppressed T2-weighted MR image of the lumbar spine (L4–5)

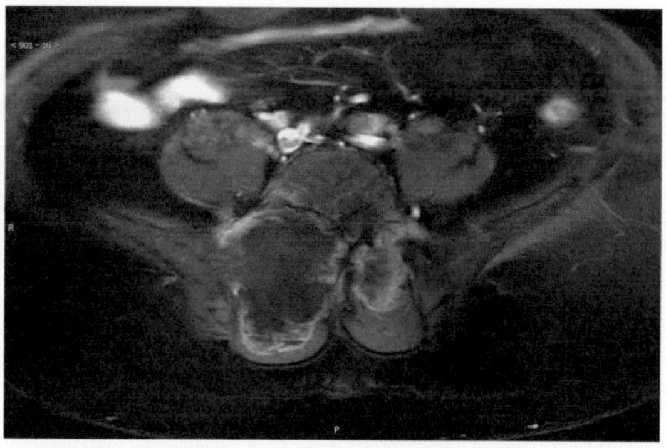

Fig. 20.10 Axial post-contrast fat-suppressed T1-weighted MR image of the lumbar spine (L4–5)

20.4 Description and Discussion from Residents

CT images demonstrated bone destruction of the bilateral posterior elements of L5 with a large lobulated soft tissue mass with relative homogenous high density, of CT value 194 HU. High-density lesion noted on non-contrast CT images suggesting of osteoblastoma or fibrous lesion. The mass showed isointense signal on T1-weighted MR images and iso to slightly high signal on T2-weighted images, with peripheral enhancement. MR findings are suggestive of fibrous or osteogenic pathology, and the enhancement pattern not supportive of aggressive lesion. Given the above findings, our top consideration is osteoblastoma and with fibrous lesion in the differential diagnosis.

20.5 Analysis and Comments from Professor Cheng Xiao-Guang

Patient was a young male. Non-contrast CT images showed high-density lesion along the bilateral facet joints of L5. Both gout and tumoral calcinosis can have these findings. Non-contrast MR images added no useful information for diagnosis. On the post-contrast images, there was peripheral enhancement and central no enhancement. Two important characteristics of the current case: (1) bilateral involvements of the facet joints, neoplastic process can be excluded, and (2) high density noted on non-contrast CT images, commonly seen in tophi with gout and tumoral calcinosis. Peripheral enhancement noted on the post-contrast MR images, whereas usually no enhancement with tophi, so my top consideration is tumoral calcinosis. Imaging diagnosis of bone tumor or tumor-like lesion usually depends on combining CT and MR images together, such as the current case; it would be very challenging to just based on the MR images alone for the diagnosis.

20.6 Diagnosis

Gout.

Suggested Reading

Anaya JEC, Coelho SRN, Taneja AK, et al. Differential diagnosis of facet joint disorders. Radiographics. 2021;41(2):543–58.

Wendling D, Prati C, Hoen B, et al. When gout involves the spine: five patients including two inaugural cases. Joint Bone Spine. 2013;80(6):656–9.

21 Schwannoma: Case 21

21.1 Medical History

Patient is a 45-year-old male. He suffered back pain for over a year with left lower extremity pain and numbness for 3 months.

21.2 Physical Examination

No abnormalities.

21.3 Imaging Findings

21.3.1 CT Imaging (Figs. 21.1, 21.2, 21.3, 21.4, 21.5, and 21.6)

CT images of the lumbar spine demonstrated soft tissue mass in the central canal around L5 level with homogeneous density and clear margin and secondary absorption around the vertebral body and extending from the left L5-S1 neuroforamen with close relationship to the S1 nerve root.

21.3.2 MR Imaging (Figs. 21.7, 21.8, 21.9, 21.10, 21.11, and 21.12)

MR images of the lumbar spine demonstrated iso-intense T1 signal and heterogeneous T2 signal within the central canal at the L5 level with internal multiple septations and multiple fluid-

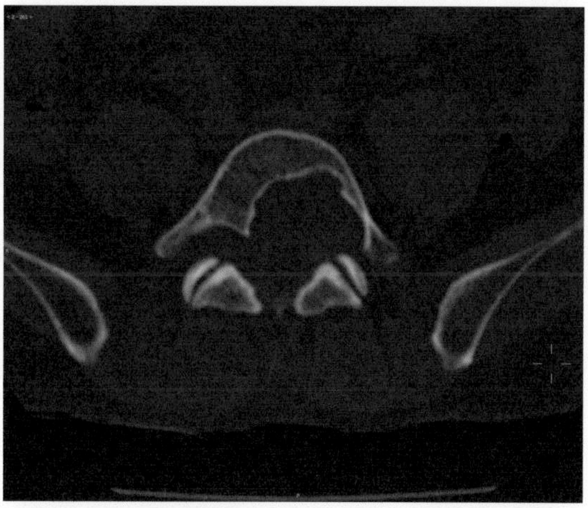

Fig. 21.1 Axial CT image of the lumbar spine in bone window (L5 level)

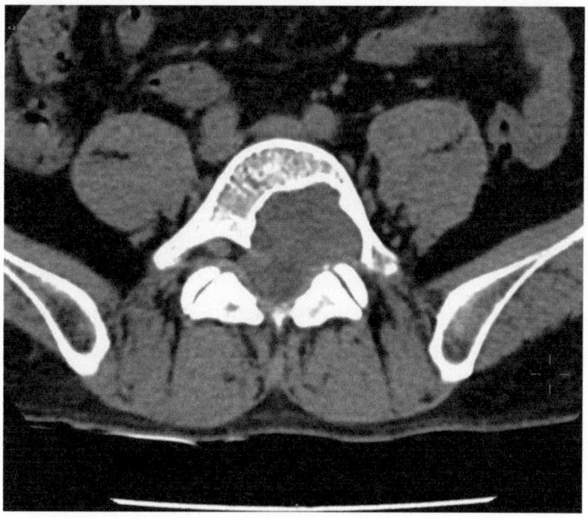

Fig. 21.2 Axial CT image of the lumbar spine in soft tissue window (L5 level)

X. Cheng et al., *Imaging of Bone Tumors in Axial Bones*,
https://doi.org/10.1007/978-981-95-2262-0_21

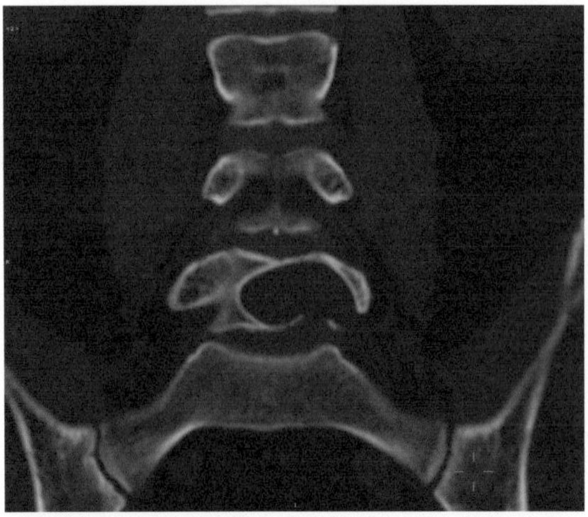

Fig. 21.3 Coronal CT image of the lumbar spine in bone window

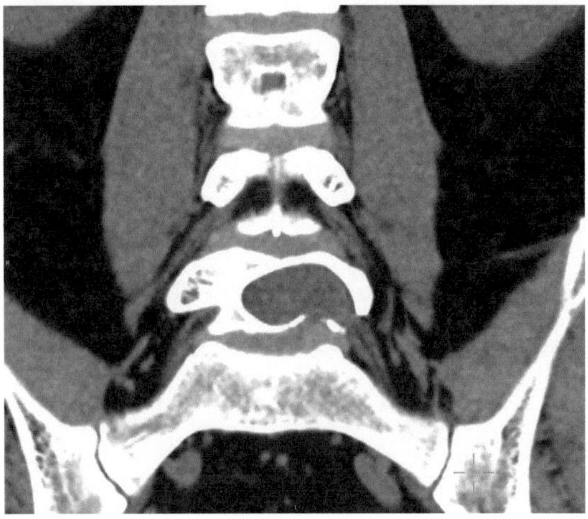

Fig. 21.4 Coronal CT image of the lumbar spine in soft tissue window

fluid levels. The lesion extended along the left L5-S1 neuroforamen with close relationship to the S1 nerve root and extending anteriorly with bone absorption of the vertebral body and mass effect upon the dura with marked narrowing of the canal. Avid peripheral enhancement was noted.

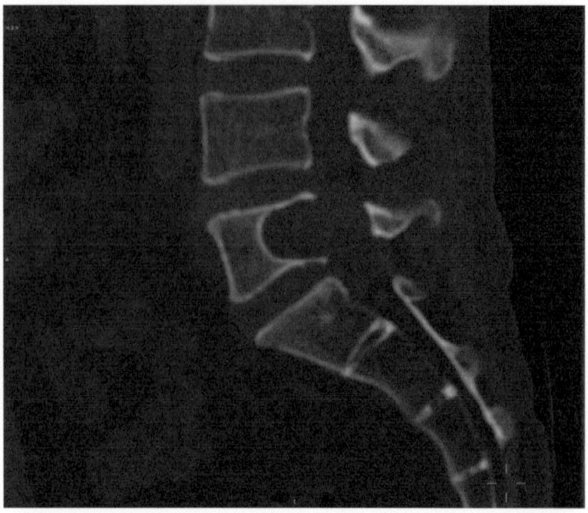

Fig. 21.5 Sagittal CT image of the lumbar spine in bone window

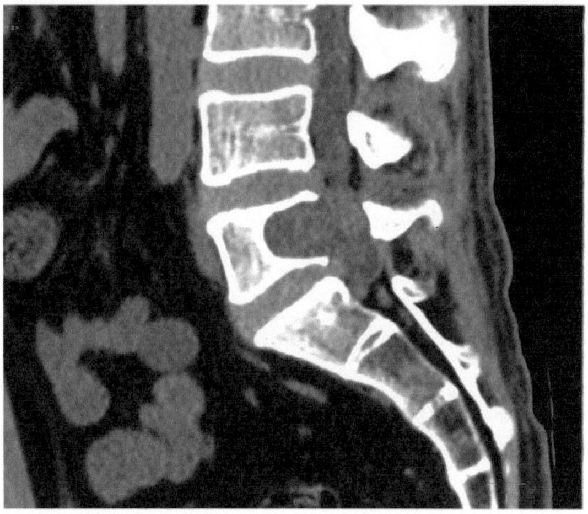

Fig. 21.6 Sagittal CT image of the lumbar spine in soft tissue window

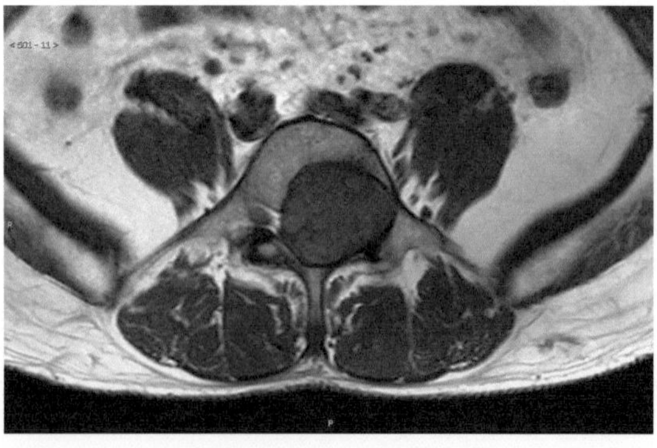

Fig. 21.7 Axial T1-weighted MR image of the lumbar spine

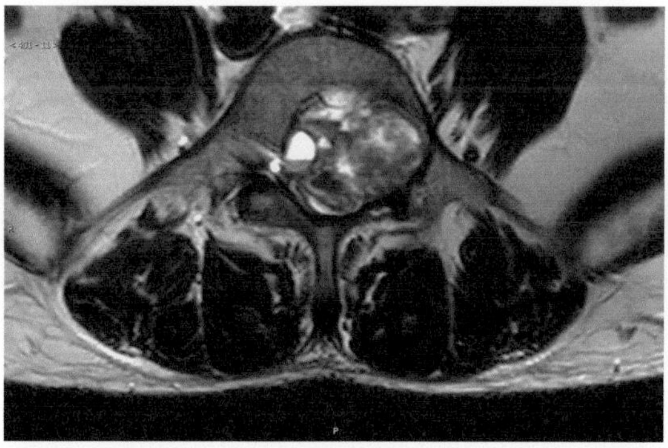

Fig. 21.8 Axial T2-weighted MR image of the lumbar spine (L4–5)

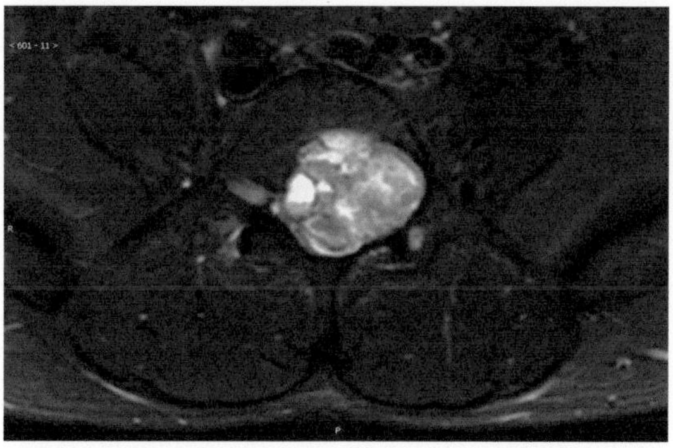

Fig. 21.9 Axial fat-suppressed T2-weighted MR image of the lumbar spine

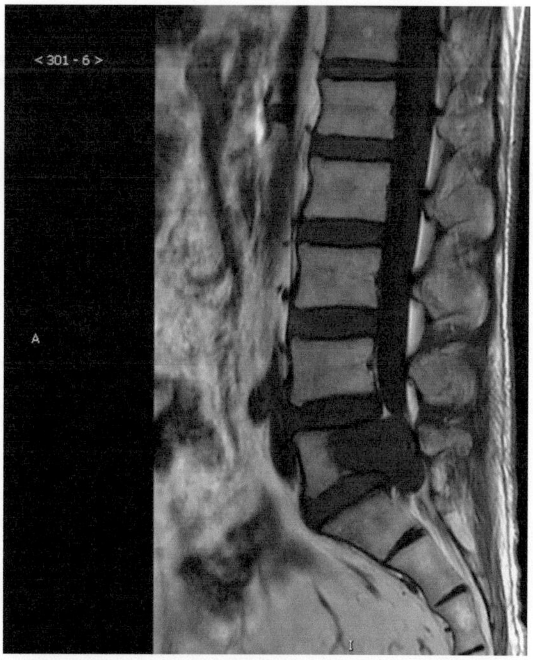

Fig. 21.10 Sagittal T1-weighted MR image of the lumbar spine

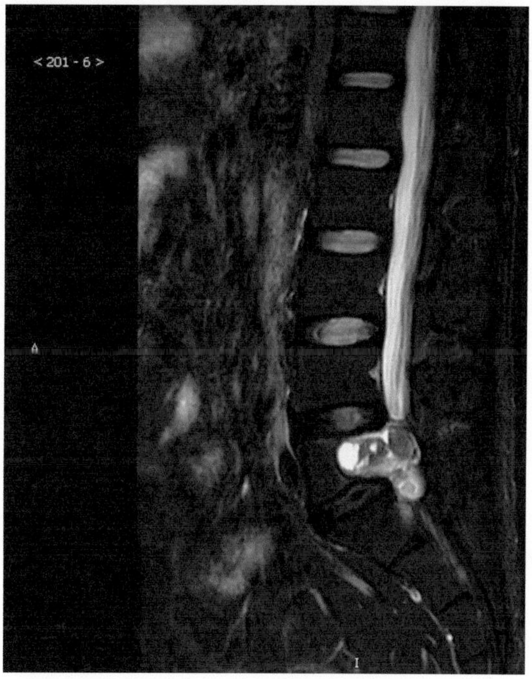

Fig. 21.11 Sagittal fat-suppressed T2-weighted MR image of the lumbar spine

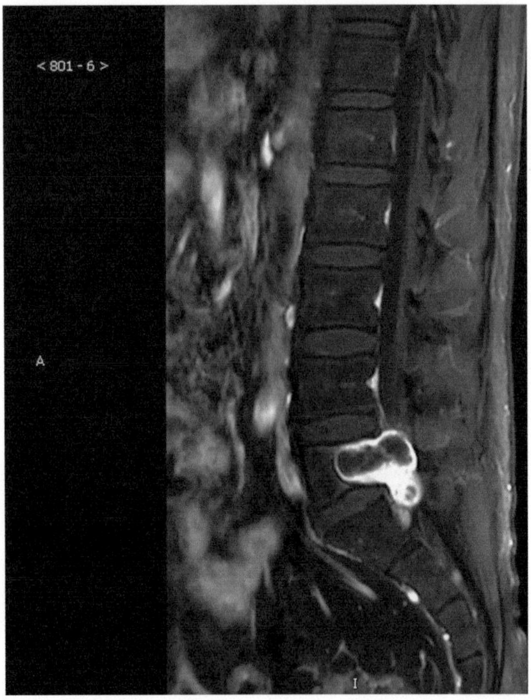

Fig. 21.12 Sagittal post-contrast fat-suppressed T1-weighted MR image of the lumbar spine

21.4 Description and Discussion from Residents

CT images demonstrated a space occupying lesion in the central canal at the L5 level with bone absorption of the vertebral body from compression with peripheral sclerosis. There was secondary enlargement of the left L5-S1 neuroforamen, suggesting a benign neurogenic tumor, such as schwannoma. MR images showed iso-intense T1 signal but slightly high signal on the right with heterogenous T2 signal and multiple fluid-fluid levels. There was a smooth margin with peripheral enhancement. MR images suggested cystic changes and hemorrhage within the lesion, again supporting schwannoma. Differential diagnosis includes lesions arising from bone, such as aneurysmal bone cyst.

21.5 Analysis and Comments from Professor Cheng Xiao-Guang

Patient is a middle-aged male. CT images showed bone destruction of L5 vertebral body with clear margin and peripheral sclerosis and no periosteal shell of reactive bone. With spinal lesion, we need to decide where the lesion arose from, the central canal or vertebral body first, and then pay attention to the relationship with the neuroforamen. There was thickening of the left S1 nerve root compared to the right with enlargement of the left neuroforamen with soft tissue mass extending along the neuroforamen. Single lesion, clear margin, and peripheral sclerosis, all suggesting a benign neoplasm. MR images showed cystic nature of the lesion with enhancements along the walls of the cysts. We need to realize that MR images commonly only have a supportive role in diagnosing bone tumors. It is not the main tool. Especially, we can't totally rely on MR scans for enhancement; mostly we should base that on CT images. Overall, my top consideration is a benign peripheral nerve sheath tumor compressing the vertebral body. Differential diagnosis includes lesions arising from the vertebral body, such as aneurysmal bone cyst.

21.6 Diagnosis

Schwannoma.

Suggested Reading

Tuan HX, Hung ND, Khuong NH, et al. Vestibular schwannoma with fluid-fluid levels mimicking aneurysm bone cyst. Radiol Case Rep. 2023;18(3):1079–83.

Wang YQ, Hu JX, Yang SM, et al. Intraosseous schwannoma of the mobile spine: a report of twenty cases. Eur Spine J. 2018;27(12):3092–104.

Zadeh FS, Azhideh A, Mantilla JG, et al. Imaging features of intraosseous schwannoma: a case series and review of the literature. Diagnostics (Basel). 2023;13(9):1610.

Tuberculous Spondylitis: Case 22

22

22.1 Medical History

Patient is a 61-year-old female. She had breast cancer surgery about 9 months ago followed by chemotherapy for eight cycles. She was diagnosed with neck lymph node tuberculosis about 4 months ago with antituberculosis therapy for 2 months. She was seen at the outpatient clinic for L5-S1 lesion about 2 months ago.

22.2 Physical Examination

Not done.

22.3 Imaging Findings

22.3.1 CT Imaging (Figs. 22.1, 22.2, 22.3, 22.4, 22.5, 22.6, and 22.7)

CT images demonstrated continuous bone destruction of both L5 and S1 vertebral bodies with peripheral sclerosis and adjacent soft tissue swelling with central low density. Patchy high densities were noted within the regions of the bone destruction. There was narrowing of the central canal. Peripheral enhancement was noted.

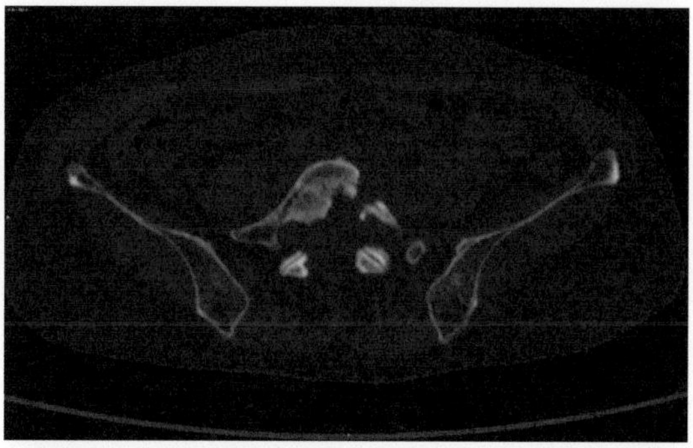

Fig. 22.1 Axial CT image of the sacrum in bone window (L5 level)

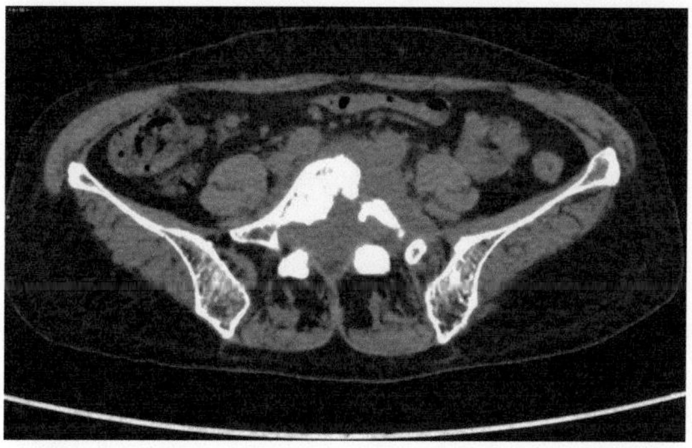

Fig. 22.2 Axial CT image of the sacrum in soft tissue window (L5 level)

X. Cheng et al., *Imaging of Bone Tumors in Axial Bones*,
https://doi.org/10.1007/978-981-95-2262-0_22

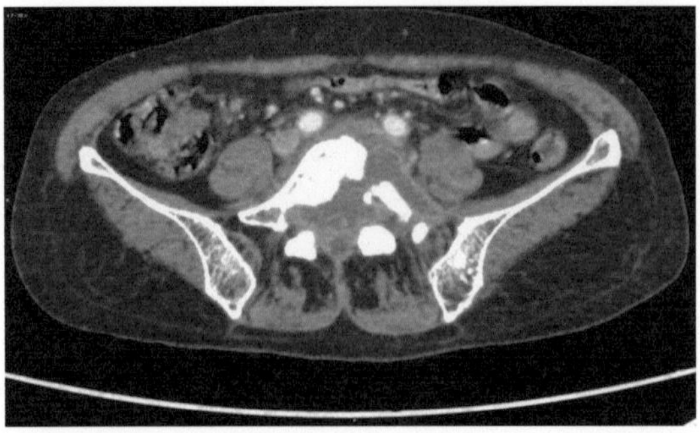

Fig. 22.3 Axial post-contrast CT image of the sacrum in soft tissue window (L5 level)

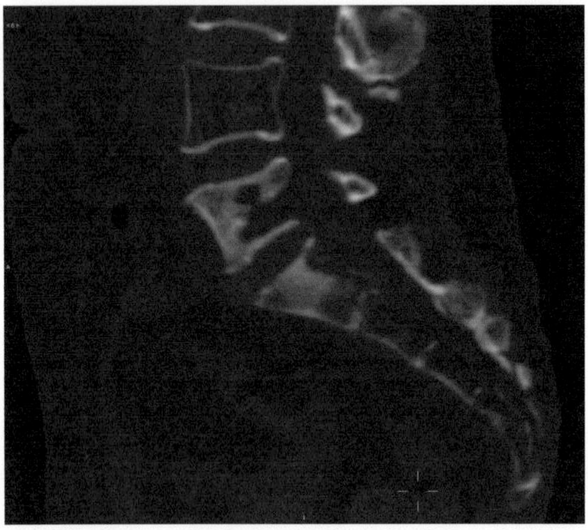

Fig. 22.4 Sagittal CT image of the sacrum in bone window

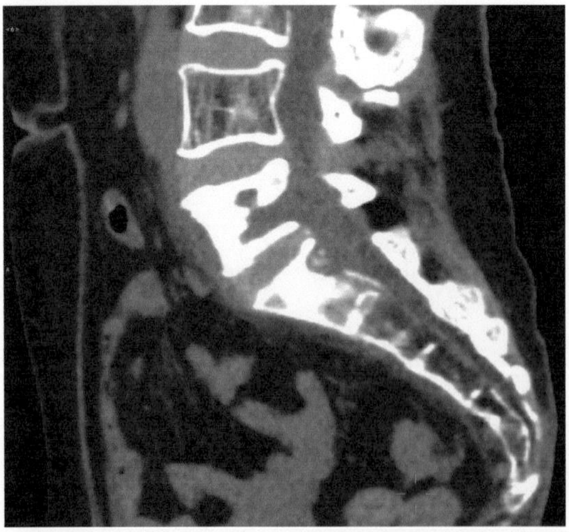

Fig. 22.5 Sagittal CT image of the sacrum in soft tissue window

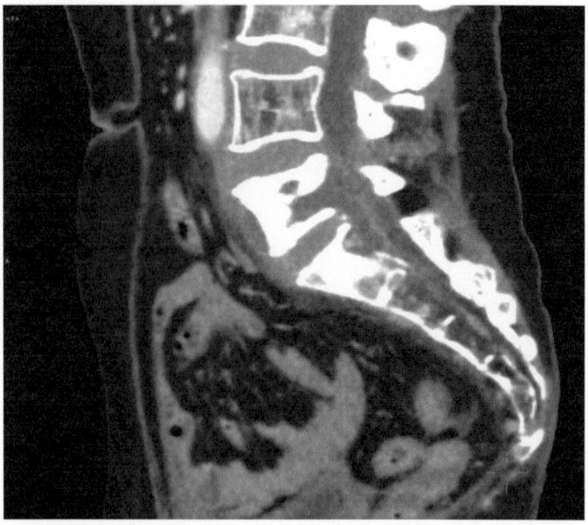

Fig. 22.6 Sagittal post-contrast CT image of the sacrum in soft tissue window

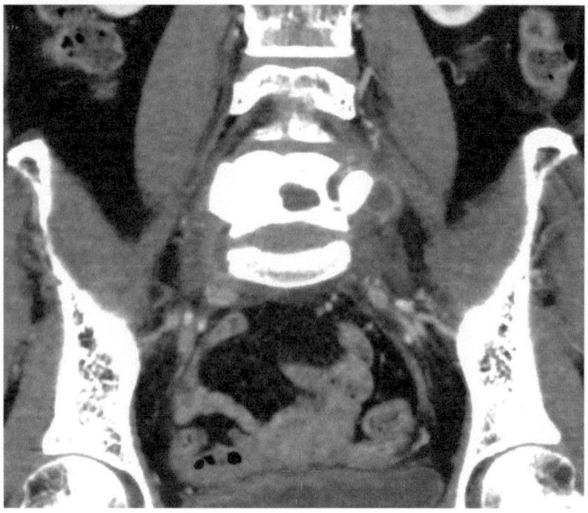

Fig. 22.7 Coronal post-contrast CT image of the sacrum in soft tissue window

22.3.2 MR Imaging (Figs. 22.8, 22.9, 22.10, 22.11, 22.12, 22.13, and 22.14)

MR images of the sacrum demonstrated bone destruction of the L5, S1 vertebral bodies, and also the superior S2 vertebral body with heterogeneous signals. On T2-weighted sequences, central slightly low T2 signal and peripheral high signal were noted. The bone destruction was communicated by disruption of the posterior cortices with some extension anteriorly. There were

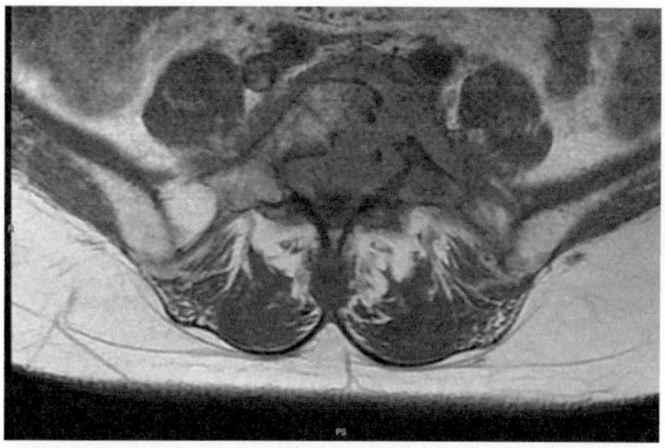

Fig. 22.8 Axial T1-weighted MR image of the lumbar spine (L5 level)

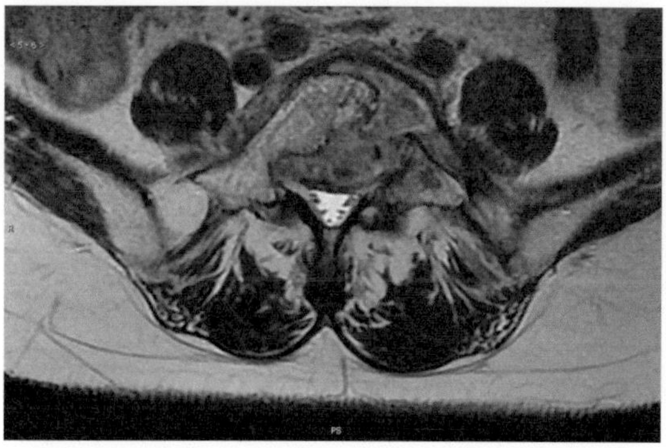

Fig. 22.9 Axial T2-weighted MR image of the lumbar spine (L5 level)

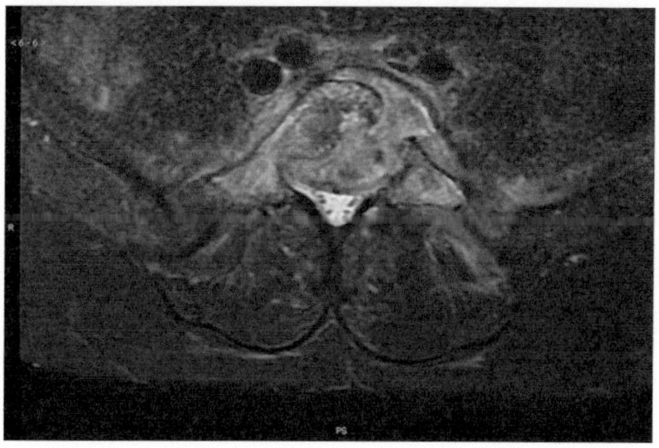

Fig. 22.10 Axial fat-suppressed T2-weighted MR image of the lumbar spine (L5 level)

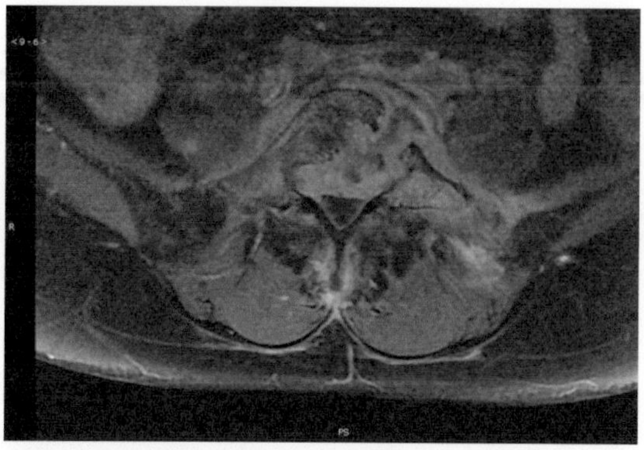

Fig. 22.11 Axial post-contrast fat-suppressed T1-weighted MR image of the lumbar spine (L5)

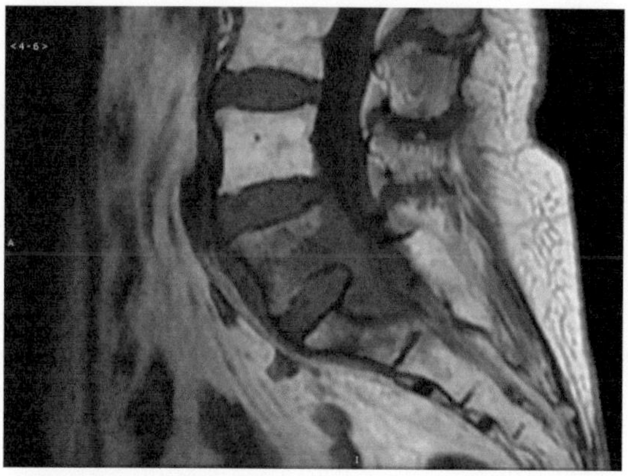

Fig. 22.12 Sagittal T1-weighted MR image of the lumbar spine

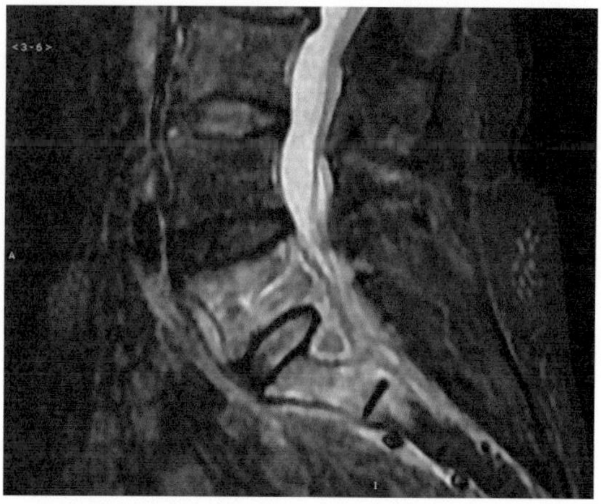

Fig. 22.13 Sagittal fat-suppressed T2-weighted MR image of the lumbar spine

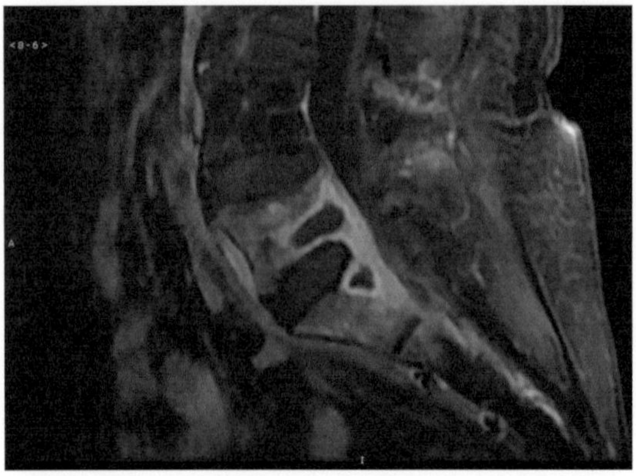

Fig. 22.14 Sagittal post-contrast fat-suppressed T1-weighted MR image of the lumbar spine

surrounding bone marrow edema and soft tissue edema. Peripheral enhancement noted with the central cystic portion showed no enhancement.

22.4 Description and Discussion from Residents

CT images showed lytic destruction of the L5 and S1 vertebral bodies with surrounding soft tissue swelling and extending beyond the vertebral bodies to the left anteriorly. There was peripheral sclerosis with preserved intervertebral disc spaces and peripheral enhancement. MR images demonstrated isointense T1 signal and heterogeneous high T2 signal and diffuse adjacent soft tissue edema. Given the above findings and the provided history, our top consideration is tuberculosis. There was no narrowing of the intervertebral disc spaces but with increased signal at the disc of L5-S1, indicating inflammatory changes of the disc. Metastatic disease from breast cancer is the differential diagnosis.

22.5 Analysis and Comments from Professor Cheng Xiao-Guang

Patient is a middle-aged female. CT images showed L5 and S1 bone destruction with adjacent soft tissue changes and peripheral reactive sclerosis around the bone destruction and preserved intervertebral disc spaces. MR images showed the inflammatory nature of the lesion: adjacent soft tissue edema, abscess inside the canal, and peripheral enhancement along the abscess wall. My top consideration is infectious processes, such as tuberculosis.

22.6 Diagnosis

Tuberculous spondylitis.

Suggested Reading

Abid W, Ladeb MF, Chidambaranathan N, et al. Imaging of musculoskeletal tuberculosis. Skeletal Radiol. 2024; https://doi.org/10.1007/s00256-023-04556-5.

Kilborn T, Rensburg PJ, Candy S. Pediatric and adult spinal tuberculosis: imaging and pathophysiology. Neuroimaging Clin N Am. 2015;25(2):209–31.

Moorthy S, Prabhu NK. Spectrum of MR imaging findings in spinal tuberculosis. AJR Am J Roentgenol. 2002;179(4):979–83.

23 Aneurysmal Bone Cyst: Case 23

23.1 Medical History

Patient is a 10-year-old girl. She started to suffer from back pain around the waist without clear causes about 9 months ago. She noticed a mass at the waist about 4 months ago and was seen at a local hospital with unknown treatment and no relief of symptoms. She had focal resection biopsy of the lesion about 2 months ago.

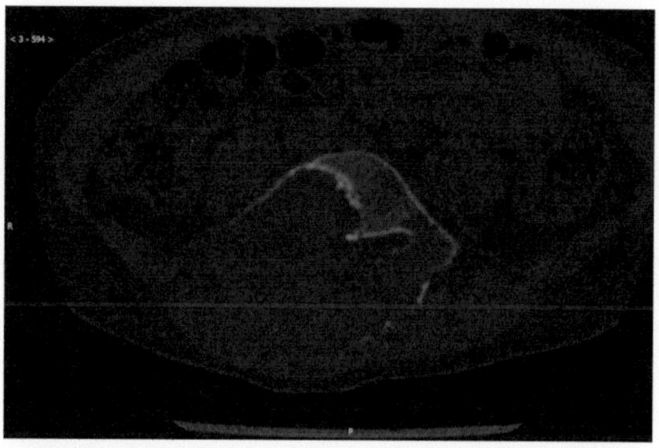

Fig. 23.1 Axial CT image of the lumbar spine in bone window (L5 level)

23.2 Physical Examination

There is a protruding mass around the right waist with a 3 cm long scar from prior surgery.

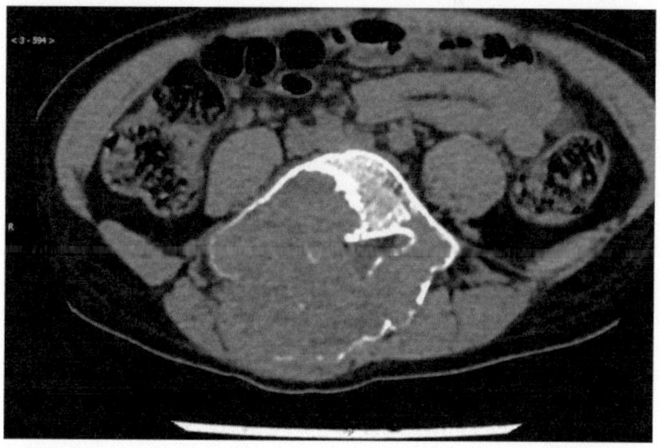

Fig. 23.2 Axial CT image of the lumbar spine in soft tissue window (L5 level)

23.3 Imaging Findings

23.3.1 CT Imaging (Figs. 23.1, 23.2, 23.3, 23.4, 23.5, and 23.6)

CT images of the lumbar spine demonstrated bone lytic destruction of L5, S1 vertebral bodies, and the posterior elements with expansile changes with clear margin. There were medullary peripheral sclerosis and discontinuous shell of reactive bone. There were multiple fluid-fluid levels with scattered calcifications around the septations. Peripheral and septation enhancements were noted. There was narrowing of the central canal of the corresponding levels.

X. Cheng et al., *Imaging of Bone Tumors in Axial Bones*,
https://doi.org/10.1007/978-981-95-2262-0_23

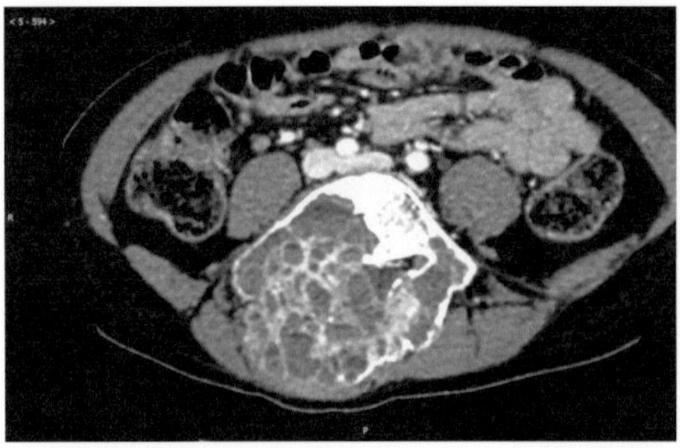

Fig. 23.3 Axial post-contrast CT image of the lumbar spine in soft tissue window (L5 level)

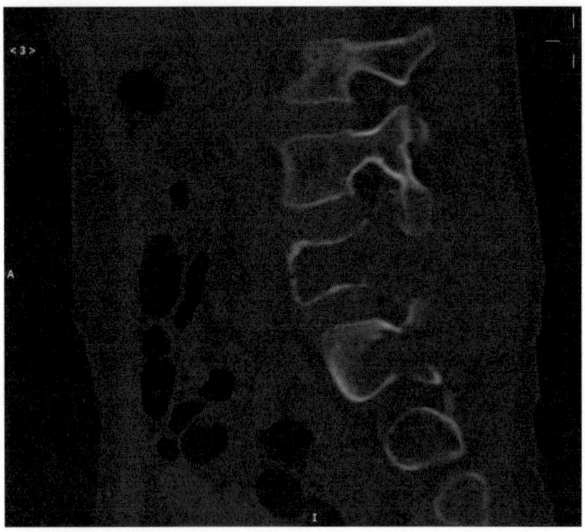

Fig. 23.4 Sagittal CT image of the lumbar spine in bone window

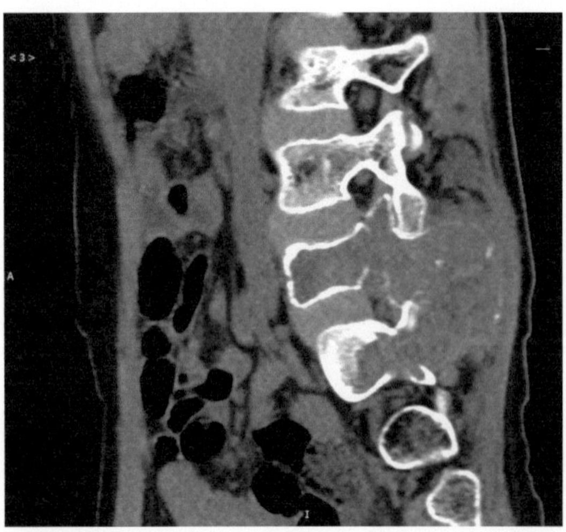

Fig. 23.5 Sagittal CT image of the lumbar spine in soft tissue window

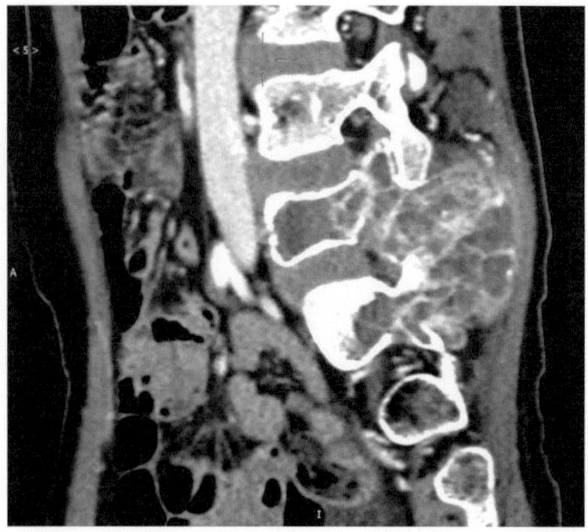

Fig. 23.6 Sagittal post-contrast CT image of the lumbar spine in soft tissue window

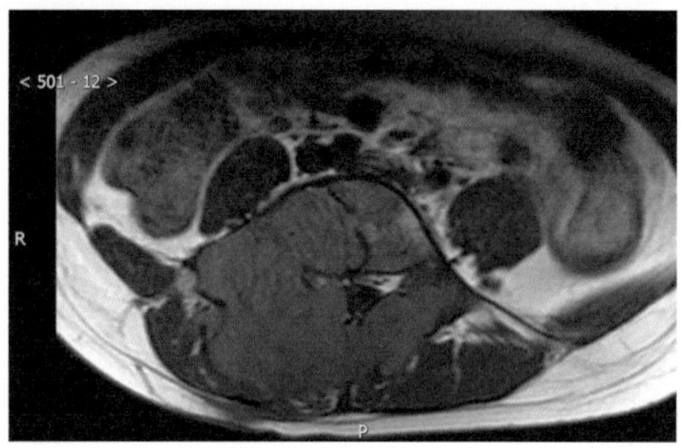

Fig. 23.7 Axial T1-weighted MR image of the lumbar spine (L5 level)

23.3.2 MR Imaging (Figs. 23.7, 23.8, 23.9, 23.10, 23.11, and 23.12)

MR images of the lumbar spine demonstrated expansile bone destruction of the L5 vertebral body and posterior elements and S1 vertebral body on the right and posterior elements. There were low signals of medullary sclerosis and peripheral shell. Multiple fluid-fluid levels noted internally with septations. Enhancements along the septations and periphery noted. There was narrowing of the spinal canal at L5 with compression of the right nerve root.

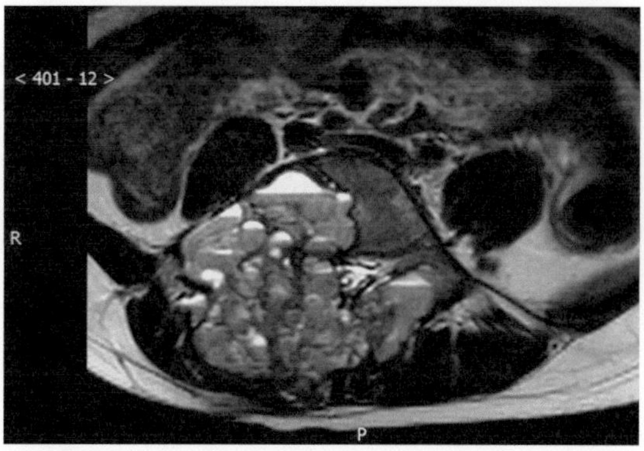

Fig. 23.8 Axial T2-weighted MR image of the lumbar spine (L5 level)

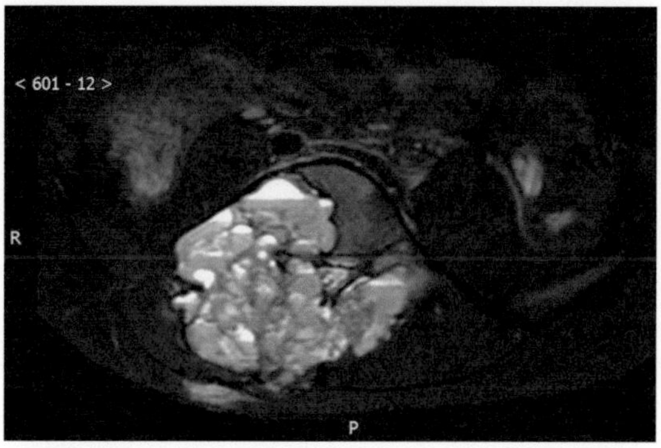

Fig. 23.9 Axial fat-suppressed T2-weighted MR image of the lumbar spine (L5 level)

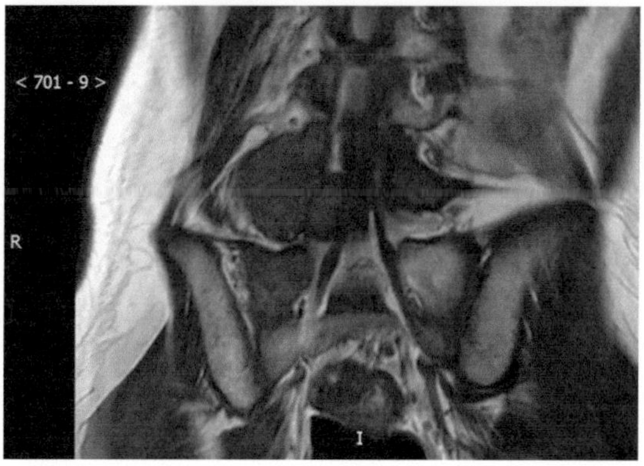

Fig. 23.10 Coronal T1-weighted MR image of the lumbar spine

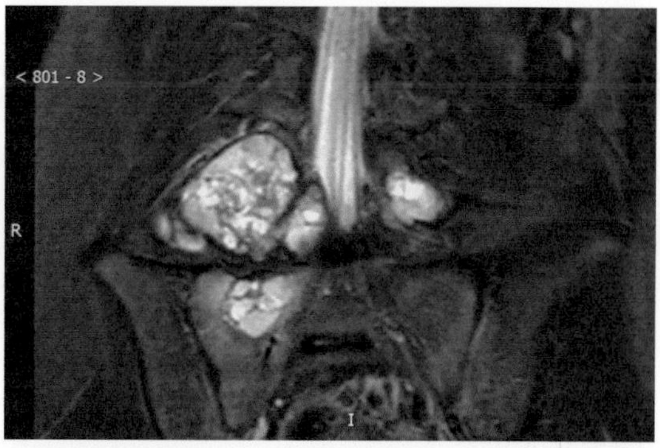

Fig. 23.11 Coronal fat-suppressed T2-weighted MR image of the lumbar spine

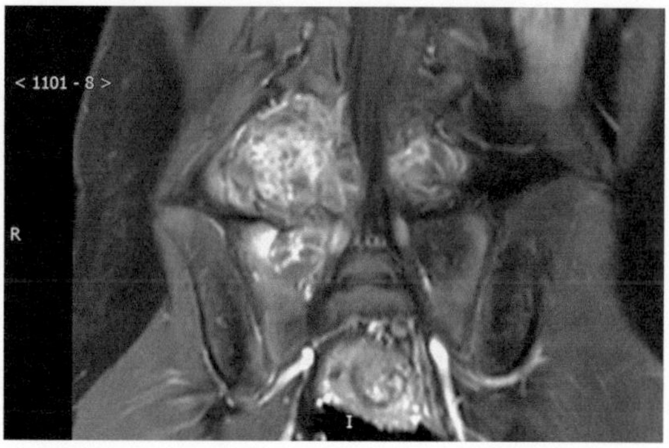

Fig. 23.12 Coronal post-contrast fat-suppressed T1-weighted MR image of the lumbar spine

23.4 Description and Discussion from Residents

This was a pediatric patient. CT images showed lytic bone destruction of L5, S1 vertebral bodies and posterior elements with clear margin, and peripheral medullary sclerosis and peripheral bone shell and heterogenous densities of the soft tissue mass. There were multiple fluid-fluid levels and ridges noted with avid peripheral and septation enhancements. Our top consideration is aneurysmal bone cyst (ABC). However, with too much septations noted with avid enhancement, telangiectatic osteosarcoma needs to be excluded. Additionally, secondary aneurysmal bone cyst is also in the differential diagnosis. The lesion showed focal high T1 signal on the MR images, suggesting hemorrhage. Multiple fluid-fluid levels noted on the T2-weighted images with small solid components. Peripheral and septation avid enhancements were also seen. The above findings are most suggestive of aneurysmal bone cyst with telangiectatic osteosarcoma in the differential diagnosis.

23.5 Analysis and Comments from Professor Cheng Xiao-Guang

Patient is a 10-year-old child. There was expansile bone destruction of the L5 vertebral body and posterior elements with clear margin and discontinued bone shell. There was involvement of the sacrum, indicating some degree of invasiveness of the lesion. Internal multiple fluid-fluid levels noted on the CT images with avid peripheral and septation enhancements. These features were more apparent in the MR images. Overall, my consideration is aneurysmal bone cyst. Currently, the consensus is that aneurysmal bone cyst is a true neoplasm and what used to be called "secondary aneurysmal bone cyst" should be termed as ABC-like changes or multicystic changes. There were some features of invasiveness of the current lesion, and telangiectatic osteosarcoma needs to be excluded.

23.6 Diagnosis

Aneurysmal bone cyst.

Suggested Reading

Ariyaratne S, Jenko N, Iyengar KP, et al. Primary benign neoplasms of the spine. Diagnostics (Basel). 2023;13(12):2006.

Sayago LR, Remondino RG, Tello CA, et al. Aneurysmal bone cysts of the spine in children: a review of 18 cases. Global Spine J. 2020;10(7):875–80.

Simple Bone Cyst: Case 24

24

24.1 Medical History

Patient is a 42-year-old male. He was seen at the outpatient clinic for a sacral lesion for 7 years.

24.2 Physical Examination

No abnormalities.

24.3 Imaging Findings

24.3.1 Radiograph (Fig. 24.1)

Radiograph of the bony pelvis showed suspected bone destruction around the right sacral ala with peripheral sclerosis.

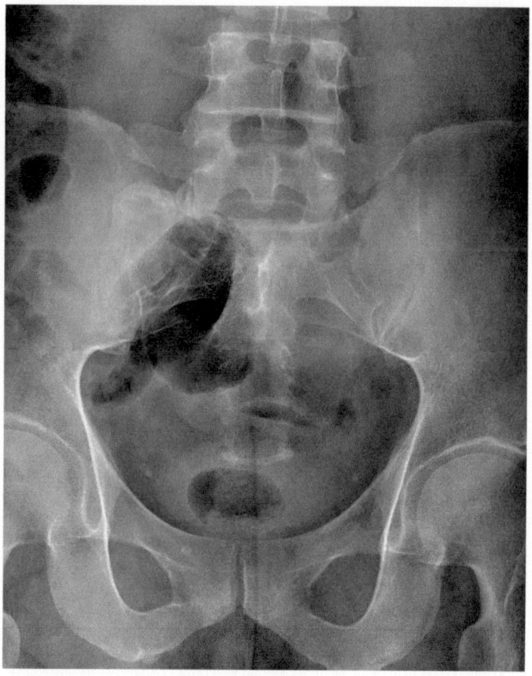

Fig. 24.1 Frontal view of the bony pelvis

24.3.2 CT Imaging (Figs. 24.2, 24.3, 24.4, 24.5, 24.6, and 24.7)

CT images of the bony pelvis demonstrated lytic bone destruction around the right sacral ala at S1 with clear margin and peripheral sclerosis. Internal density of the lesion was with CT value of 42 HU, with mild heterogeneous enhancement and post-contrast CT value of 66 HU. The lesion did not involve the neuroforamen.

X. Cheng et al., *Imaging of Bone Tumors in Axial Bones*,
https://doi.org/10.1007/978-981-95-2262-0_24

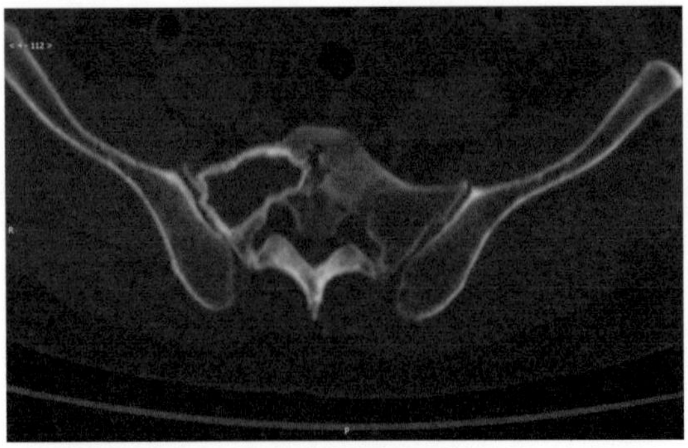

Fig. 24.2 Axial CT image of the bony pelvis in bone window

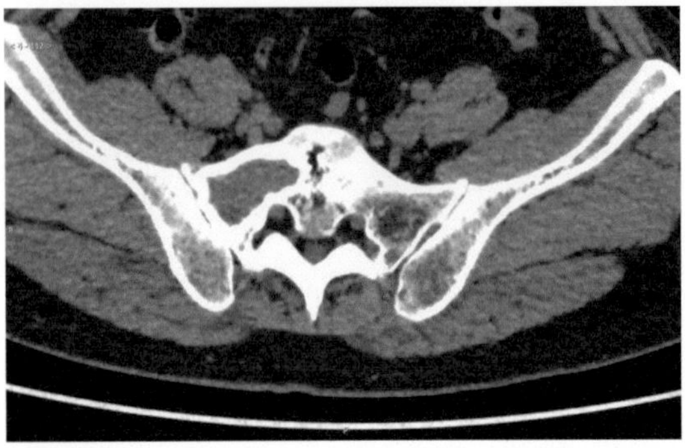

Fig. 24.3 Axial CT image of the bony pelvis in soft tissue window

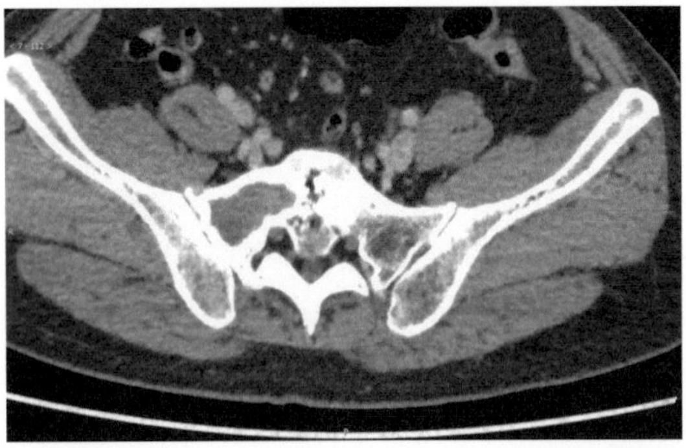

Fig. 24.4 Axial post-contrast CT image of the bony pelvis in soft tissue window

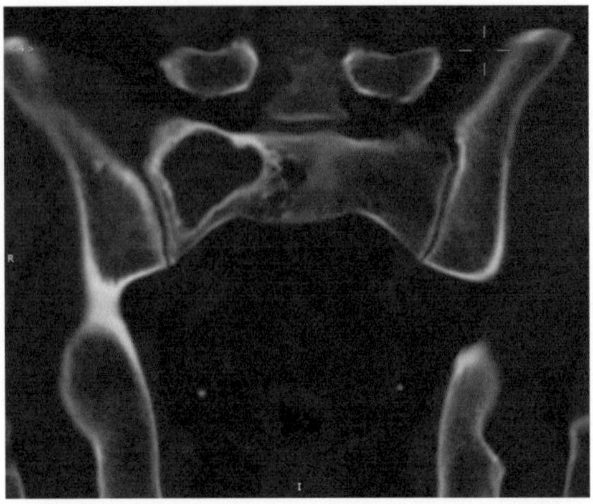

Fig. 24.5 Coronal CT image of the bony pelvis in bone window

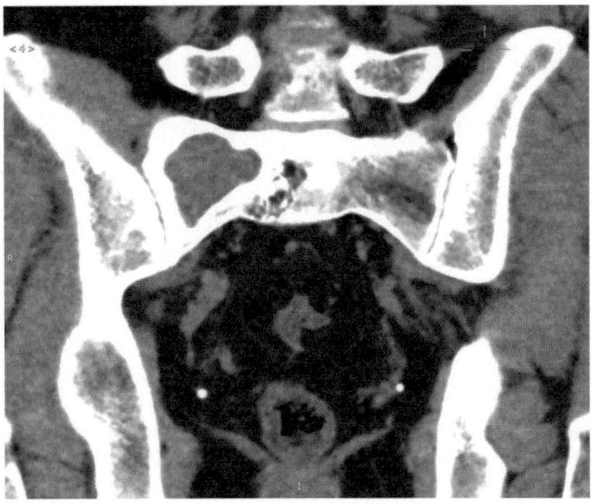

Fig. 24.6 Coronal CT image of the bony pelvis in soft tissue window

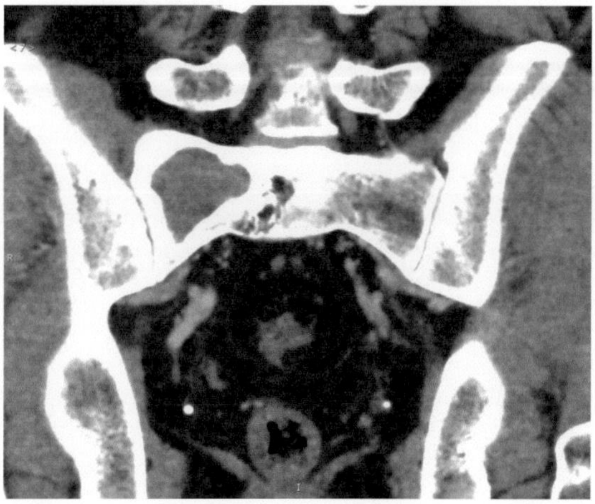

Fig. 24.7 Coronal post-contrast CT image of the bony pelvis in soft tissue window

24.4 Description and Discussion from Residents

There was suspicious low density at right sacral ala with peripheral sclerosis on the radiograph. CT images showed bone destruction of the right sacral ala with clear peripheral sclerosis and no associated soft tissue mass or involvement of the adjacent neuroforamen. No avid enhancement was noted. Without the provided history, our consideration would be fibrous dysplasia. However, the patient is with long history and no clear treatment history; benign lesions such as simple bone cyst or aneurysmal bone cyst can have similar changes after treatment (non-complete bone repair), should be in the differential diagnosis. It is hard to differentiate between internal cysts and solid components based on CT images alone; further evaluation with MR images is needed.

24.5 Analysis and Comments from Professor Cheng Xiao-Guang

The radiograph showed suspicious low densities of the right sacral ala. Bone destruction at right sacral ala noted on the CT images with clear margin, peripheral sclerosis, and internal heterogenous densities but without calcification. There was no involvement of the neuroforamen or spinal canal. No enhancement was noted. Overall, my consideration is benign processes such as fibrous dysplasia and aneurysmal bone cyst.

24.6 Diagnosis

Simple bone cyst.

Suggested Reading

Llauger J, Palmer J, Amores S, et al. Primary tumors of the sacrum: diagnostic imaging. AJR Am J Roentgenol. 2000;174(2):417–24.

Sambri A, Fiore M, Giannini C, et al. Primary tumors of the sacrum: imaging findings. Curr Med Imaging. 2022;18(2):170–86.

25 Ewing Sarcoma: Case 25

25.1 Medical History

Patient is a 9-year-old girl. She complained of intermittent pain along the left gluteal and back of the left proximal thigh without clear causes about 4 years ago. No radiation of the pain with self-reported relief from oral milk. She did not seek formal treatment. She had a sudden episode of pain about 1 month ago and found of mass in the spinal canal.

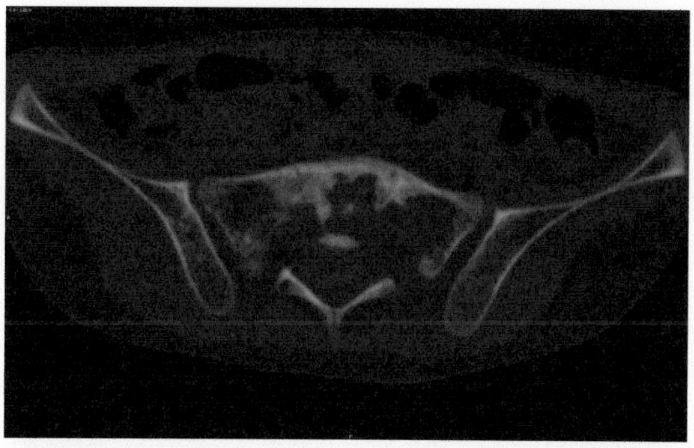

Fig. 25.1 Axial CT image of the sacrum in bone window (S1 level)

25.2 Physical Examination

Not done.

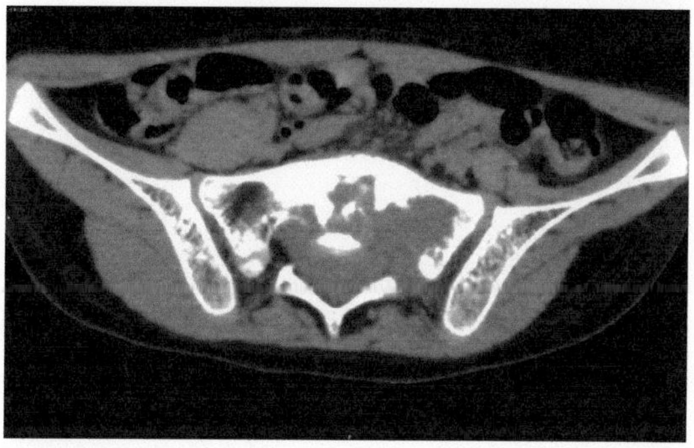

Fig. 25.2 Axial CT image of the sacrum in soft tissue window (S1 level)

25.3 Imaging Findings

25.3.1 CT Imaging (Figs. 25.1, 25.2, 25.3, 25.4, 25.5, 25.6, and 25.7)

CT images of the sacrum demonstrated bone destruction at S1and S2 with soft tissue mass in the spinal canal from L5 to S2 and involving the bilateral S1/S2 neuroforamens with protrusion anteriorly into the pelvis. There was avid heterogenous enhancement.

X. Cheng et al., *Imaging of Bone Tumors in Axial Bones*,
https://doi.org/10.1007/978-981-95-2262-0_25

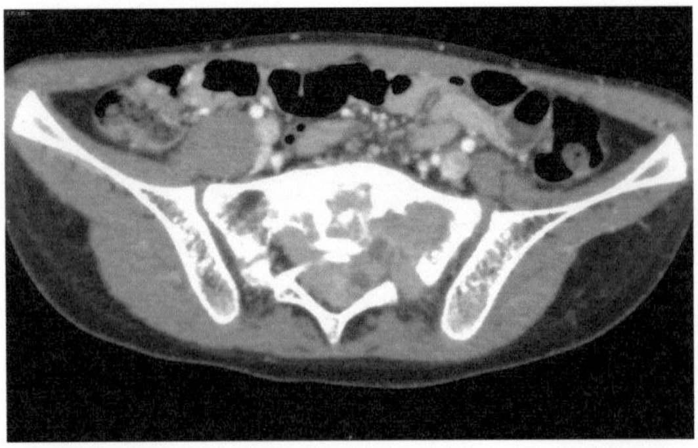

Fig. 25.3 Axial post-contrast CT image of the sacrum in soft tissue window (S1 level)

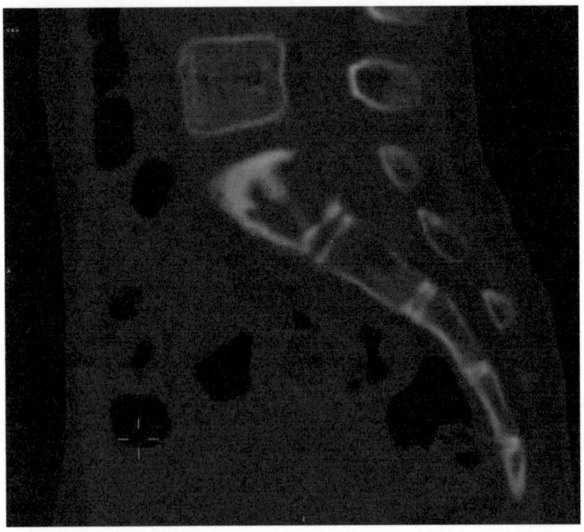

Fig. 25.4 Sagittal CT image of the sacrum in bone window

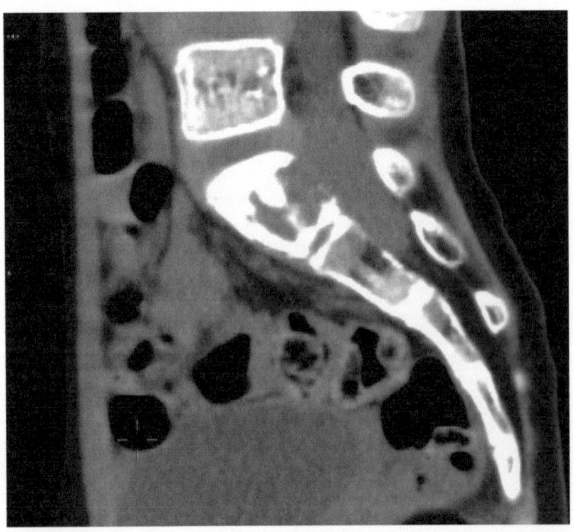

Fig. 25.5 Sagittal CT image of the sacrum in soft tissue window

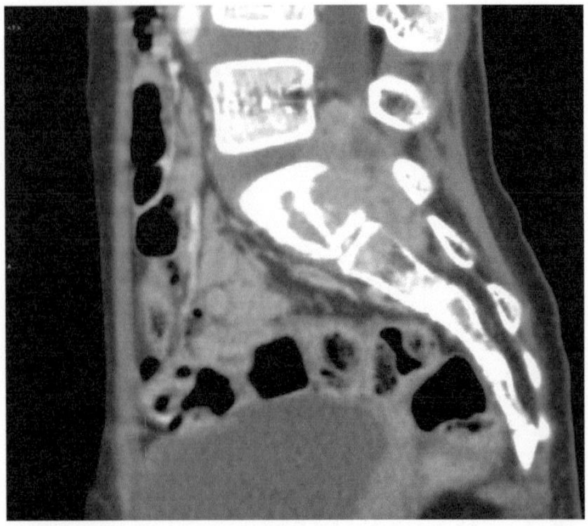

Fig. 25.6 Sagittal post-contrast CT image of the sacrum in soft tissue window

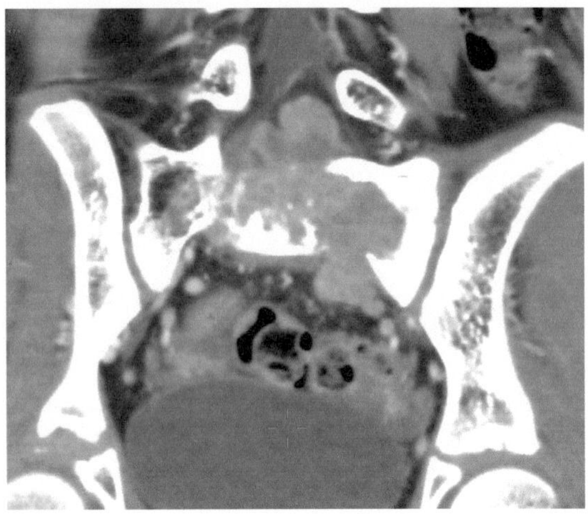

Fig. 25.7 Coronal post-contrast CT image of the sacrum in soft tissue window

25.3.2 MR Imaging (Figs. 25.8, 25.9, 25.10, and 25.11)

MR images of the sacrum demonstrated bone destruction of S1 and S2 with soft tissue mass at the spinal canal of L5 to S2 levels. There were involvements of the bilateral S1/S2 neuroforamen with anterior protrusion to the pelvis. The lesion demonstrated relatively homogeneous isointense T1 signal and slightly high T2 signal. The lesion had an indistinct margin. Heterogeneous avid enhancement was noted.

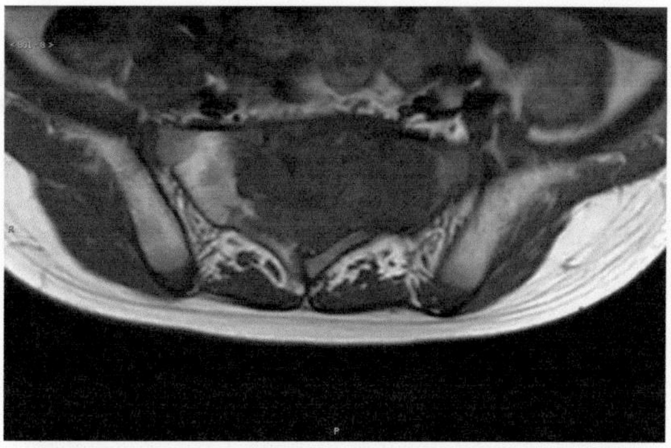

Fig. 25.8 Axial T1-weighted MR image of the sacrum (S1 level)

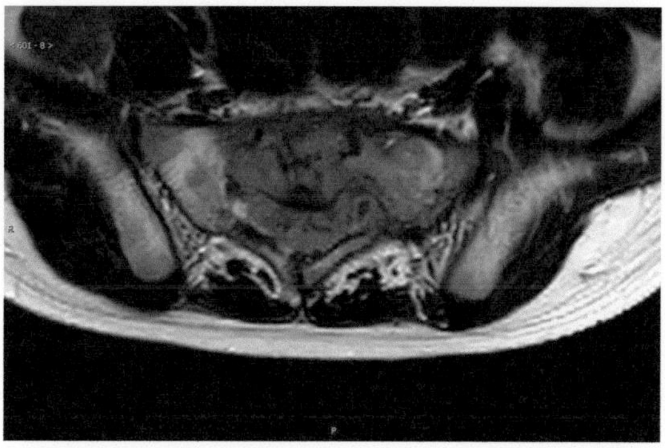

Fig. 25.9 Axial T2-weighted MR image of the sacrum (S1 level)

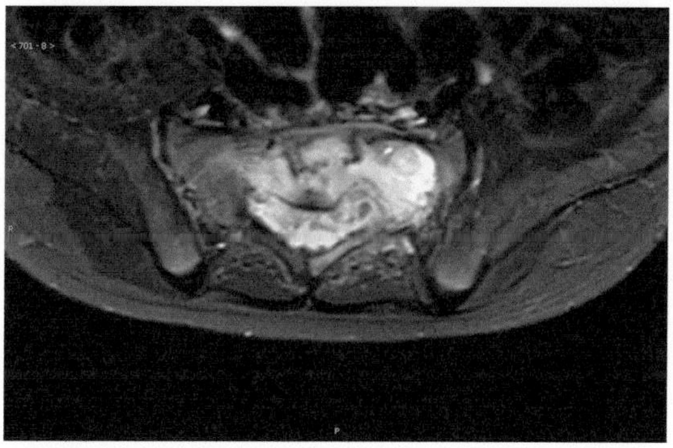

Fig. 25.10 Axial fat-suppressed T2-weighted MR image of the sacrum (S1 level)

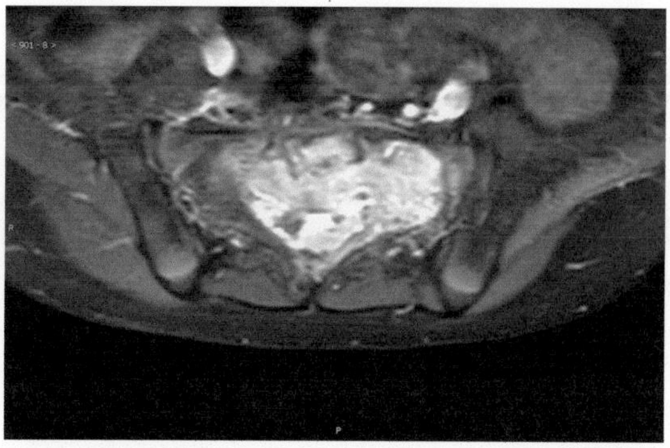

Fig. 25.11 Axial post-contrast fat-suppressed T1-weighted MR image of the sacrum (S1 level)

25.4 Description and Discussion from Residents

CT images showed ill-defined lytic destruction of the sacrum with irregular margin and focal sclerosis and without periosteal reaction. There was disruption of the cortex posteriorly with soft tissue mass extending into the spinal canal and protruding anteriorly to the pelvis. There was internally a very small number of high densities, which could be calcification or residual bone. Heterogeneous enhancements were noted. Given the provided history, our top consideration is low-grade malignant tumor, such as neurogenic tumor. The differential diagnosis includes osteosarcoma, Ewing sarcoma, and lymphoma. The lesion demonstrated isointense T1 signal and heterogeneous high T2 signal and no fatty component and heterogeneous avid enhancement, supporting malignant neoplasm. Aside from the above diagnoses, given the avid enhancement, hemangioendothelioma is also in the differential diagnosis.

25.5 Analysis and Comments from Professor Cheng Xiao-Guang

Patient was a child. CT images showed bone destruction of the sacrum with disruption of some of the cortex; high densities anteriorly of osteogenic changes could be from neoplastic bone formation or reactive sclerosis. With neoplastic bone formation, there is usually cloud-like high densities inside of the bone destruction. Reactive sclerosis usually occurs at the periphery of the bone destruction. Findings of current case favor reactive sclerosis. Additionally, the soft tissue mass noted extending to the spinal canal. MR images demonstrated the extent of the disease better than the CT images with little contribution at narrowing down the diagnosis. The image findings support the lesion as a malignant neoplasm at superior sacrum in a pediatric patient. Ewing sarcoma is the most common one that fits this criterion. Hemangioendothelioma could be in the differential diagnosis, however without specific imaging findings to support it.

25.6 Diagnosis

Ewing sarcoma.

Suggested Reading

Ilaslan H, Sundaram M, Unni KK, et al. Primary Ewing's sarcoma of the vertebral column. Skeletal Radiol. 2004;33(9):506–13.

Sambri A, Fiore M, Giannini C, et al. Primary tumors of the sacrum: imaging findings. Curr Med Imaging. 2022;18(2):170–86.

Osteosarcoma: Case 26

26

26.1 Medical History

Patient is a 14-year-old girl. She had bilateral lower extremities pain without clear inciting events about 1 year ago, with numbness around the gluteal regions and needle point sensation around the left heel. Her symptoms worsened in the past 1 month with incontinence.

26.2 Physical Examination

Pain around the sacrococcygeal region with point tenderness. There were decreased muscle tones of both lower extremities with decreased shallow sensation distally. There was anal sphincter relaxation, loss sensation at the perineal area, and decreased reflex of the Achilles tendon.

26.3 Imaging Findings

26.3.1 CT Imaging (Figs. 26.1, 26.2, 26.3, 26.4, 26.5, and 26.6)

CT images of the sacrum demonstrated bone destruction with spiculated periosteal reaction and surrounding soft tissue mass with heterogeneous densities and ill-defined margin. There were peripheral and internal septal like enhancements.

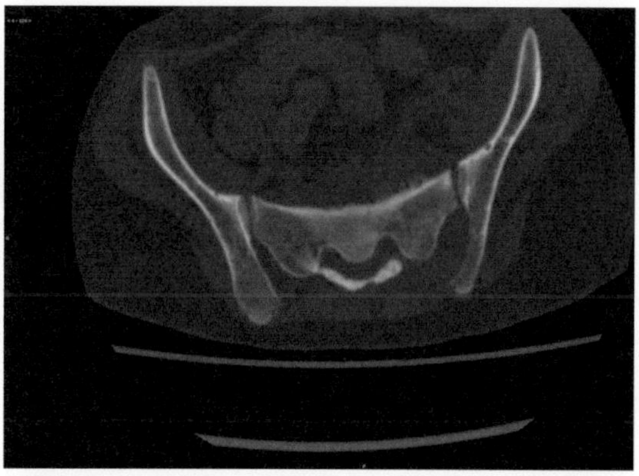

Fig. 26.1 Axial CT image of the sacrum in bone window (S1 level)

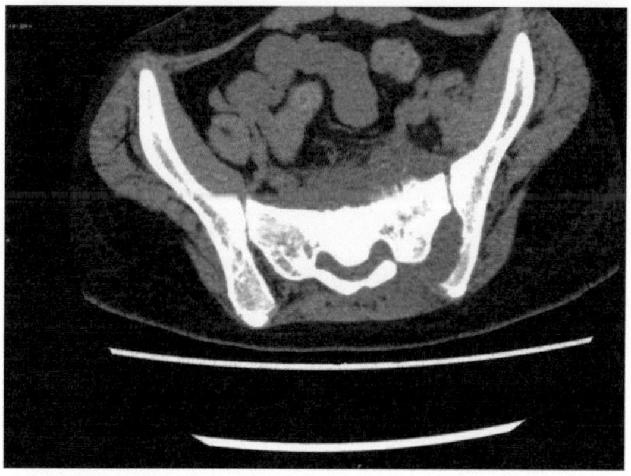

Fig. 26.2 Axial CT image of the sacrum in soft tissue window (S1 level)

X. Cheng et al., *Imaging of Bone Tumors in Axial Bones*,
https://doi.org/10.1007/978-981-95-2262-0_26

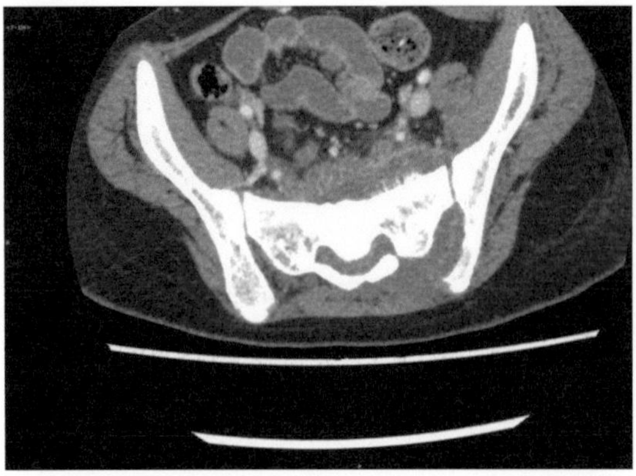

Fig. 26.3 Axial post-contrast CT image of the sacrum in soft tissue window (S1 level)

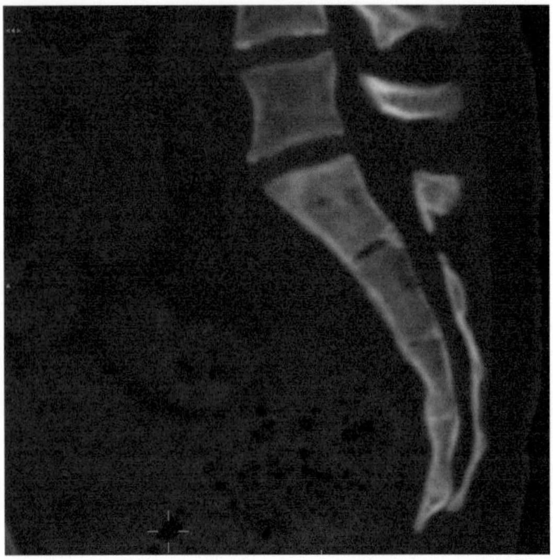

Fig. 26.4 Sagittal CT image of the sacrum in bone window

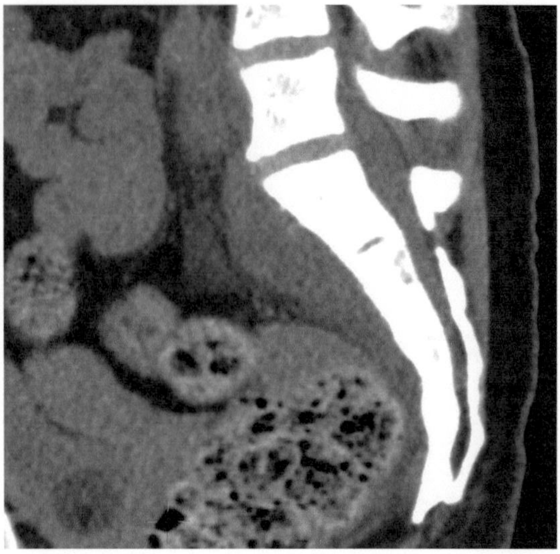

Fig. 26.5 Sagittal CT image of the sacrum in soft tissue window

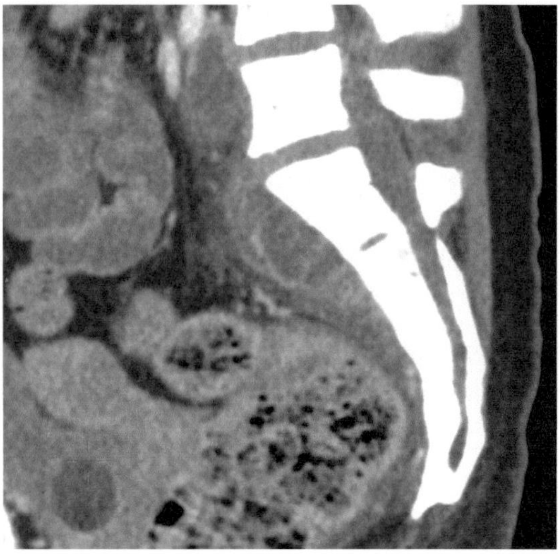

Fig. 26.6 Sagittal post-contrast CT image of the sacrum in soft tissue window

26.3.2 MR Imaging (Figs. 26.7, 26.8, 26.9, 26.10, 26.11, and 26.12)

MR images of the sacrum demonstrated bone destruction of the sacrum with surrounding soft tissue mass as iso to low T1, high T2 signals. The lesion affected from L5 to coccyx level and involving the prevertebral soft tissues. It extended posteriorly affecting spinal canal from L5 to S5 level and bilateral spinal erector muscles with surrounding soft tissue edema. There was heterogeneous avid enhancement, more peripherally.

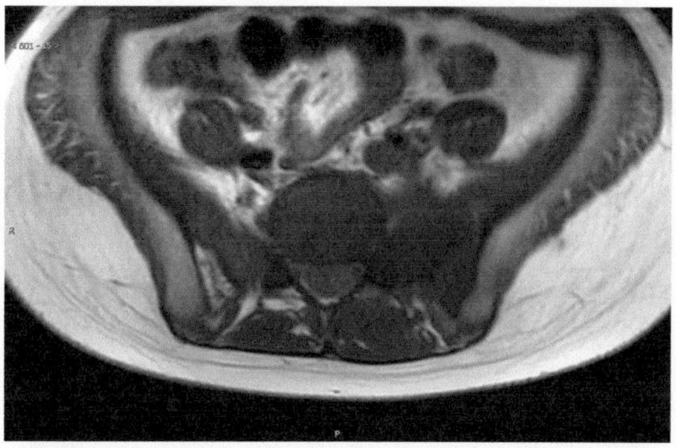

Fig. 26.7 Axial T1-weighted MR image of the sacrum (S1 level)

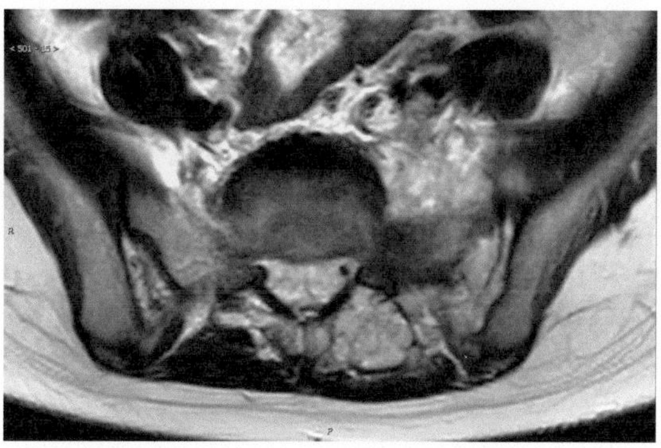

Fig. 26.8 Axial T2-weighted MR image of the sacrum (S1 level)

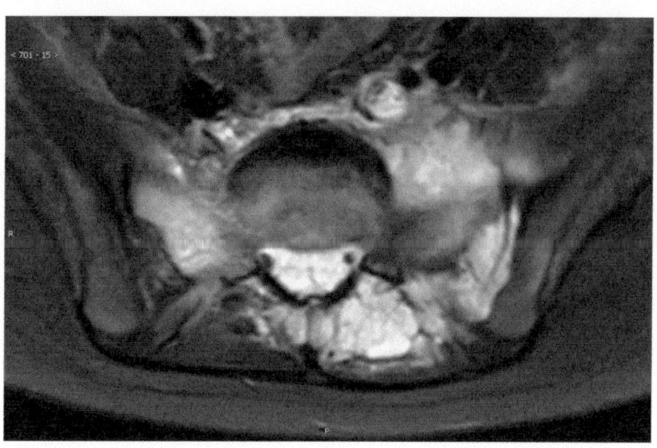

Fig. 26.9 Axial fat-suppressed T2-weighted MR image of the sacrum (S1 level)

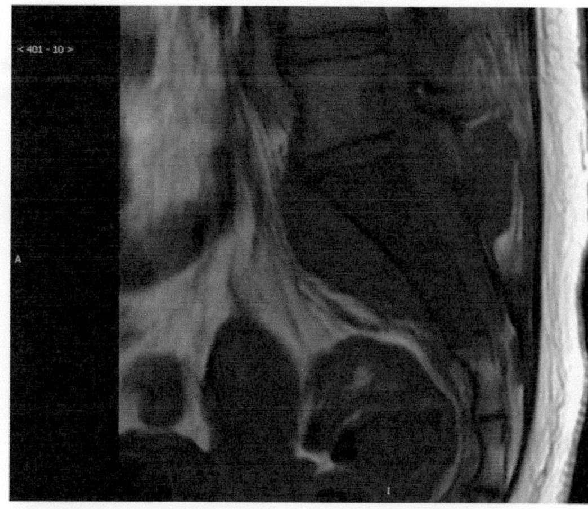

Fig. 26.10 Sagittal T1-weighted MR image of the sacrum

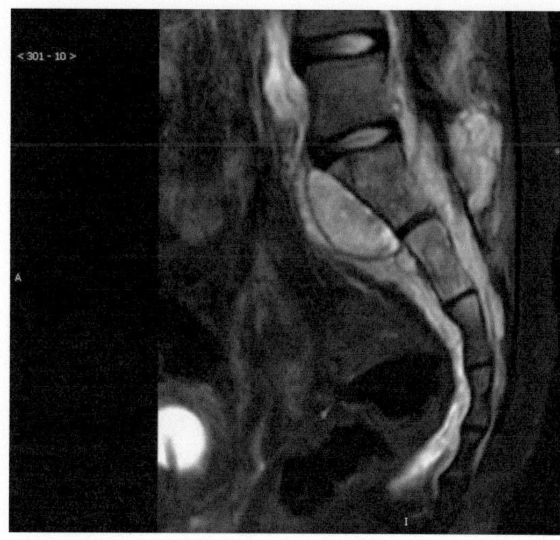

Fig. 26.11 Sagittal fat-suppressed T2-weighted MR image of the sacrum

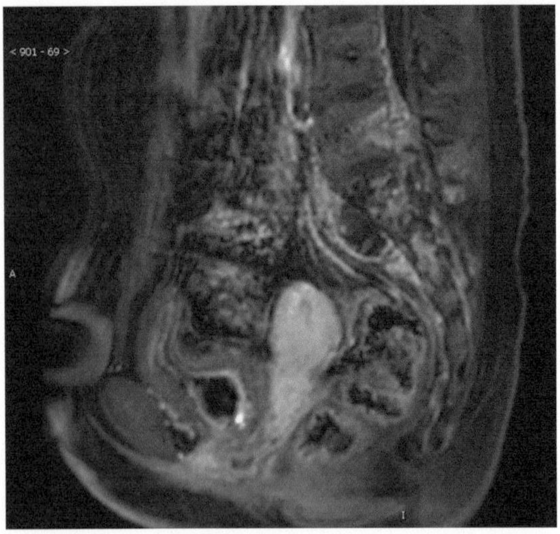

Fig. 26.12 Sagittal post-contrast fat-suppressed T1-weighted MR image of the sacrum

26.4 Description and Discussion from Residents

CT images showed sacrum destruction with large soft tissue mass. The bone destruction was relatively occult with spiculated periosteal reaction along the anterior sacrum. The soft tissue mass affected a large area including the left sacroiliac joint, sacral canal, and ventral aspect of the sacrum. Avid heterogeneous enhancement noted and more peripherally. Given the patient's age, our top consideration is Ewing sarcoma. MR images showed the affected area more extensive than the CT images with more apparent soft tissue mass. Sacrum and presacral soft tissue and sacral canal were all involved. The bone destruction and soft tissue mass showed iso to low T1 signal and high T2 signal with heterogeneous avid enhancement, all supporting the diagnosis of Ewing sarcoma. With clear margin of the soft tissue mass and involvement of the sacral canal, neurogenic tumor is included in the differential diagnosis.

26.5 Analysis and Comments from Professor Cheng Xiao-Guang

Patient was an adolescent. CT images showed large soft tissue mass around the sacrum and no apparent bone destruction, easily misdiagnosed as soft tissue tumor; thus we need to be careful at making the diagnosis. The soft tissue mass surrounded the sacrum with heterogenous enhancement. Neoplasm with these kinds of image findings that are most common in pediatric and adolescent population is Ewing sarcoma. Osteosarcoma is in the differential diagnosis; however, sacrum is not a common site for osteosarcoma. Additionally, there is usually tumoral bone formation with osteosarcoma, not consistent with the current case. MR images showed low T1 signal in sacrum and coccyx with large surrounding soft tissue mass, indicating "permeated destruction" of bone. All these findings support high degree of malignancy and most commonly as Ewing sarcoma in pediatric/adolescent patients. Peripheral enhancement noted without central enhancement could be related to fast tumor growth and lack of blood supply in the center of the lesion.

26.6 Diagnosis

Osteosarcoma.

Suggested Reading

Ilaslan H, Sundaram M, Unni KK, et al. Primary vertebral osteosarcoma: imaging findings. Radiology. 2004;230(3):697–702.

Sambri A, Fiore M, Giannini C, et al. Primary tumors of the sacrum: imaging findings. Curr Med Imaging. 2022;18(2):170–86.

27 Solidary Fibrous Tumor of Bone: Case 27

27.1 Medical History

Patient is a 36-year-old female. She experienced right thigh pain about 11 months ago without clear causes with symptoms worsening at night. She received local analgesic treatment with short-term recovery. About 5 months ago, the symptoms worsened with pain around sacrococcygeal region and restricted activities. She had a history of "meningioma resection" 6 years ago and "resection for meningioma recurrence" about 2 years ago. She takes Depakine (sodium valproate) for anti-epilepsy therapy.

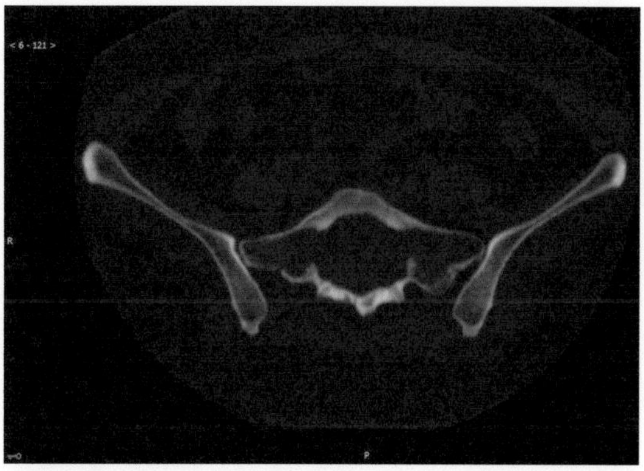

Fig. 27.1 Axial CT image of the sacrum in bone window (S1 level)

27.2 Physical Examination

Decreased sensation around the lower sacrococcygeal region. Muscle strength of both lower extremities III–IV and unsteady gait.

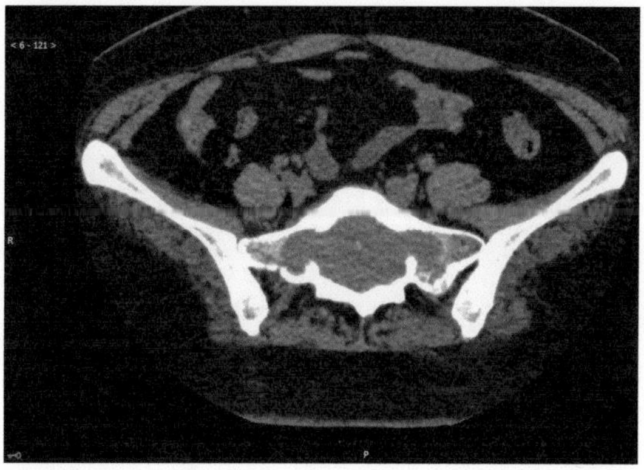

Fig. 27.2 Axial CT image of the sacrum in soft tissue window (S1 level)

27.3 Imaging Findings

27.3.1 CT Imaging (Figs. 27.1, 27.2, 27.3, 27.4, 27.5, 27.6, and 27.7)

CT images of the sacrum demonstrated bone destruction of S1 and S2 vertebral bodies with clear margin and focal peripheral sclerosis. The soft tissue mass extended beyond the posterior

X. Cheng et al., *Imaging of Bone Tumors in Axial Bones*,
https://doi.org/10.1007/978-981-95-2262-0_27

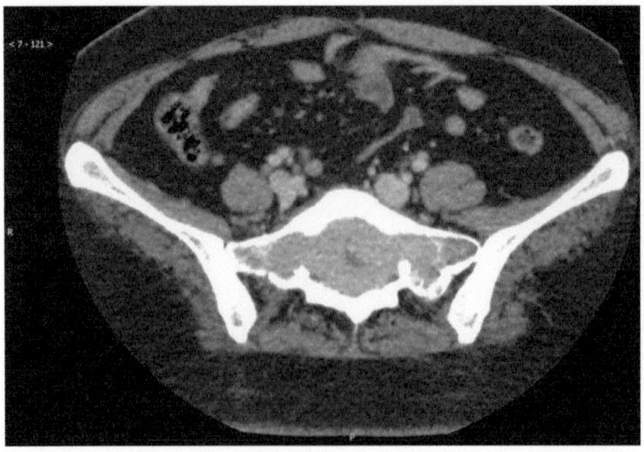

Fig. 27.3 Axial post-contrast CT image of the sacrum in soft tissue window (S1 level)

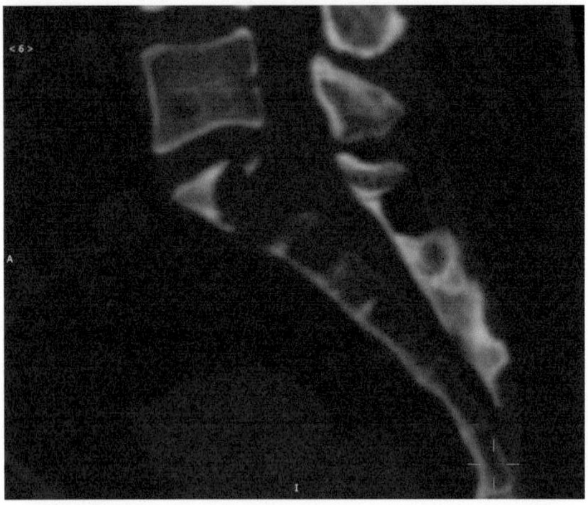

Fig. 27.4 Sagittal CT image of the sacrum in bone window

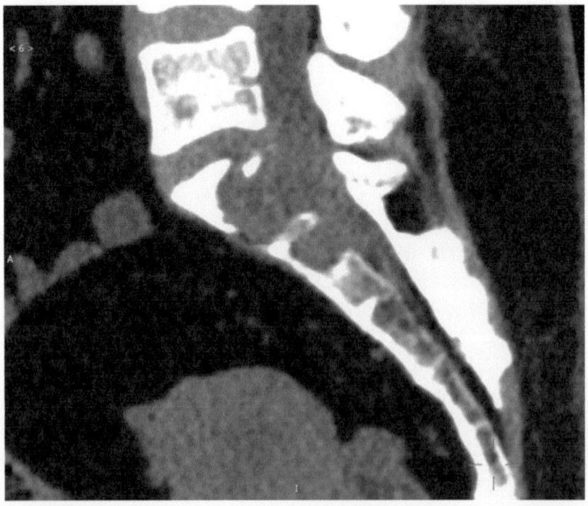

Fig. 27.5 Sagittal CT image of the sacrum in soft tissue window

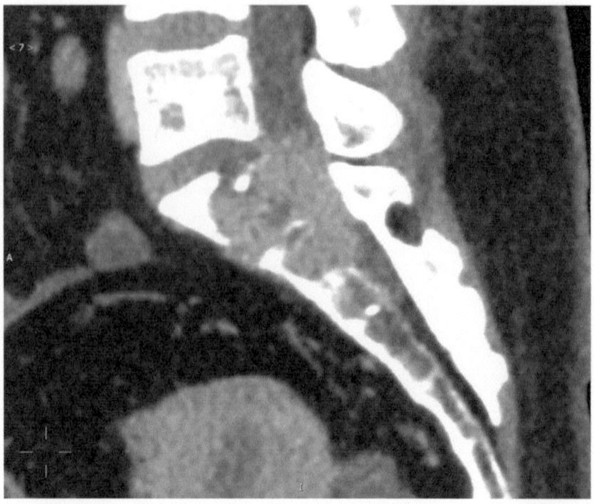

Fig. 27.6 Sagittal post-contrast CT image of the sacrum in soft tissue window

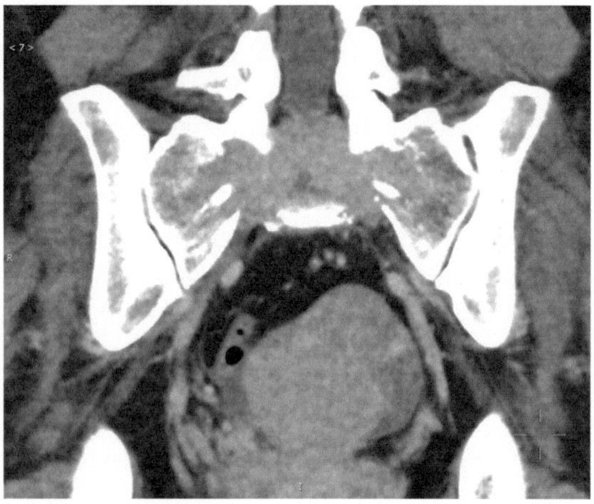

Fig. 27.7 Coronal post-contrast CT image of the sacrum in soft tissue window

cortex of the sacrum, involving the spinal canal. Heterogeneous enhancement noted with large area of avid enhancement. There was smaller bone destruction in the L5 vertebral body with avid enhancement.

27.3.2 MR Imaging (Figs. 27.8, 27.9, 27.10, 27.11, 27.12, and 27.13)

MR images of the sacrum demonstrated bone destruction of S1 and S2 with soft tissue mass extending to the spinal canal. The lesion demon-

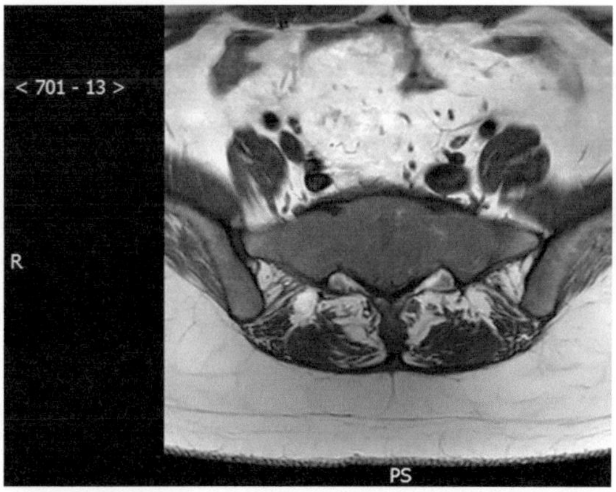

Fig. 27.8 Axial T1-weighted MR image of the sacrum (S1 level)

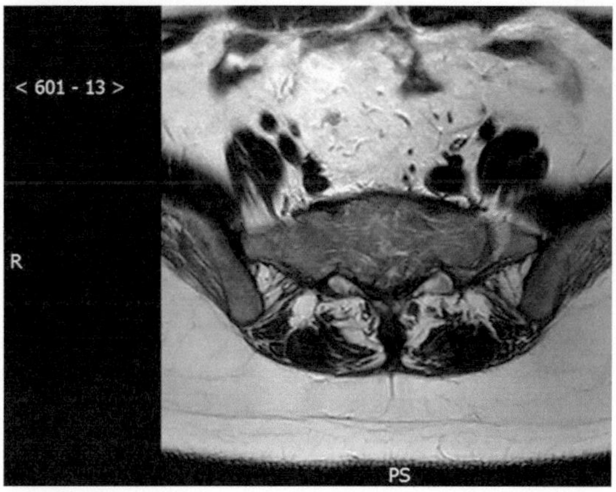

Fig. 27.9 Axial T2-weighted MR image of the sacrum (S1 level)

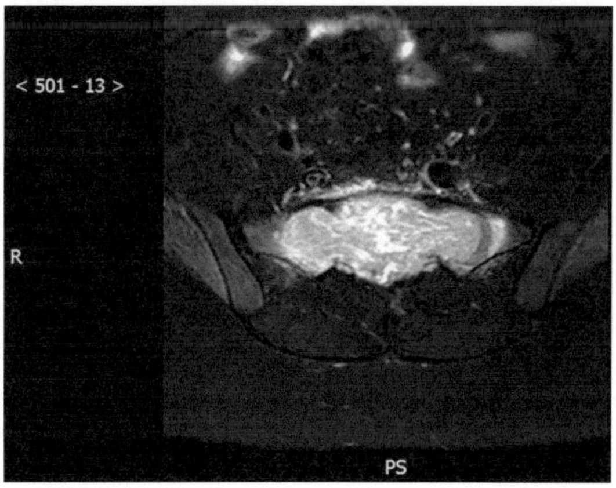

Fig. 27.10 Axial fat-suppressed T2-weighted MR image of the sacrum (S1 level)

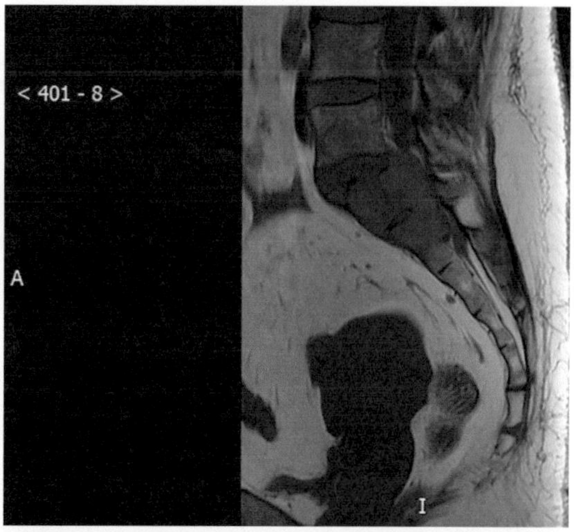

Fig. 27.11 Sagittal T1-weighted MR image of the sacrum

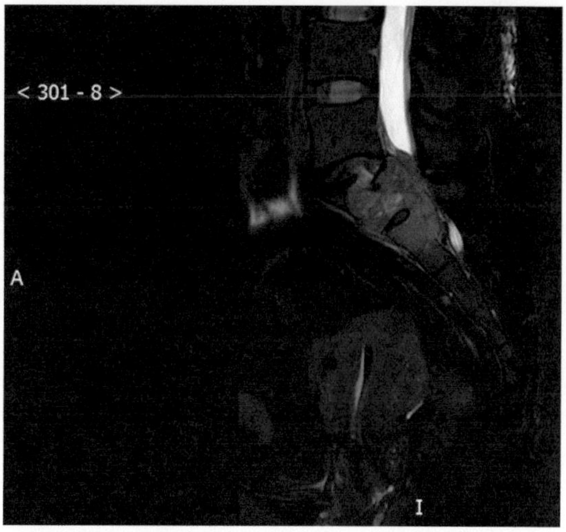

Fig. 27.12 Sagittal fat-suppressed T2-weighted MR image of the sacrum

strated predominantly slightly high T2 signal with internal multiple linear much higher signals with avid enhancement. Preserved signal noted at the S1–2 disc. There was small focus of abnormal signal inside of the L5 vertebral body with avid enhancement.

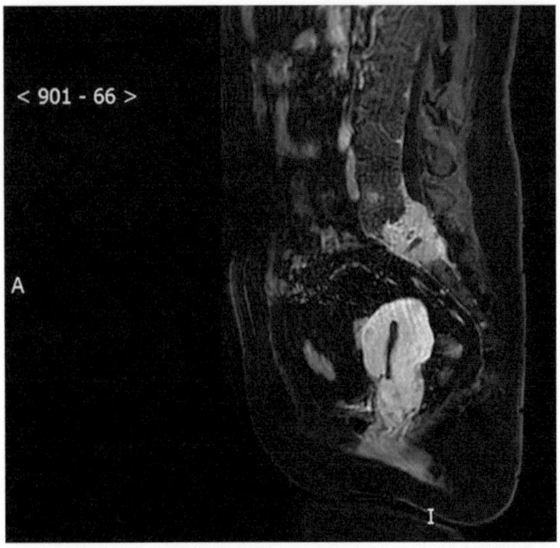

Fig. 27.13 Sagittal post-contrast fat-suppressed T1-weighted MR image of the sacrum

27.4 Description and Discussion from Residents

CT images showed expansive lytic bone destruction of S1 and S2 vertebral bodies with clear margin. The lesion appeared in the center, with symmetric involvements of bilateral sacral alae with relatively preserved cortex. Soft tissue mass extended to the spinal canal causing narrowing with avid enhancement. Overall, we favor nonaggressive lesion. MR images also demonstrated expansile growth of the lesion. Soft tissue mass focally extended beyond the posterior cortex. The lesion showed heterogeneous signal, with slightly high T2 signal with avid enhancement. Lesions commonly involving the sacrum are chordoma, giant cell tumor of bone, and neurogenic tumors. Chordoma usually involves the lower sacrum and the other two usually involve the superior sacrum. Neurogenic tumors are usually asymmetrical with widening of the sacral canal. Thus, our top consideration is giant cell tumor of bone.

27.5 Analysis and Comments from Professor Cheng Xiao-Guang

Patient is a young female. CT images showed bone destruction of S1 and S2 with preserved disc, indicating neoplasm. The lesion involved superior sacrum with mild expansile appearance and homogeneous density and avid enhancement, all features supporting the diagnosis of giant cell tumor of bone. However, there was a very mild expansile appearance and not clear peripheral bone shell of the posterior soft tissue mass. Additionally, there was focal lesion in the L5 vertebral body. Thus, I can't exclude more aggressive entities, such as lymphoma or metastatic lesion.

27.6 Diagnosis

Solidary fibrous tumor of bone.

Suggested Reading

Musyoki FN, Nahal A, Powell TI. Solitary fibrous tumor: an update on the spectrum of extrapleural manifestations. Skeletal Radiol. 2012;41(1):5–13.

Sambri A, Fiore M, Giannini C, et al. Primary tumors of the sacrum: imaging findings. Cur Med Imaging. 2022;18(2):170–86.

Giant Cell Tumor of Bone: Case 28

28

28.1 Medical History

Patient is a 33-year-old male. He started to experience soreness and pain at posterior lower extremities bilaterally with urinary frequency about 2 months ago without a clear reason. The symptoms worsened with activities and improved with rest.

28.2 Physical Examination

Not done.

28.3 Imaging Findings

28.3.1 Radiograph (Figs. 28.1 and 28.2)

Radiographs of the sacrum demonstrated expansile lytic bone destruction of S2 vertebral body with thinning of the cortex.

28.3.2 CT Imaging (Figs. 28.3, 28.4, 28.5, 28.6, 28.7, 28.8, and 28.9)

CT images of the sacrum demonstrated expansile lytic bone destruction of S2 vertebral body with homogeneous density, no peripheral scle-

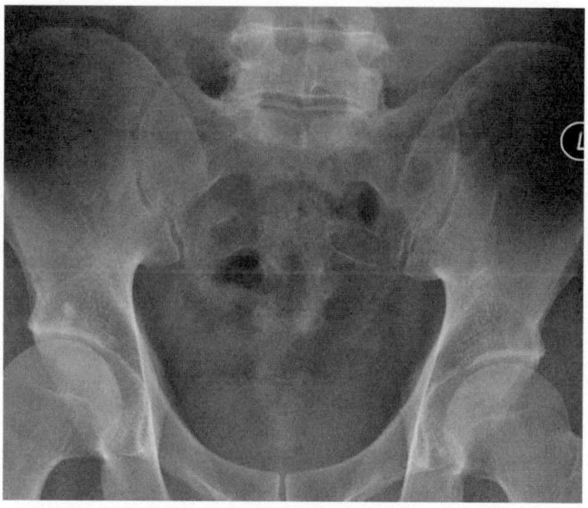

Fig. 28.1 Frontal view of the sacrum

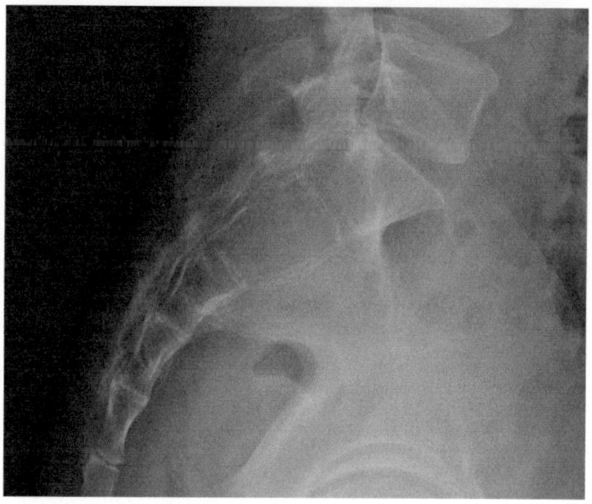

Fig. 28.2 Lateral view of the sacrum

X. Cheng et al., *Imaging of Bone Tumors in Axial Bones*,
https://doi.org/10.1007/978-981-95-2262-0_28

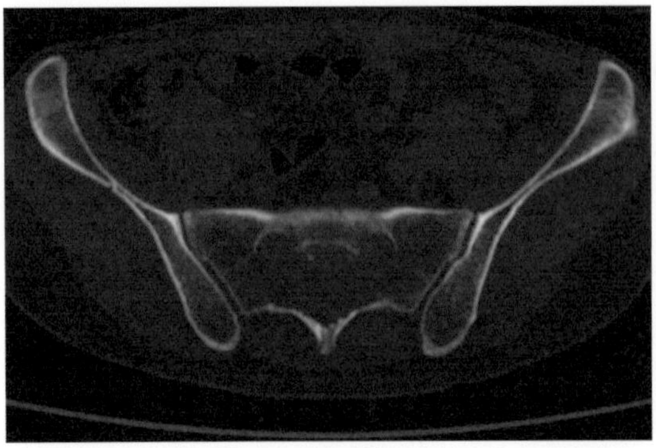

Fig. 28.3 Axial CT image of the sacrum in bone window (S2 level)

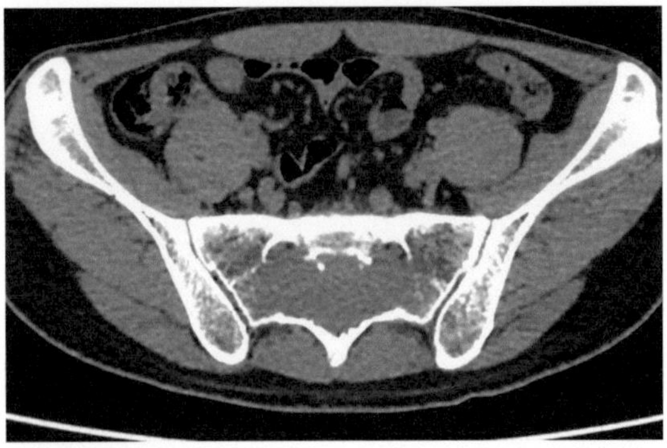

Fig. 28.4 Axial CT image of the sacrum in soft tissue window (S2 level)

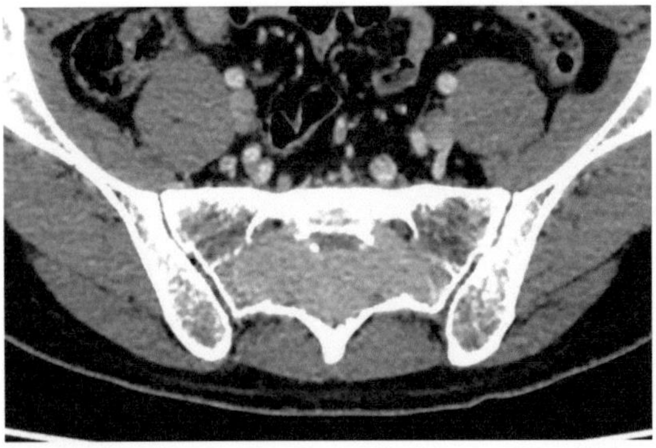

Fig. 28.5 Axial post-contrast CT image of the sacrum in soft tissue window (S2 level)

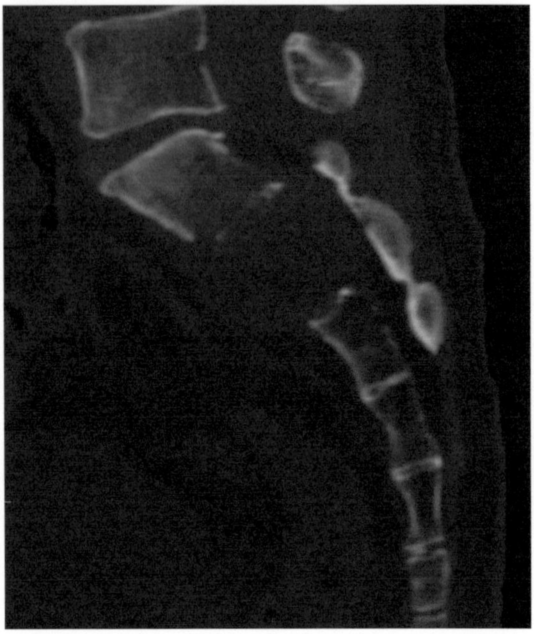

Fig. 28.6 Sagittal CT image of the sacrum in bone window

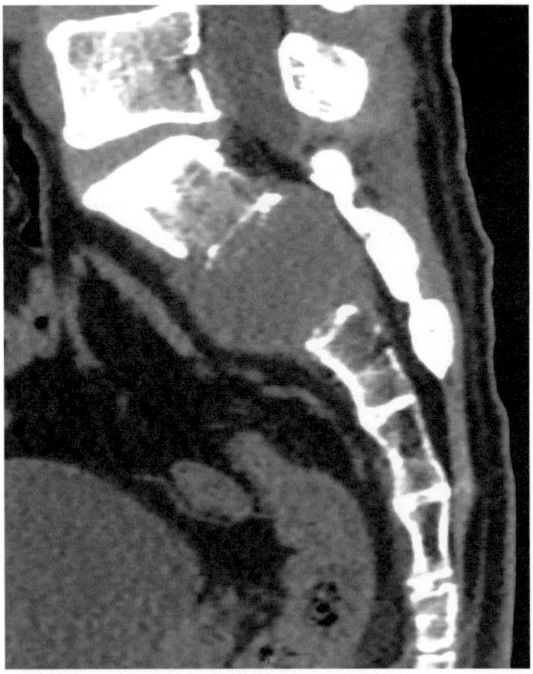

Fig. 28.7 Sagittal CT image of the sacrum in soft tissue window

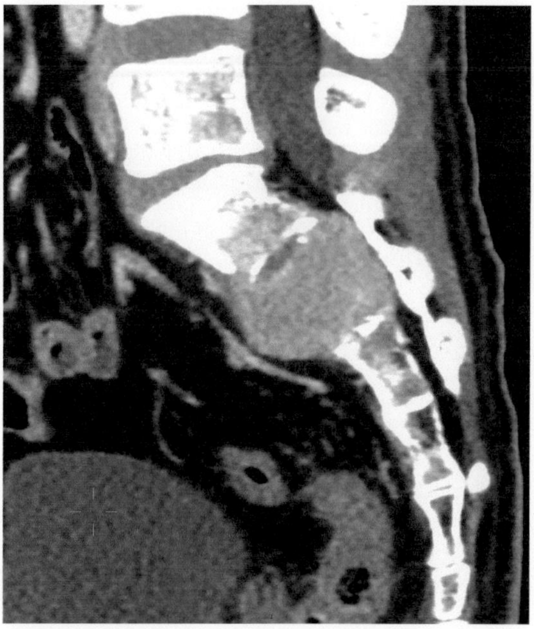

Fig. 28.8 Sagittal post-contrast CT image of the sacrum in soft tissue window

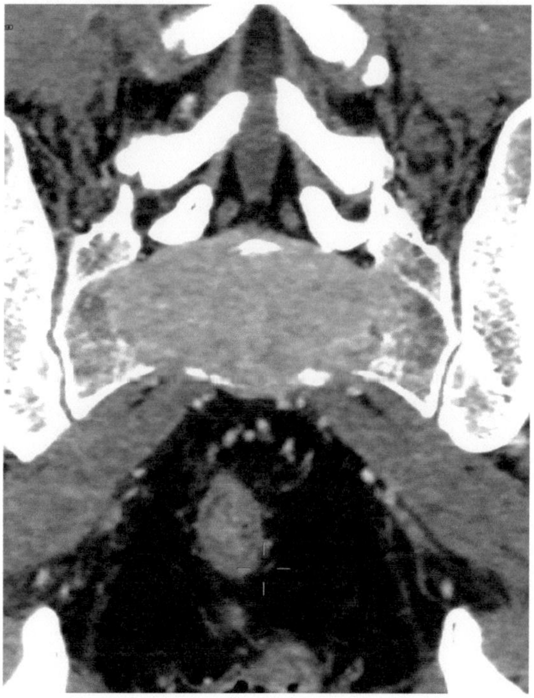

Fig. 28.9 Coronal post-contrast CT image of the sacrum in soft tissue window

rosis, and indistinct border. There was thinning of the cortex with focal disruption, compression of the sacral canal posteriorly, and avid enhancement.

28.4 Description and Discussion from Residents

Patient is a middle-aged man. Radiographs showed expansile and lytic bone destruction of the S2 vertebral body with thinning of the cortex. CT images showed the lesion at the center of S2 vertebral body with internal homogeneous soft tissue densities and no calcification with thinning of the cortex without peripheral sclerosis. The lesion extended peripherally involving the sacral canal with compression to the cauda equina, which could explain patient's clinical symptoms. There was no enlargement of the sacral neuroforamen. Avid homogeneous enhancement noted. Given patient's age, our top consideration is giant cell tumor of bone. Differential diagnosis is neurogenic tumor, which commonly is asymmetric, with cystic component and hemorrhage causing heterogeneous densities with less avid enhancement compared to giant cell tumor of bone and usually with enlargement of the sacral neuroforamen.

28.5 Analysis and Comments from Professor Cheng Xiao-Guang

Radiographs showed decreased density of S2 vertebral body with expansile changes. CT images showed expansile and lytic bone destruction of S2 vertebral body with soft tissue mass and clear margin, peripheral bone shell, and no enlargement of the sacral neuroforamen. Avid enhancement was noted. Given patient's age, diagnosis is giant cell tumor of bone, with typical imaging presentation.

28.6 Diagnosis

Giant cell tumor of bone.

Suggested Reading

Bukata SV, Blay JY, Rutkowski P, et al. Denosumab treatment for giant cell tumor of the spine including the sacrum. Spine (Phila Pa 1976). 2021;46(5):277–84.

Si MJ, Wang CS, Ding XY, et al. Differentiation of primary chordoma, giant cell tumor and schwannoma of the sacrum by CT and MRI. Eur J Radiol. 2013;82(12):2309–15.

29 Conventional Chordoma: Case 29

29.1 Medical History

Patient is a 68-year-old female. She started to experience sacrococcygeal pain without clear causes about 1 year ago and symptoms worsened with supine position. Radiograph examination at that time showed no abnormalities. The pain worsened and she started to develop frequent urination, difficulty defecating, and thinning of the stool, no blood noted.

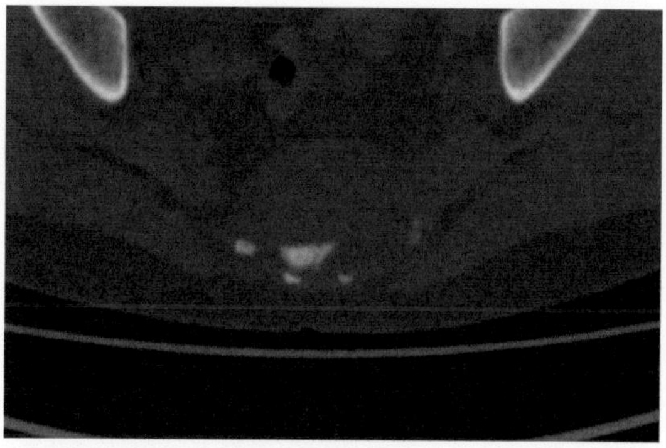

Fig. 29.1 Axial CT image of the sacrococcygeal region in bone window

29.2 Physical Examination

Point tenderness around the sacrococcygeal region, pain on percussion.

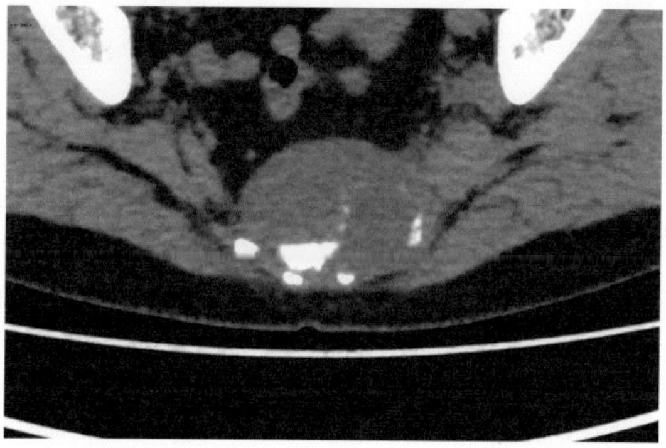

Fig. 29.2 Axial CT image of the sacrococcygeal region in soft tissue window

29.3 Imaging Findings

29.3.1 CT Imaging (Figs. 29.1, 29.2, 29.3, 29.4, 29.5, 29.6, and 29.7)

CT images of the sacrum and coccyx demonstrated lytic bone destruction of sacrum and coccyx with anterior soft tissue mass and internal irregular calcifications. The lesion showed a clear margin, involving the posterior sacral canal with linear mild enhancement.

X. Cheng et al., *Imaging of Bone Tumors in Axial Bones*,
https://doi.org/10.1007/978-981-95-2262-0_29

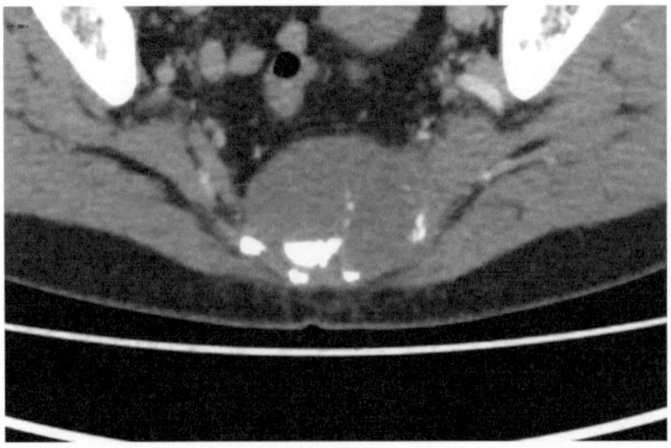

Fig. 29.3 Axial post-contrast CT image of the sacrococcygeal region in soft tissue window

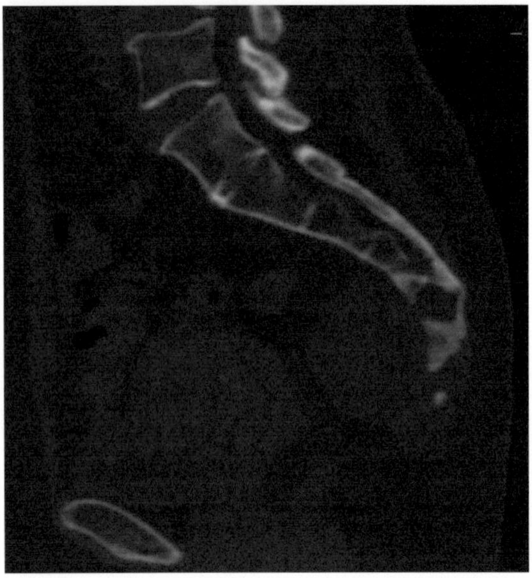

Fig. 29.4 Sagittal CT image of the sacrococcygeal region in bone window

29.3.2 MR Imaging (Figs. 29.8, 29.9, 29.10, and 29.11)

MR images of the sacrum demonstrated lytic bone destruction of lower sacrum and superior coccyx with soft tissue mass and extending to the sacral canal and pelvis with predominant high T2 signal and patchy high T1 signal, and with adjacent soft tissue edema. Avid and heterogeneous enhancements noted of the soft tissue mass. The fat plane between the lesion and rectum was preserved.

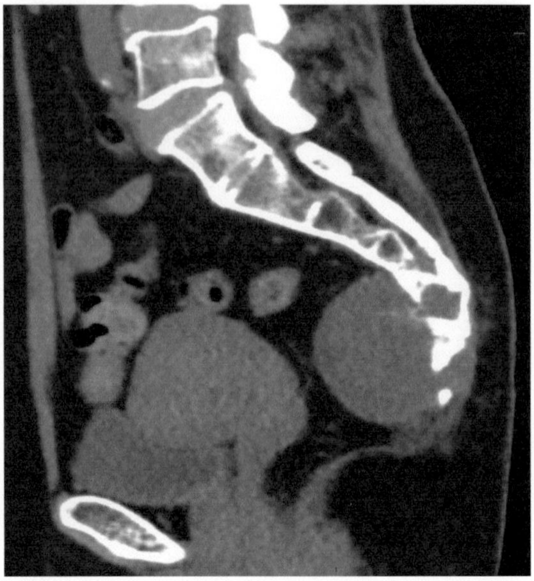

Fig. 29.5 Sagittal CT image of the sacrococcygeal region in soft tissue window

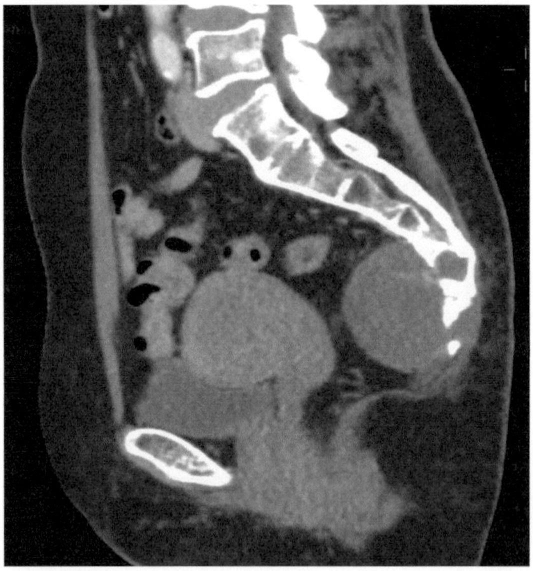

Fig. 29.6 Sagittal post-contrast CT image of the sacrococcygeal region in soft tissue window

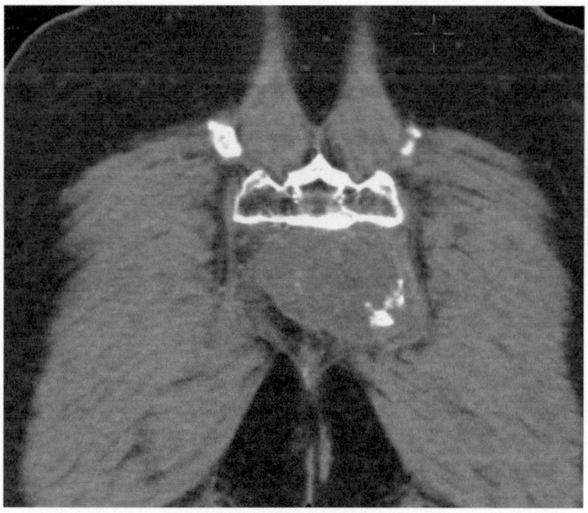

Fig. 29.7 Coronal post-contrast CT image of the sacrococcygeal region in soft tissue window

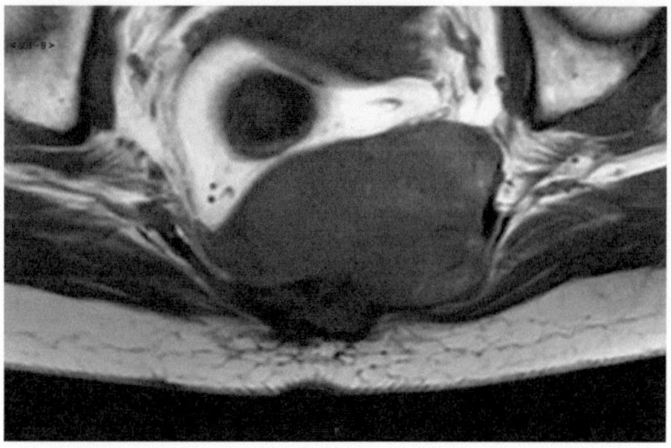

Fig. 29.8 Axial T1-weighted MR image of the sacrum (lower sacrum)

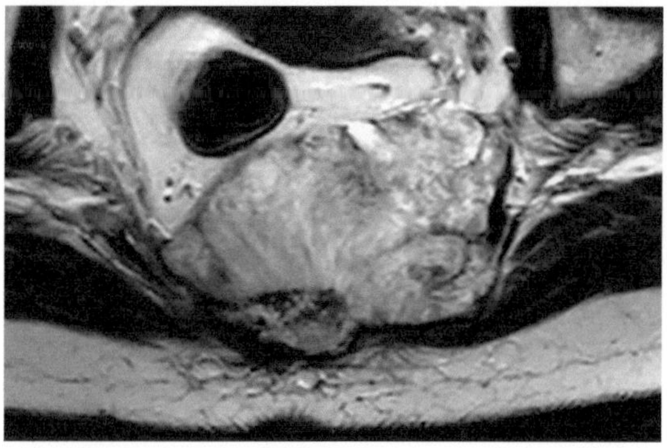

Fig. 29.9 Axial T2-weighted MR image of the sacrum (lower sacrum)

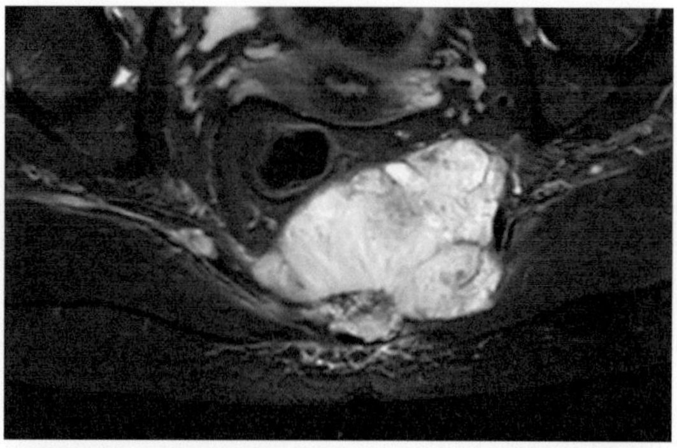

Fig. 29.10 Axial fat-suppressed T2-weighted MR image of the sacrum (lower sacrum)

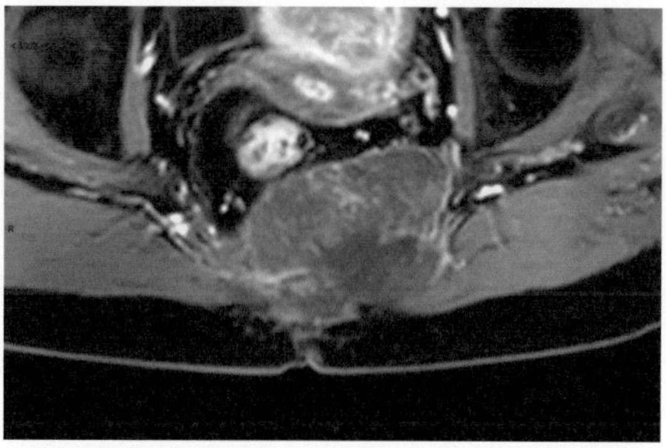

Fig. 29.11 Axial post-contrast fat-suppressed T1-weighted MR image of the sacrum (lower sacrum)

29.4 Description and Discussion from Residents

Patient was an older female. CT images showed lytic bone destruction of S5 vertebral body and coccyx. Soft tissue mass extended to the pelvis with heterogeneous densities, overall, slightly lower than the muscle with internal multiple punctate calcifications. Multiple internal linear mild enhancements noted. Overall, the findings are typical of chordoma. MR images showed heterogeneous signal of the mass with patchy high T1 signal and predominant high T2 signal and internal low linear signal, indicating mucinous and fibrous tissues, with heterogeneous enhancement. The diagnosis is chordoma. Chordoma usually affects patients of 40–80 years old and commonly affects cranial and caudal portion of the spine. About 50% of chordoma affects sacrum and coccyx, 35% affects clivus, and 15% affects elsewhere. The soft tissue mass can reach an average of about 10 cm and commonly with cystic changes and calcifications. Other neoplasm commonly affects the sacrum and coccyx include (1) giant cell tumor of bone, most commonly affects patients of 20–40 years old and usually affects proximal sacrum, and (2) neurogenic tumor, usually asymmetric with enlargement of the sacral neuroforamen. Neither is consistent with the current case.

29.5 Analysis and Comments from Professor Cheng Xiao-Guang

The patient was an older female. CT images showed bone destruction of sacrum and coccyx with anterior large soft tissue mass with heterogeneous densities and internal multiple calcifications and no avid enhancement. MR images showed bone destruction with sclerosis and heterogeneous signal of the soft tissue mass. The diagnosis is chordoma in a characteristic location with typical imaging findings. There are not many differential diagnoses. In rare occasions, chondrosarcoma can affect the sacral and coccyx with similar imaging findings as chordoma, difficult to differentiate. Other neoplasm that commonly affects the sacrum includes giant cell tumor of bone, which usually affects superior sacrum in young patients with expansile bone destruction and avid enhancement, very different from chordoma.

29.6 Diagnosis

Conventional chordoma.

Suggested Reading

Farsad K, Kattapuram SV, Sacknoff R, et al. Sacral chordoma. Radiographics. 2009;29(5):1525–30.

Sambri A, Fiore M, Giannini C, et al. Primary tumors of the sacrum: imaging findings. Curr Med Imaging. 2022;18(2):170–86.

30 Malignant Peripheral Nerve Sheath Tumor of Bone: Case 30

30.1 Medical History

Patient is a 39-year-old female. She started to experience needle pricking like pain at the back without clear causes about 4 months ago. There was radiation of the pain to the right lateral thigh and lateral lower leg and lateral ankle. The pain was intermittent and relieved by rest without night pain.

30.2 Physical Examination

No recorded.

30.3 Imaging Findings

30.3.1 Radiograph (Fig. 30.1)

The radiograph demonstrated suspicious circular low-density area in the right iliac adjacent to the sacroiliac joint.

30.3.2 CT Imaging (Figs. 30.2, 30.3, 30.4, 30.5, 30.6, and 30.7)

CT images of the bony pelvis demonstrated focal lytic bone destruction of the right iliac near the sacroiliac joint without clear margin and no peripheral sclerosis. The soft tissue mass extruded beyond the cortex to both sides. There was mild enhancement in the peripheral without apparent enhancement centrally.

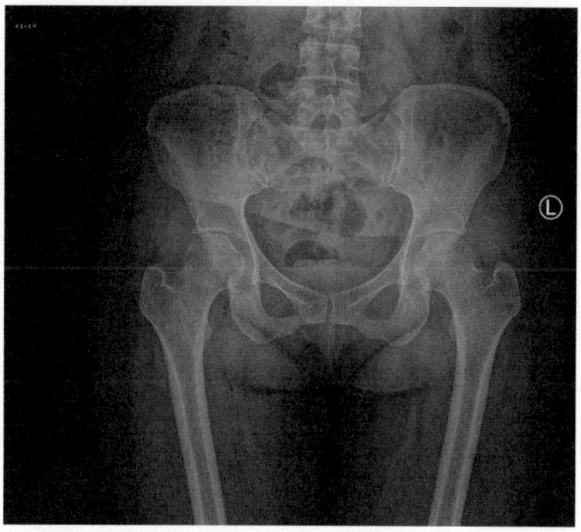

Fig. 30.1 Frontal view of the bony pelvis

30.3.3 MR Imaging (Figs. 30.8, 30.9, 30.10, 30.11, 30.12, 30.13, and 30.14)

MR images of the bony pelvis demonstrated bone destruction of right iliac with internal iso T1 signal and heterogeneous high T2 signal with cortical disruption and associated soft tissue mass with peritumoral edema. Apparent circular avid enhancement noted.

X. Cheng et al., *Imaging of Bone Tumors in Axial Bones*,
https://doi.org/10.1007/978-981-95-2262-0_30

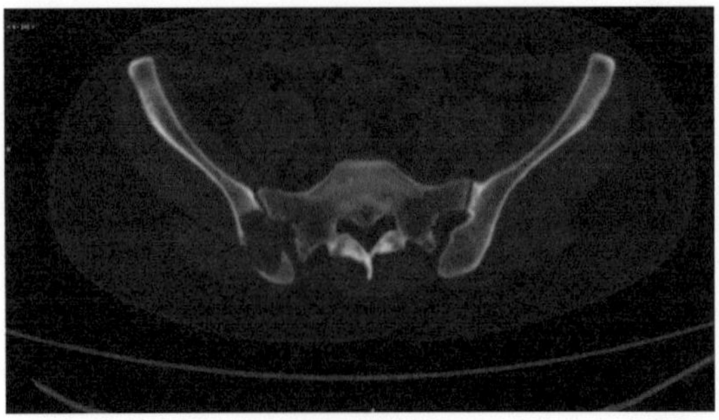

Fig. 30.2 Axial CT image of the bony pelvis in bone window

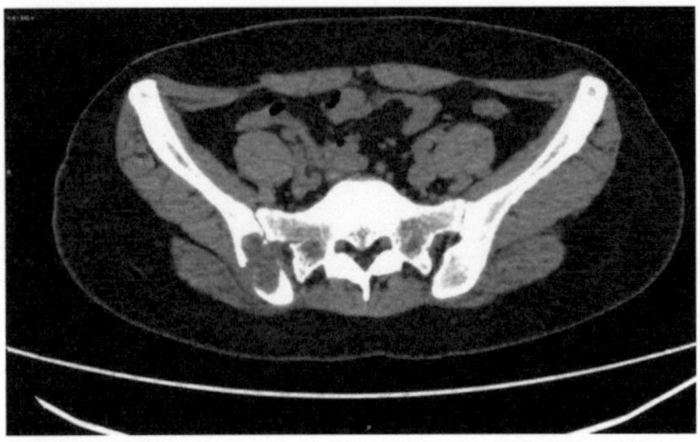

Fig. 30.3 Axial CT image of the bony pelvis in soft tissue window

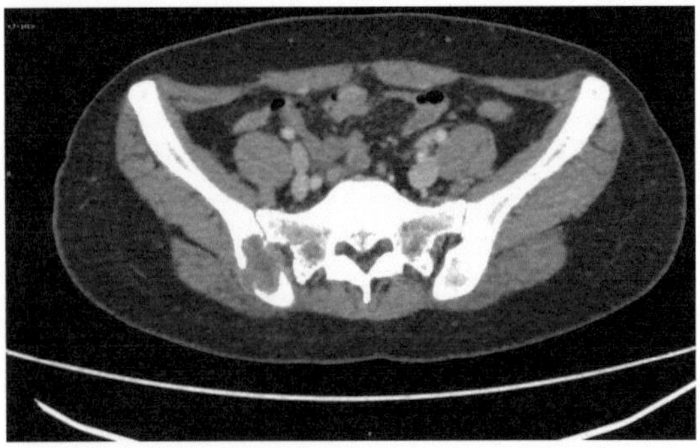

Fig. 30.4 Axial post-contrast CT image of the bony pelvis in soft tissue window

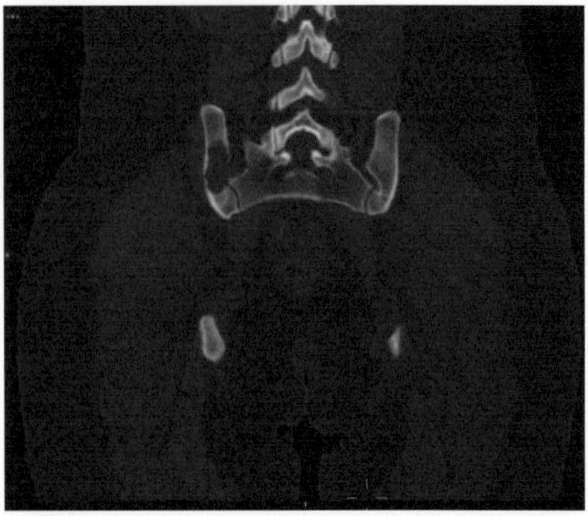

Fig. 30.5 Coronal CT image of the bony pelvis in bone window

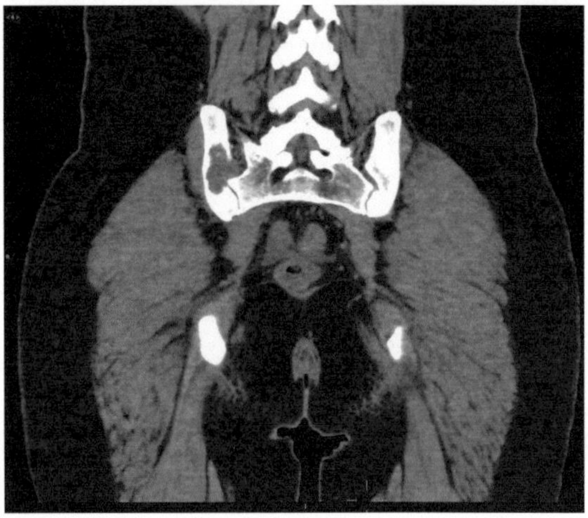

Fig. 30.6 Coronal CT image of the bony pelvis in soft tissue window

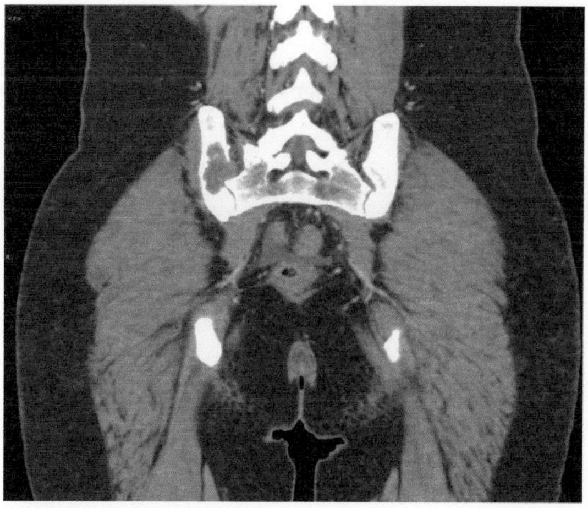

Fig. 30.7 Coronal post-contrast CT image of the bony pelvis in soft tissue window

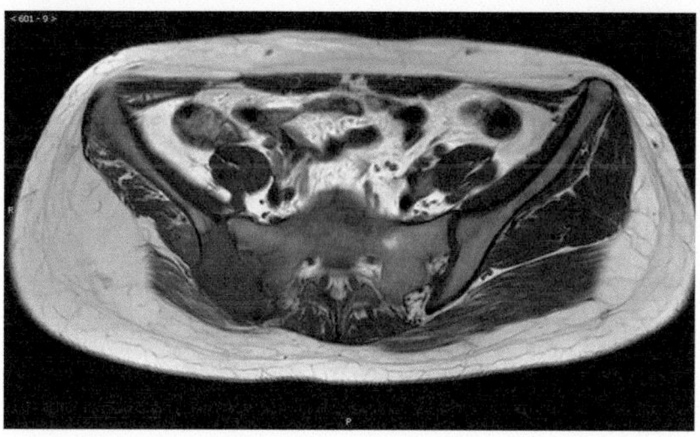

Fig. 30.8 Axial T1-weighted MR image of the bony pelvis

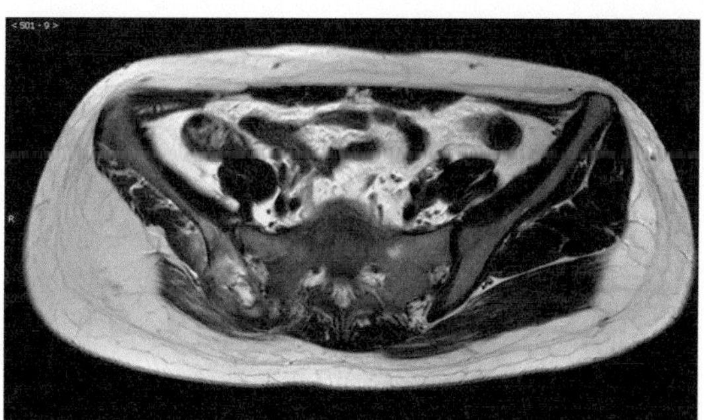

Fig. 30.9 Axial T2-weighted MR image of the bony pelvis

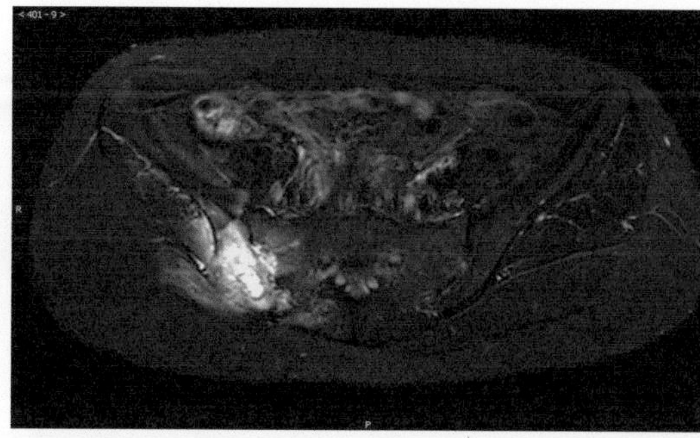

Fig. 30.10 Axial fat-suppressed T2-weighted MR image of the bony pelvis

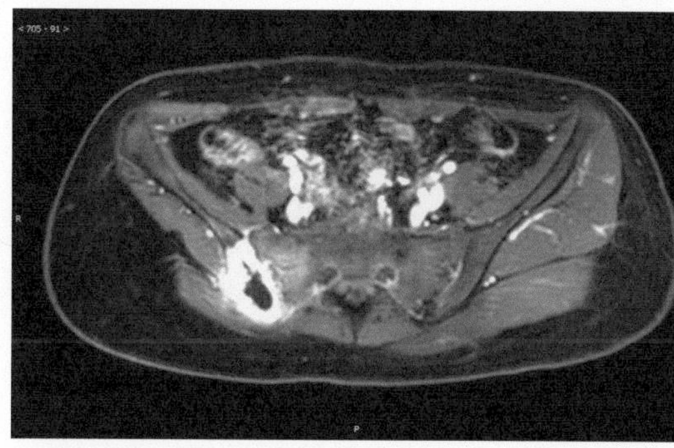

Fig. 30.11 Axial post-contrast fat-suppressed T1-weighted MR image of the bony pelvis

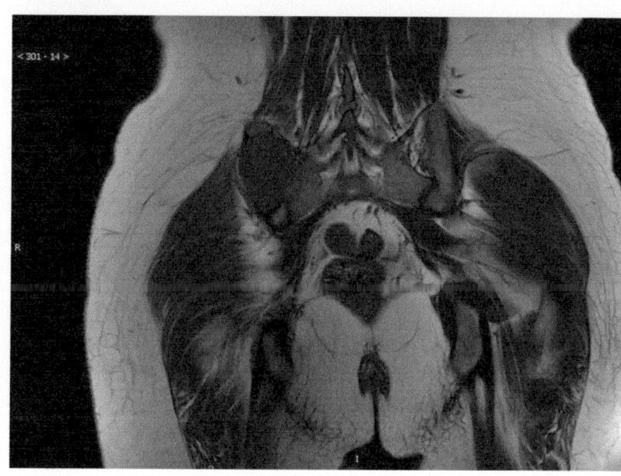

Fig. 30.12 Coronal T1-weighted MR image of the bony pelvis

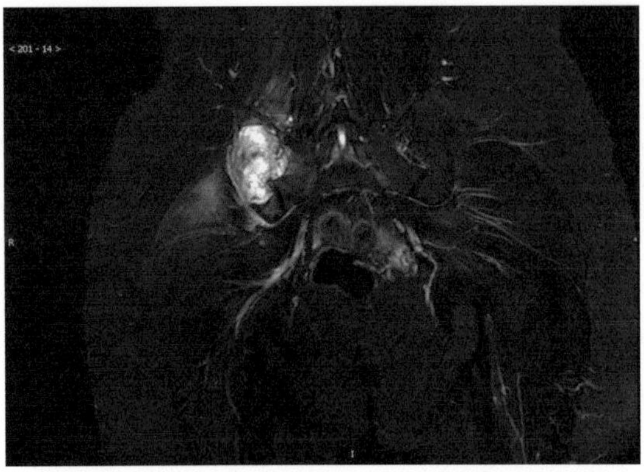

Fig. 30.13 Coronal fat-suppressed T2-weighted MR image of the bony pelvis

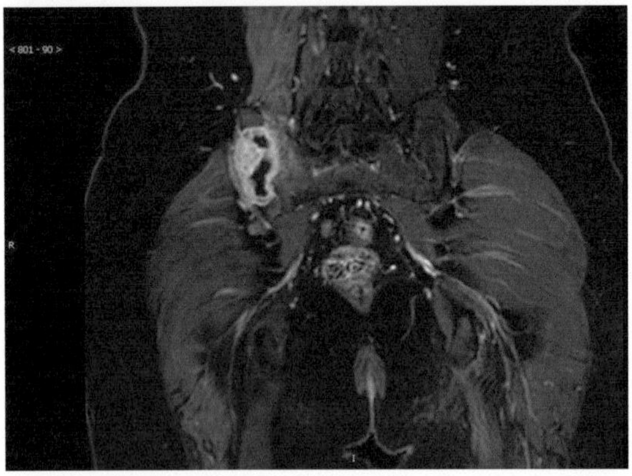

Fig. 30.14 Coronal post-contrast fat-suppressed T1-weighted MR image of the bony pelvis

30.4 Description and Discussion from Residents

The radiograph showed no apparent abnormalities. CT images demonstrated bone destruction of the right iliac with suspicious decreased bone density of the adjacent sacrum could be a process of the sacroiliac joint pathology. Small septations noted in the lesion with focal cortical break and soft tissue mass with mild heterogeneous enhancement, suggesting a malignant process. On the MR images, the signal of the sacrum is normal (not affected), low signal septations noted inside lesion with peritumoral edema and peripheral avid enhancement with central no enhancement, highly suggesting malignant tumor.

30.5 Analysis and Comments from Professor Cheng Xiao-Guang

The patient is a middle-aged female. Radiograph showed focal heterogeneous density in the right iliac adjacent to the sacroiliac joint. CT images showed bone destruction of right iliac with internal heterogeneous densities and no apparent osteogenesis or calcification. No apparent enhancement noted. There was cortical break with the soft tissue mass affecting the sacroiliac joint. The findings suggest aggressive nature of the process, and given patient's age and location of the lesion, chondrosarcoma is most common. However, there was no apparent calcification, not typical of chondrosarcoma. MR images showed focal cystic signal with apparent high signal on fat-suppressed T2-weighted sequences with apparent adjacent soft tissue edema and circular peripheral enhancement and no enhancement centrally. This case is challenging for diagnosis, based on above findings; the differential diagnosis includes (1) eosinophilic granuloma, most based on apparent inflammation in the surrounding tissues, (2) chondrosarcoma, but no apparent chondroid matrix, and (3) Aneurysmal bone cyst, no significant expansile nature of the lesion. Current case demonstrated strong aggressiveness of the process without characteristic imaging feature, thus challenging.

30.6 Diagnosis

Malignant peripheral nerve sheath tumor of bone (with heterologous differentiation).

Suggested Reading

Lang N, Liu XG, Yuan HS. Malignant peripheral nerve sheath tumor in spine: imaging manifestations. Clin Imaging. 2012;36(3):209–15.

Yu YH, Wu JT, Ye J, et al. Radiological findings of malignant peripheral nerve sheath tumor: reports of six cases and review of literature. World J Surg Oncol. 2016;14:142.

Chondromyxoid Fibroma: Case 31 31

31.1 Medical History

Patient is a 44-year-old male. He has right lower back and thigh pain for 3 years with worsening symptoms and right iliac lesion noted in the last 6 weeks.

31.2 Physical Examination

No recorded in hospital system.

31.3 Imaging Findings

31.3.1 Radiograph (Fig. 31.1)

Radiograph of the pelvis demonstrated lytic bone destruction of the right iliac wing with clear margin and peripheral sclerosis.

31.3.2 CT Imaging (Figs. 31.2, 31.3, 31.4, 31.5, 31.6, 31.7, and 31.8)

CT images of the bony pelvis demonstrated mild expansile and lytic bone destruction of the right iliac wing with distinct border and very thin bone shell peripherally and internal rather homogenous soft tissue densities. Peripheral enhancement with internal scattered patchy enhancements noted.

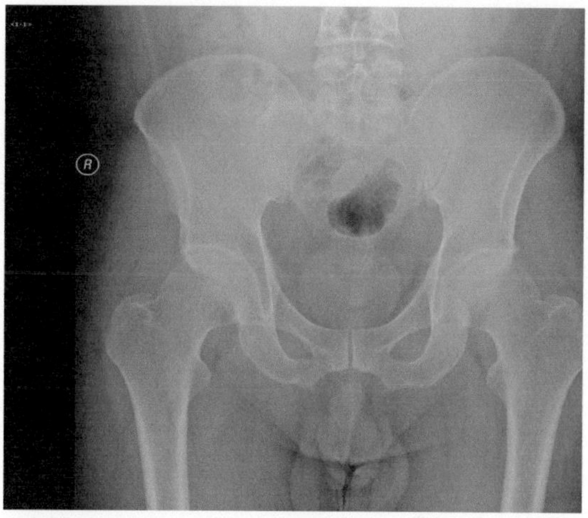

Fig. 31.1 Frontal view of pelvis

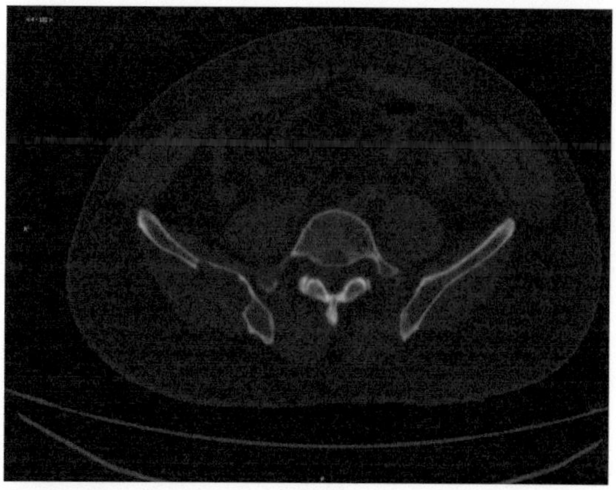

Fig. 31.2 Axial CT image of the bony pelvis in bone window

X. Cheng et al., *Imaging of Bone Tumors in Axial Bones*,
https://doi.org/10.1007/978-981-95-2262-0_31

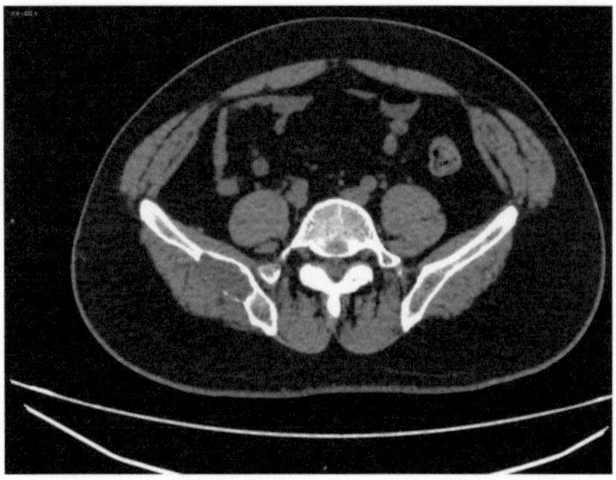

Fig. 31.3 Axial CT image of the bony pelvis in soft tissue window

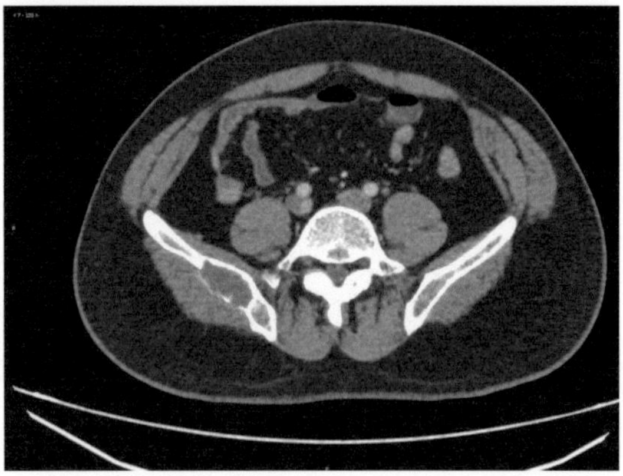

Fig. 31.4 Axial post-contrast CT image of the bony pelvis in soft tissue window

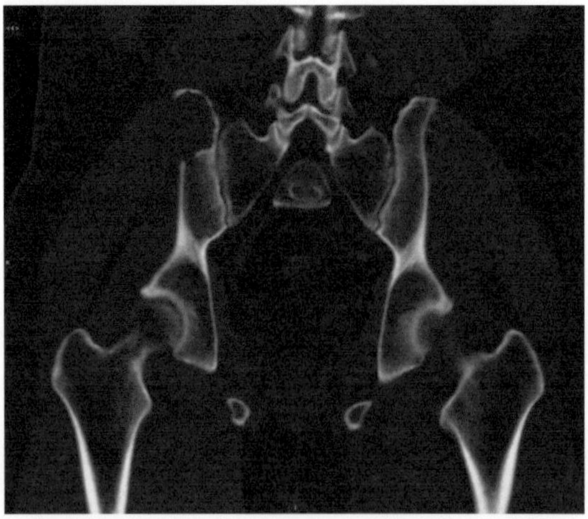

Fig. 31.5 Coronal CT image of the bony pelvis in bone window

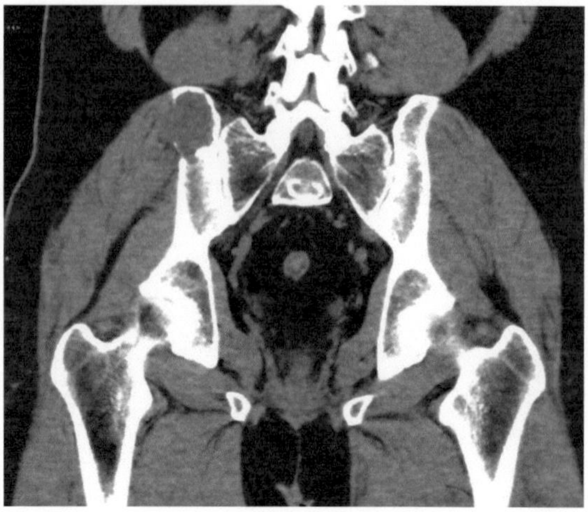

Fig. 31.6 Coronal CT image of the bony pelvis in soft tissue window

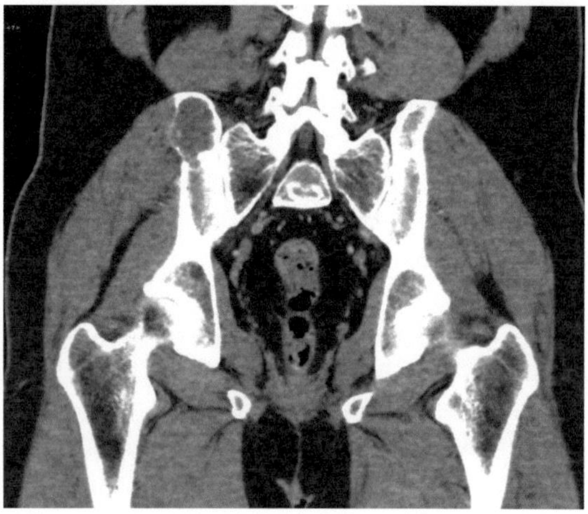

Fig. 31.7 Coronal post-contrast CT image of the bony pelvis in soft tissue window

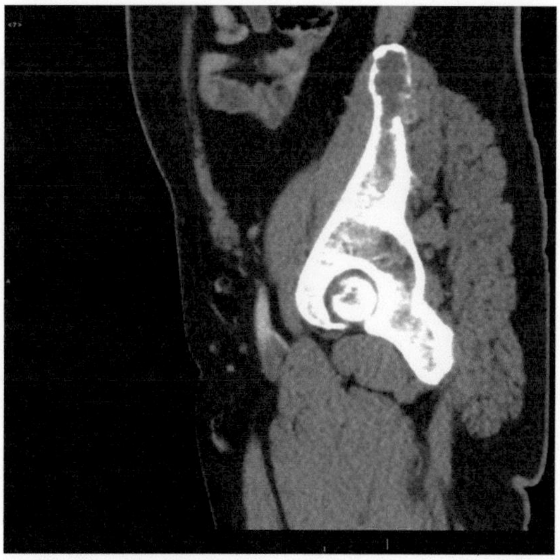

Fig. 31.8 Sagittal post-contrast CT image of the bony pelvis in soft tissue window

31.4 Description and Discussion from Residents

The radiograph showed oval low-density destruction at the right iliac wing with clear margin and peripheral mild sclerosis. CT images demonstrated focal lytic bone destruction of the right iliac wing with internal homogeneous densities and no peripheral sclerosis or periosteal reaction. There appeared to be focal cortical disruption and mild external protrusion of the soft tissue component and mild peripheral enhancement. Overall, we favor a malignant process, such as chondrosarcoma.

31.5 Analysis and Comments from Professor Cheng Xiao-Guang

Patient was a middle-aged male. The radiograph showed bone destruction at the right iliac wing with clear margin. CT images demonstrated a mild expansile lytic bone destruction with relatively continuous shell of reactive sclerosis, without much enhancement. With solitary bone destruction of the right iliac wing in a middle-aged man, the most common process is chondrosarcoma. However, no apparent chondroid matrix noted of the current case, not consistent with chondrosarcoma. This could be related to the small size of the lesion. Aneurysmal bone cyst is in the differential diagnosis. However, the lesion did not demonstrate typical expansile appearance and no obvious cystic components noted, not supporting this diagnosis. Given the above imaging findings, overall, I favor a benign or low-grade malignant lesion and further evaluation with MRI would be helpful.

31.6 Diagnosis

Chondromyxoid fibroma.

Suggested Reading

Alsford S, Low S, Mistry A. Chondromyxoid fibroma of the iliac bone: a brief radiological review. BMJ Case Rep. 2022;15(11):e251363.

Cappelle S, Pans S, Sciot R. Imaging features of chondromyxoid fibroma: report of 15 cases and literature review. Br J Radiol. 2016;89(1064):20160088.

Phosphaturic Mesenchymal Tumor of Bone: Case 32

32

32.1 Medical History

Patient is a 54-year-old male. He started to suffer from right back and gluteal pain after injury about 1 month ago and found to have lesion around the right iliac. He underwent needle biopsy. The symptoms worsened afterward with rest and night pain, and not exacerbated by activities.

32.2 Physical Examination

Point tenderness around the right gluteal region.

32.3 Imaging Findings

32.3.1 Radiograph (Fig. 32.1)

Radiograph of the pelvis demonstrated mild high densities of right ilium around the sacroiliac joint with clear margin.

32.3.2 CT Imaging (Figs. 32.2, 32.3, 32.4, 32.5, 32.6, and 32.7)

CT images of the bony pelvis demonstrated lytic bone destruction of the right iliac bone with clear margin and peripheral sclerosis, with soft tissue mass extending laterally beyond the cortex. There were internal punctate and linear high densities with avid enhancement.

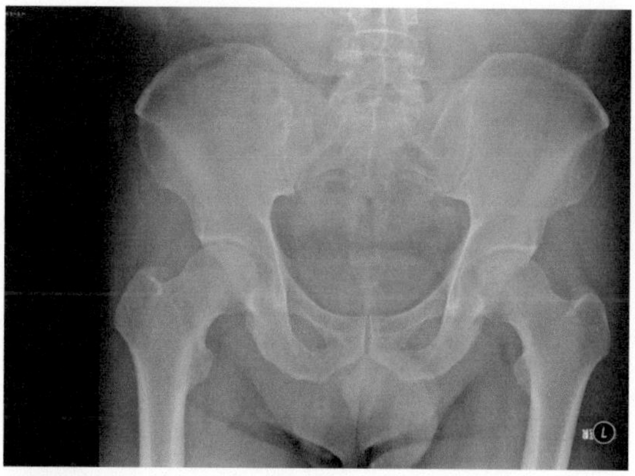

Fig. 32.1 Frontal view of pelvis

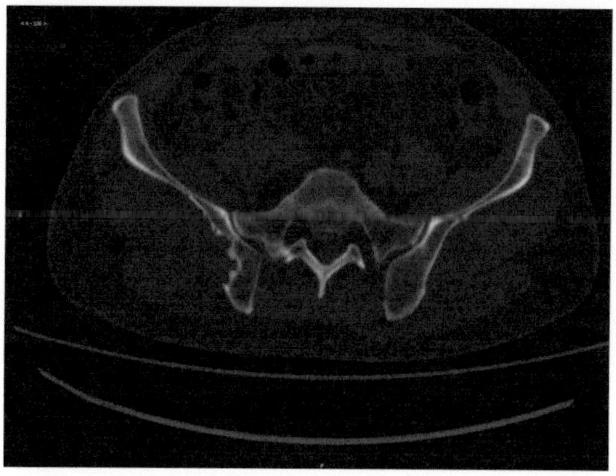

Fig. 32.2 Axial CT image of the bony pelvis in bone window

X. Cheng et al., *Imaging of Bone Tumors in Axial Bones*,
https://doi.org/10.1007/978-981-95-2262-0_32

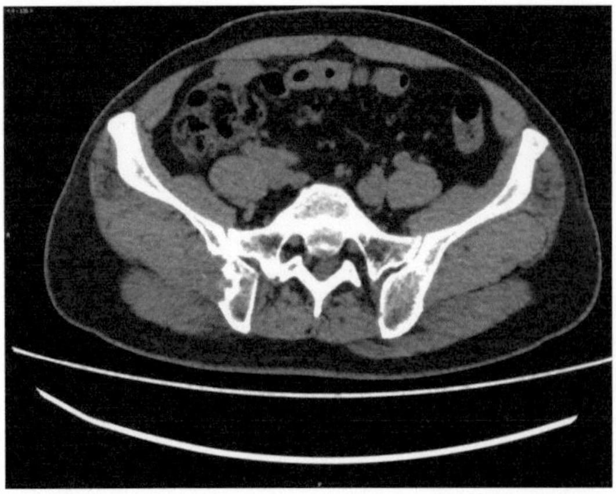

Fig. 32.3 Axial CT image of the bony pelvis in soft tissue window

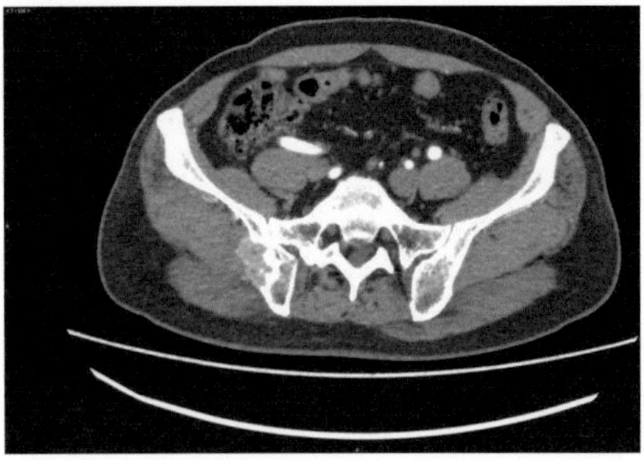

Fig. 32.4 Axial post-contrast CT image of the bony pelvis in soft tissue window

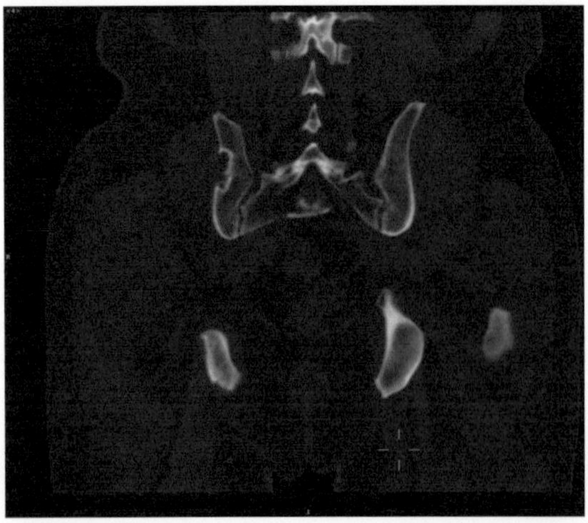

Fig. 32.5 Coronal CT image of the bony pelvis in bone window

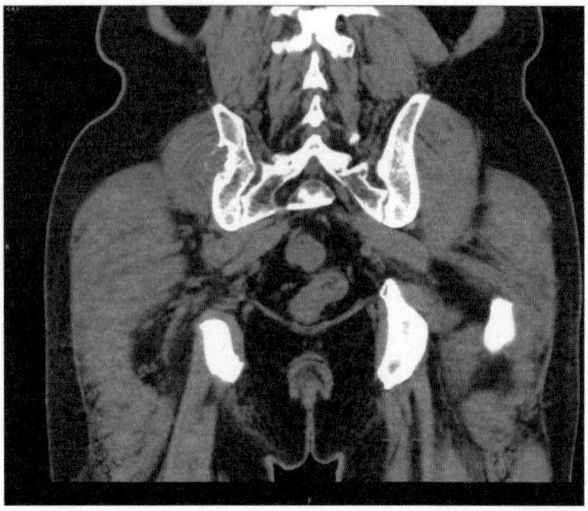

Fig. 32.6 Coronal CT image of the bony pelvis in soft tissue window

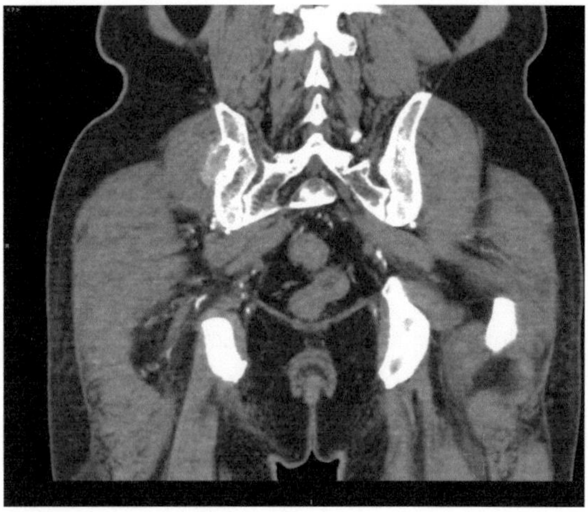

Fig. 32.7 Coronal post-contrast CT image of the bony pelvis in soft tissue window

32.3.3 MR Imaging (Figs. 32.8, 32.9, 32.10, and 32.11)

MR images showed destruction of the right ilium with peripheral mildly low signal of sclerosis and lobulated soft tissue mass extending beyond the cortex with T1 and T2 slightly low signal. There were internal punctate and linear fluid like high T2 signal. Avid enhancement noted.

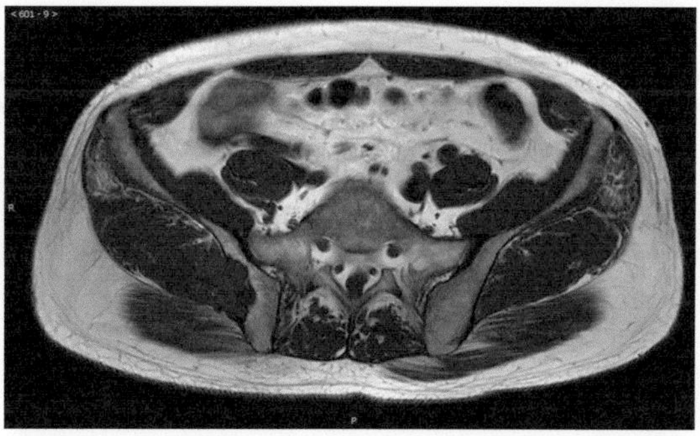

Fig. 32.8 Axial T1-weighted MR image of the bony pelvis

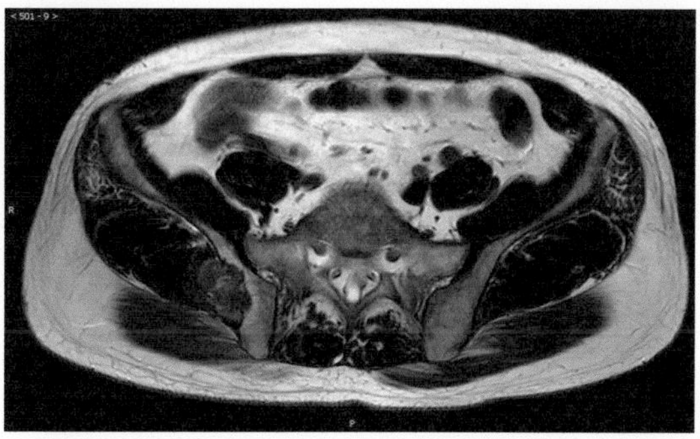

Fig. 32.9 Axial T2-weighted MR image of the bony pelvis

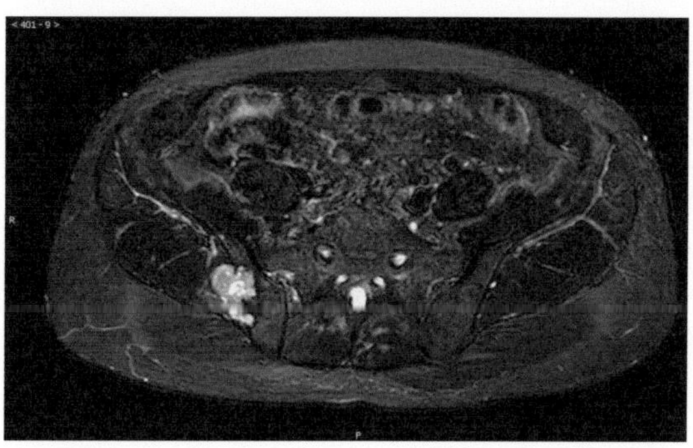

Fig. 32.10 Axial fat-suppressed T2-weighted MR image of the bony pelvis

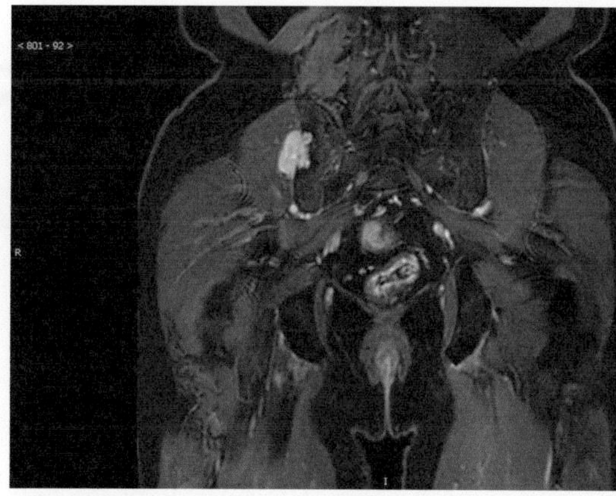

Fig. 32.11 Coronal post-contrast fat-suppressed T1-weighted MR image of the bony pelvis

32.4 Description and Discussion from Residents

The radiograph showed focal ground glass like density around the right sacroiliac joint with clear margin and peripheral sclerosis. Bone destruction of right ilium with peripheral sclerosis noted on CT images with focal compressive changes, suggestive of subperiosteal process. Avid enhancement noted of the soft tissue mass. Most of these findings support benign process. On fat-suppressed T2-weighted MR images, low signals mixed inside of the high signals, suggestive of the presence of fibrous tissue. There was no involvement of the adjacent soft tissues. Avid enhancement noted. Overall, we favor a fibrous lesion, such as fibrous dysplasia.

32.5 Analysis and Comments from Professor Cheng Xiao-Guang

Radiograph showed the right iliac lesion with well-defined margin. CT images showed the isolated lesion of the right iliac bone with clear margin medially and mild expansion laterally with thin shell. No apparent calcification or ground glass density inside of the lesion, not typical of fibrous dysplasia. Avid enhancement noted, suggesting avid blood supply. Overall, I favor a benign process. However, with the soft tissue mass extending beyond the cortex, concern is raised. The lesion was of relatively low signal on T1- and T2-weighted MR images and high signal on fat-suppressed T2-weighted sequences with soft tissue mass focally extending beyond the cortex, indicating some invasiveness of the lesion. Overall, the current case has features favor both benign and aggressive process, with contradiction and very challenging, and the diagnosis will need to be combined with pathology.

32.6 Diagnosis

Phosphaturic mesenchymal tumor of bone.

Suggested Reading

Broski SM, Folpe AL, Wenger DE, et al. Imaging features of phosphaturic mesenchymal tumors. Skeletal Radiol. 2019;48(1):119–27.

Gupta A, Kandasamy D, Sharma R, et al. Imaging characteristics of phosphaturic mesenchymal tumors. Acta Radiol. 2023;64(6):2061–73.

Gorham-Stout Disease: Case 33

33

33.1 Medical History

Patient is a 27-year-old male. He was seen at an outpatient clinic for left iliac lesion.

33.2 Physical Examination

Not recorded in hospital system.

33.3 Imaging Findings

33.3.1 Radiograph (Fig. 33.1)

Radiograph of the bony pelvis demonstrated bone deficiency around the part of the left iliac bone and left L4 vertebral body with deformity.

33.3.2 CT Imaging (Figs. 33.2, 33.3, 33.4, 33.5, 33.6, and 33.7)

CT images of the bony pelvis demonstrated deformity of left ilium, ischium, and vertebral body of L4 with atrophy and loss of bone, replaced with linear soft tissue density with ipsilateral muscles atrophy. No enhancement noted.

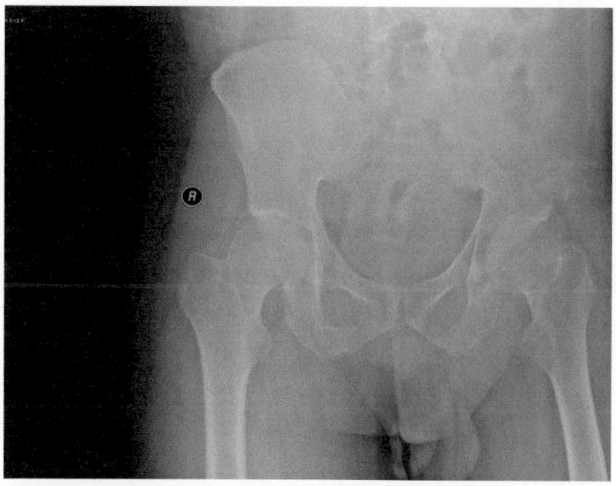

Fig. 33.1 Frontal view of pelvis

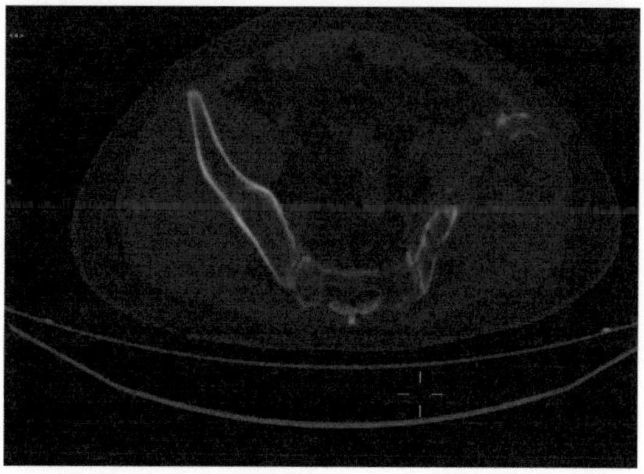

Fig. 33.2 Axial CT image of the bony pelvis in bone window

X. Cheng et al., *Imaging of Bone Tumors in Axial Bones*,
https://doi.org/10.1007/978-981-95-2262-0_33

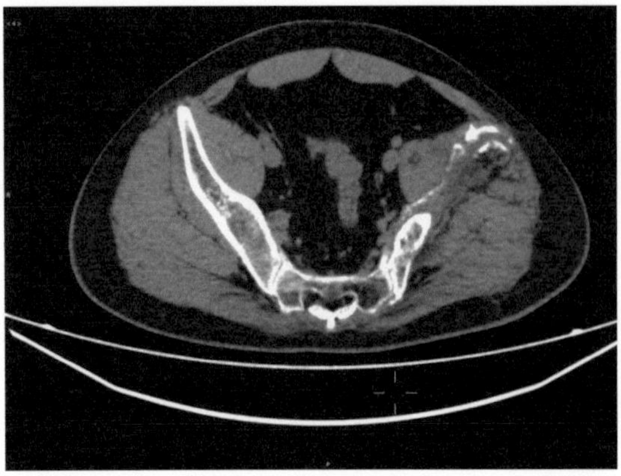

Fig. 33.3 Axial CT image of the bony pelvis in soft tissue window

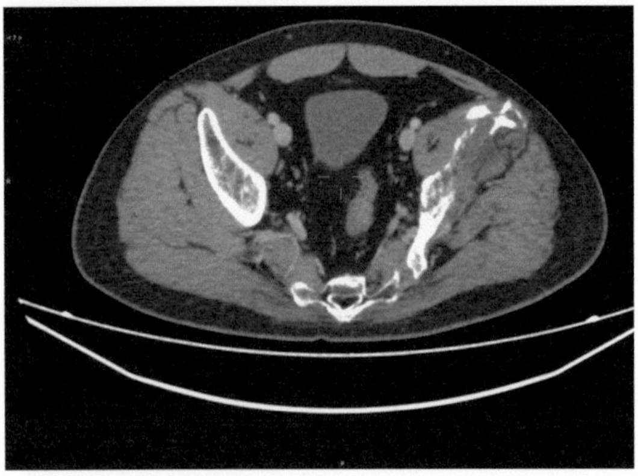

Fig. 33.4 Axial post-contrast CT image of the bony pelvis in soft tissue window

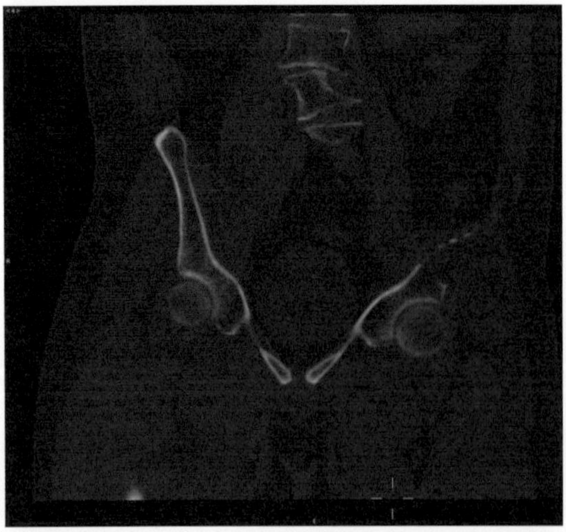

Fig. 33.5 Coronal CT image of the bony pelvis in bone window

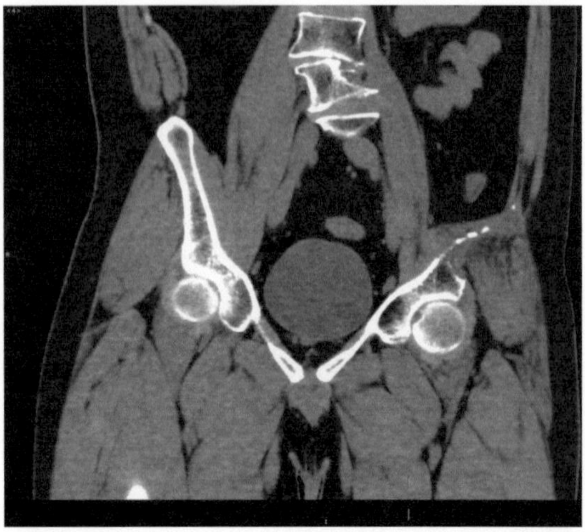

Fig. 33.6 Coronal CT image of the bony pelvis in soft tissue window

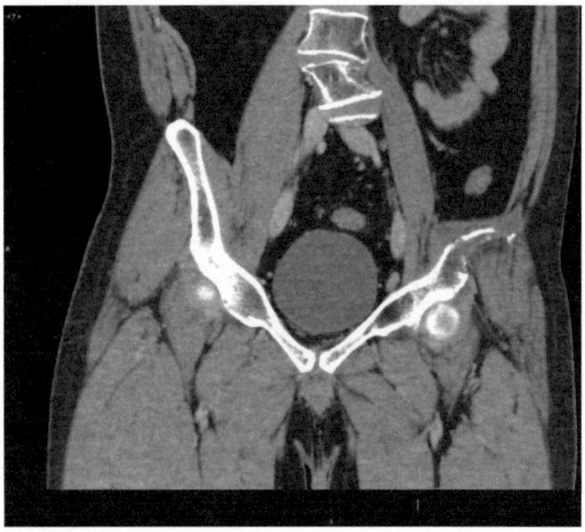

Fig. 33.7 Coronal post-contrast CT image of the bony pelvis in soft tissue window

33.4 Description and Discussion from Residents

The radiograph showed bone deficiency of left L4 vertebral body and left iliac wing with decreased bone density of left bony pelvis and left hip. The joint space of the left hip was preserved with indistinct left sacroiliac joint and decreased densities of the left gluteal muscles. CT images demonstrated disappearance of the left iliac wing with residual relatively weakened bones. There was disappearance of the left L4 vertebral body with sclerosis and cystic changes and narrowing of the intervertebral disc space. The lesion was without periosteal reaction or soft tissue mass. There was muscle atrophy of the left hip and gluteal region. No enhancement was noted. Overall, we favor vanishing bone disease (Gorham-Stout disease).

33.5 Analysis and Comments from Professor Cheng Xiao-Guang

The patient was a young male without history of surgery. Radiograph showed bone disappearance of the left L4 vertebral body and left iliac bone with overall decreased bone densities. CT images demonstrated large area of disappearance of the osseous structures of the left iliac wing and left L4 vertebral body with ipsilateral apparent muscle atrophy. These were not typical bone destruction and soft tissue mass from malignant neoplasm but more suggestive of vanishing bone disease (Gorham-Stout disease). Currently, the mechanism of this condition is not well understood. We can see hemangioma-like structures in pathology; however, some cases show fibrotic and granulation tissues. Overall, there is no characteristic pathological feature of vanishing bone disease; the diagnosis mainly relies on imaging findings.

33.6 Diagnosis

Gorham-Stout disease.

Suggested Reading

Lee Y, Lee S, Hur S, et al. The spectrum of imaging manifestations of Gorham-Stout disease: a novel dynamic contrast-enhanced MR lymphangiography. Orphanet J Rare Dis. 2023;18(1):96.

Ruggieri P, Montalti M, Angelini A, et al. Gorham-Stout disease: the experience of the Rizzoli Institute and review of the literature. Skeletal Radiol. 2011;40(11):1391–7.

34 Chondrosarcoma: Case 34

34.1 Medical History

Patient is a 50-year-old male. He suffered from lower back pain and bilateral hip pain, more on the right, starting 5 years ago without clear causes. CT exam showed narrowing of the spinal canal, and he received no therapy. He was found to have pathology around the right bony pelvis about 2 months ago.

34.2 Physical Examination

Point tenderness around the right iliac.

34.3 Imaging Findings

34.3.1 Radiograph (Fig. 34.1)

Radiograph of the pelvis showed heterogeneous density lesion around the right iliac.

34.3.2 CT Imaging (Figs. 34.2, 34.3, 34.4, 34.5, and 34.6)

CT images of the bony pelvis demonstrated bone destruction of right iliac wing with expansile growth and cortical destruction with mass. There was internal high-density septations and multiple punctate calcifications with peripheral discontinuous high-density shadow and no avid enhancement. There was focal bone destruction of the left ilium with internal fat density and peripheral sclerosis.

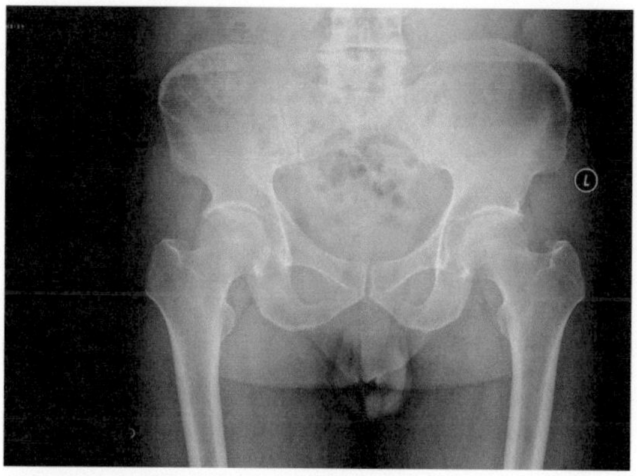

Fig. 34.1 Frontal view of the pelvis

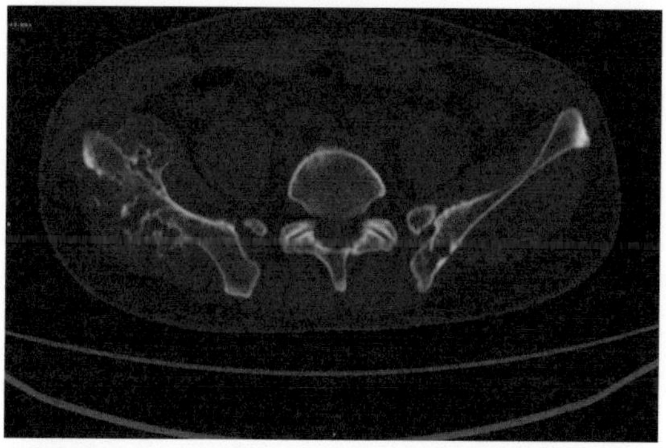

Fig. 34.2 Axial CT image of the bony pelvis in bone window

X. Cheng et al., *Imaging of Bone Tumors in Axial Bones*,
https://doi.org/10.1007/978-981-95-2262-0_34

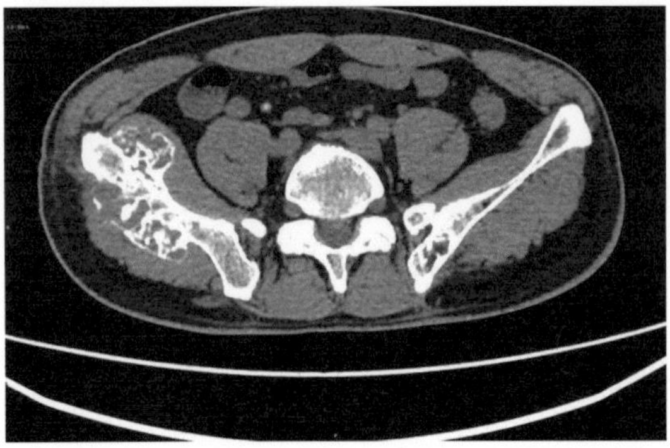

Fig. 34.3 Axial CT image of the bony pelvis in soft tissue window

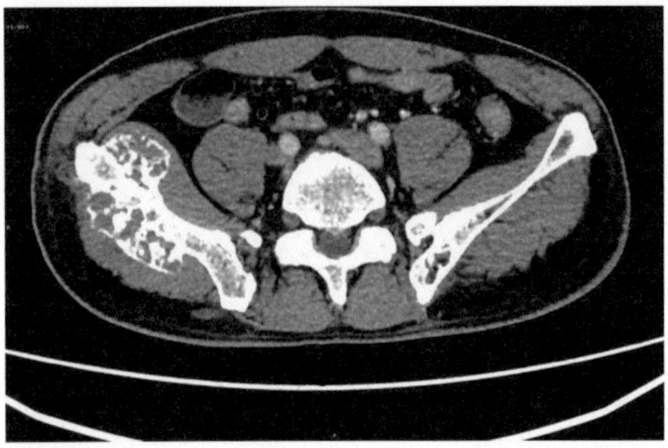

Fig. 34.4 Axial post-contrast CT image of the bony pelvis in soft tissue window

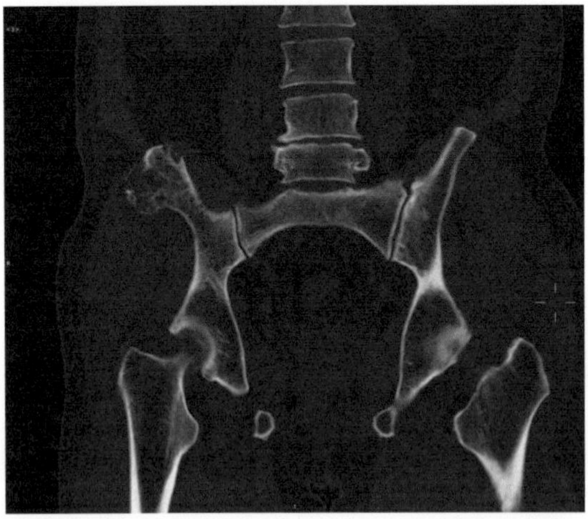

Fig. 34.5 Coronal CT image of the bony pelvis in bone window

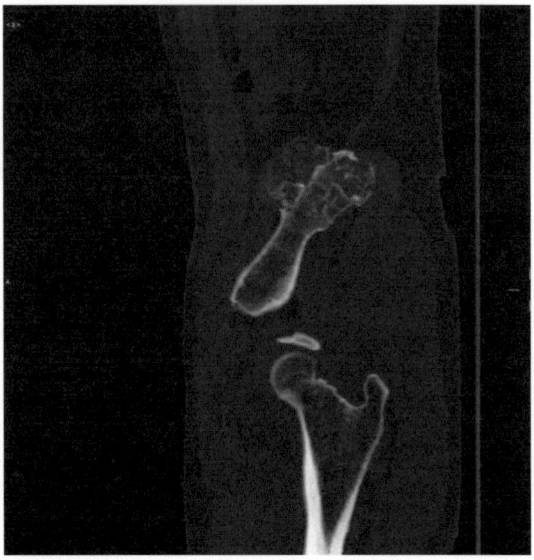

Fig. 34.6 Sagittal CT image of the bony pelvis in bone window

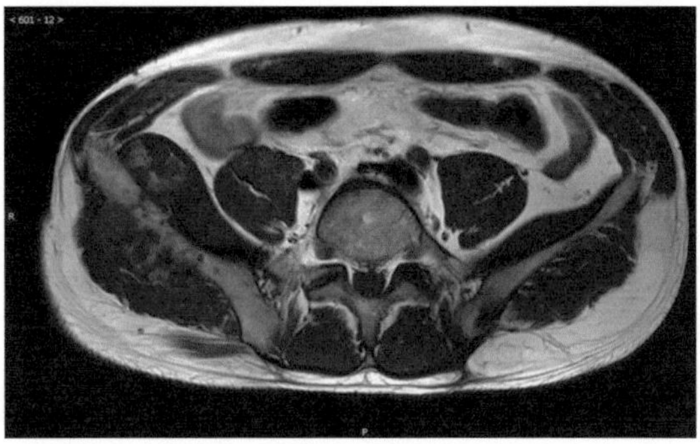

Fig. 34.7 Axial T1-weighted MR image of the bony pelvis

34.3.3 MR Imaging (Figs. 34.7, 34.8, 34.9, and 34.10)

MR images of the bony pelvis demonstrated expansile bone destruction of the right iliac wing with internal multiple foci of T2 high signal with punctate low signal and linear low-signal septations with irregular morphology. Peripheral and septation enhancement noted with punctate enhancement. There was focal bone destruction

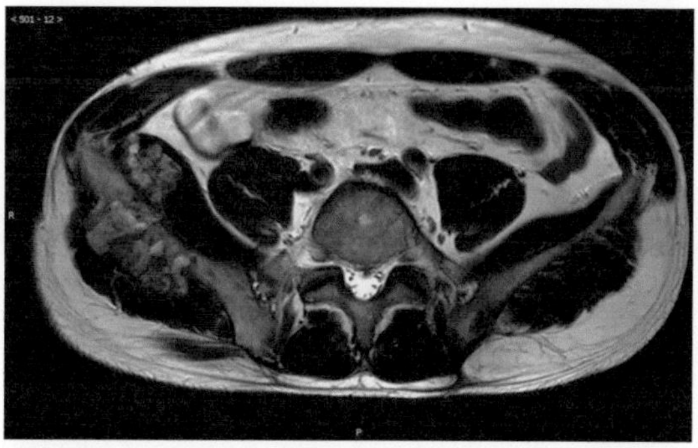

Fig. 34.8 Axial T2-weighted MR image of the bony pelvis

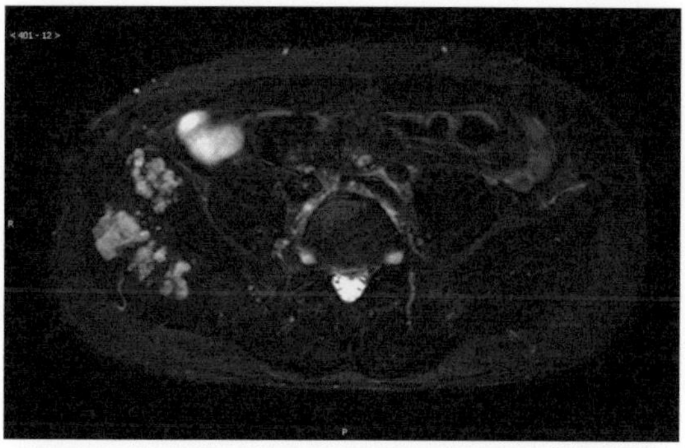

Fig. 34.9 Axial fat-suppressed T2-weighted MR image of the bony pelvis

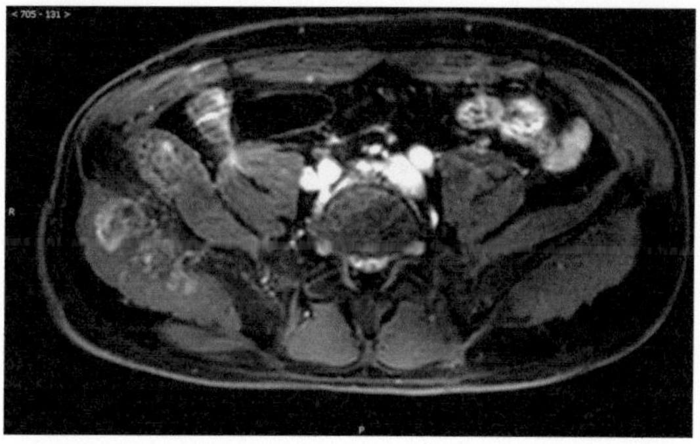

Fig. 34.10 Axial post-contrast fat-suppressed T1-weighted MR image of the bony pelvis

of the left iliac with internal fat signal and peripheral enhancement.

34.4 Description and Discussion from Residents

CT images showed expansile bone destruction of right iliac wing with focal discontinuous cortex. Punctate calcifications noted in the lesion with mild enhancement, indicating low-grade chondrosarcoma. There was bone destruction around the left iliac spine with internal low density, likely of fat, not same process as of the right iliac bone. MR images showed heterogeneous signals of the lesion with calcifications with mild and heterogeneous enhancement. Given patients age, overall, we favor low-grade chondrosarcoma.

34.5 Analysis and Comments from Professor Cheng Xiao-Guang

There was expansile bone destruction of right iliac bone with peripheral bone shell. There were heterogeneous densities within the lesion with small amount of punctate calcification and no avid enhancement. Additionally, there was very low density in the lesion, close to fat density, needing further investigation. There was linear and patchy high T1 signal in the lesion on the MR images, likely of bone structure. High signals of chondroid lobules were noted on the fat-suppressed T2-weighted images. The very low-density area on CT showed high T1 signal and low signal on fat-suppressed T2-weighted images, indicating fat component in the lesion. Native chondrosarcoma usually does not contain fat component, thus raises the consideration of malignant transformation of osteochondroma. The lesion in the left iliac spine demonstrated nonspecific image findings and increased complexity of the diagnosis.

34.6 Diagnosis

Chondrosarcoma (of the right iliac lesion).

Suggested Reading

Douis H, Saifuddin A. The imaging of cartilaginous bone tumours. II. Chondrosarcoma. Skeletal Radiol. 2013;42(5):611–26.

Kim JH, Lee SK. Classification of chondrosarcoma: from characteristic to challenging imaging findings. Cancers (Basel). 2023;15(6):1703.

Jain V, Oliveira I, Chavda A, et al. MRI differentiation of low-grade and high-grade chondrosarcoma of the shoulder girdle, chest wall and pelvis: a pictorial review based on 111 consecutive cases. Br J Radiol. 2021;94(1126):20201404.

35 Intraosseous Hemangioma: Case 35

35.1 Medical History

Patient is a 58-year-old female. She suffered from left hip pain for 27 months and worsened with restricted activities for 5 months.

35.2 Physical Examination

Restricted movement around the left hip from pain.

35.3 Imaging Findings

35.3.1 Radiograph (Fig. 35.1)

Radiograph of the pelvis showed mild expansile bone destruction of the left acetabular roof and iliac bone with internal septations.

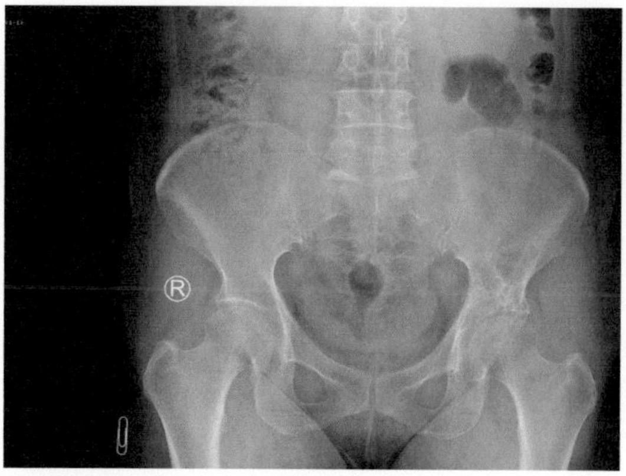

Fig. 35.1 Frontal view of the pelvis

35.3.2 CT Imaging (Figs. 35.2, 35.3, 35.4, 35.5, 35.6, and 35.7)

CT images of the bony pelvis demonstrated mild expansile bone destruction of the left acetabulum with internal multiple septations with focal grid-like changes. The lesion was well circumscribed with mild peripheral sclerosis, thinning of the cortex and suspected focal cortical disruption. No associated soft tissue mass noted. Avid heterogeneous enhancement noted.

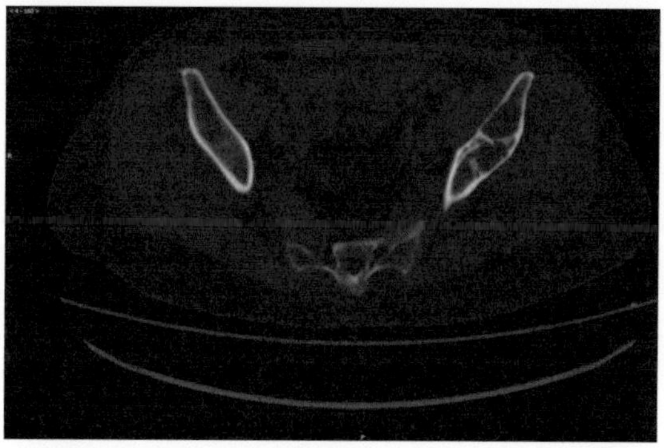

Fig. 35.2 Axial CT image of the bony pelvis in bone window

X. Cheng et al., *Imaging of Bone Tumors in Axial Bones*,
https://doi.org/10.1007/978-981-95-2262-0_35

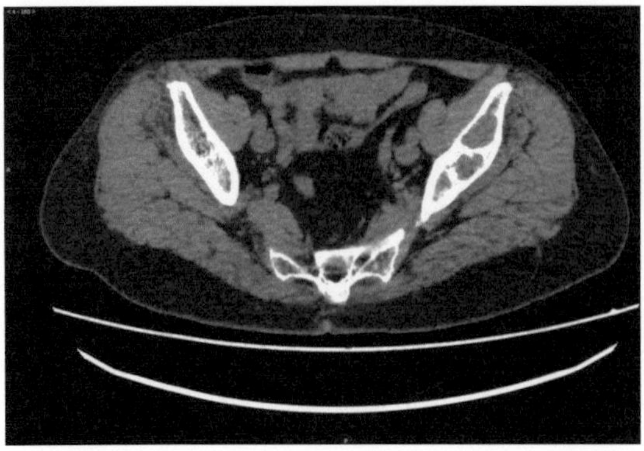

Fig. 35.3 Axial CT image of the bony pelvis in soft tissue window

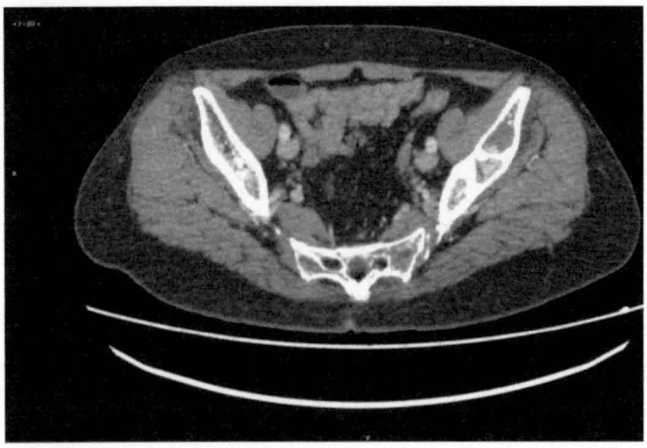

Fig. 35.4 Axial post-contrast CT image of the bony pelvis in soft tissue window

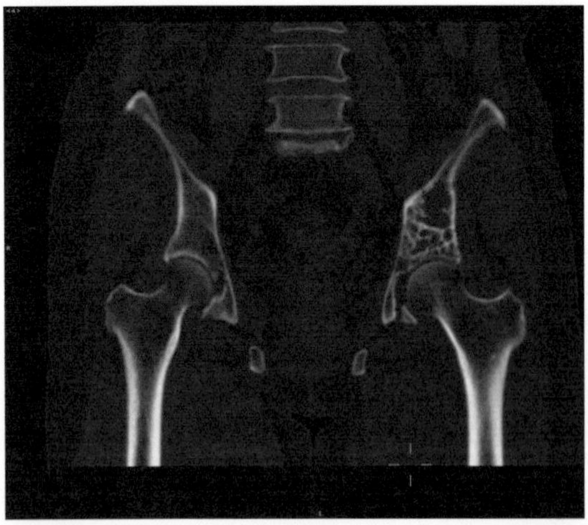

Fig. 35.5 Coronal CT image of the bony pelvis in bone window

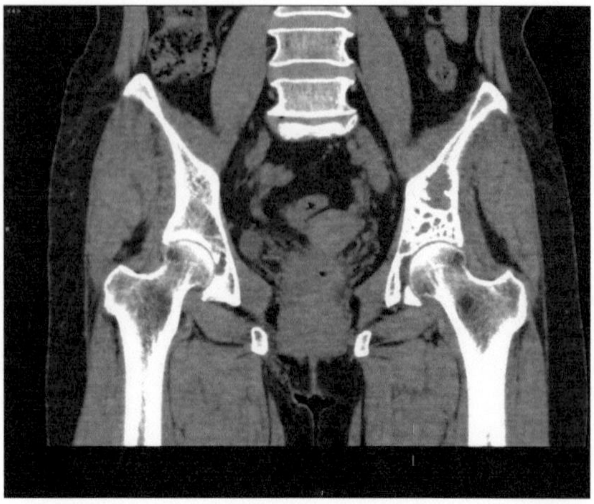

Fig. 35.6 Coronal CT image of the bony pelvis in soft tissue window

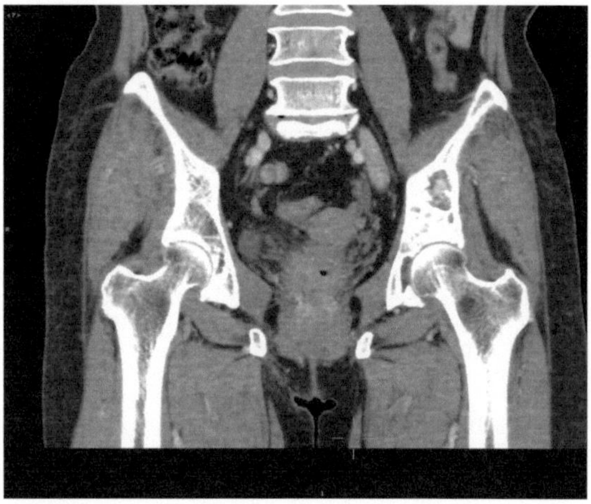

Fig. 35.7 Coronal post-contrast CT image of the bony pelvis in soft tissue window

35.4 Description and Discussion from Residents

Radiograph demonstrated mild expansile bone destruction at the junction of the left iliac wing and iliac body with internal grid-like or honeycomb-like changes. The left hip joint space was preserved. CT images showed multiple cyst-like destruction of the left acetabular roof with mild expansion and internal multiple residual bone trabeculae, focal sclerosis, and no periosteal reaction or soft tissue mass. Avid heterogeneous enhancement noted. Our top consideration is vascular tumor, such as hemangioma. Given mild expansion, fibrous dysplasia is in the differential diagnosis.

35.5 Analysis and Comments from Professor Cheng Xiao-Guang

Radiograph showed bone destruction at the left acetabular roof with slightly indistinct border and preserved left hip joint. CT images demonstrated bone destruction at the junction of the left iliac wing and iliac body. The lesion was confined to the bone with mild expansion and residual coarse bone trabeculae noted within the lesion with focal avid enhancement, all findings supporting a benign lesion. This kind of bone destruction appeared to be caused by vessels coursing through the trabecula and stimulate the trabeculae, leading to bone proliferation and enlargement. Additionally, current case is a multicentric lesion, most suggestive of a vascular tumor, such as hemangioma. Paget disease is in the differential diagnosis. However, no deformity noted of the current case, not consistent.

35.6 Diagnosis

Intraosseous hemangioma.

Suggested Reading

Ko SW, Park JG. Cavehourrnous hemangioma of the ilium mimicking aggressive malignant bone tumor with increased activity on (18)F-FDG PET/CT. Korean J Radiol. 2013;14(2):294–8.

Powell GM, Littrell LA, Broski SM, et al. Imaging features of intraosseous hemangiomas: beyond the mobile spine and calvarium. Skeletal Radiol. 2023;52(9):1739–46.

Wenger DE, Wold LE. Benign vascular lesions of bone: radiologic and pathologic features. Skeletal Radiol. 2000;29(2):63–74.

Chondroblastoma: Case 36

36

36.1 Medical History

Patient is an 18-year-old male. He suffered from left hip pain and discomfort for about a year after a fall and worsened in the last 3 months.

36.2 Physical Examination

Apparent point tenderness around the left hip, positive Patrick's test and mild restricted left hip activities.

36.3 Imaging Findings

36.3.1 Radiograph (Fig. 36.1)

Radiograph of the pelvis showed expansile bone destruction around the left acetabulum with clear margin and mild peripheral sclerosis.

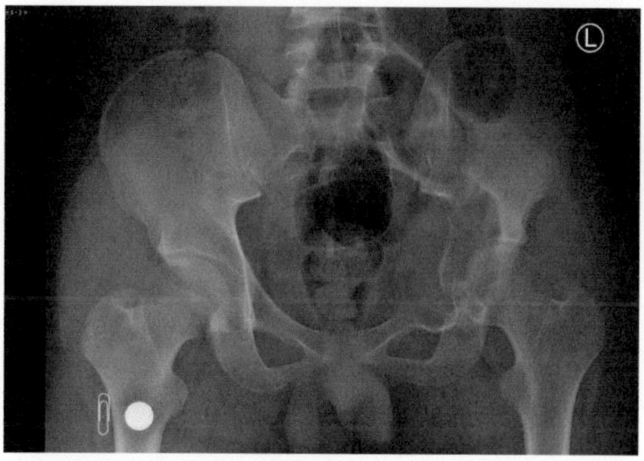

Fig. 36.1 Frontal view of the pelvis

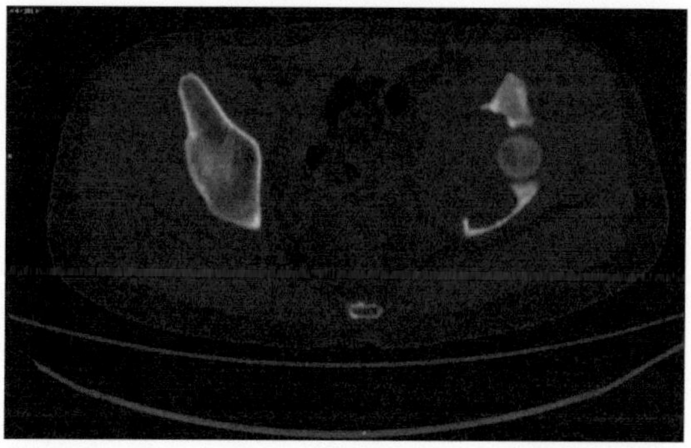

Fig. 36.2 Axial CT image of the bony pelvis in bone window

36.3.2 CT Imaging (Figs. 36.2, 36.3, 36.4, 36.5, 36.6, and 36.7)

CT images of the bony pelvis demonstrated expansile and lytic bone destruction of the left acetabulum with internal heterogeneous density and clear margin with focal cortical disruption. No associated soft tissue mass noted. Avid heterogeneous enhancement noted with internal non-enhancing cystic changes.

X. Cheng et al., *Imaging of Bone Tumors in Axial Bones*, https://doi.org/10.1007/978-981-95-2262-0_36

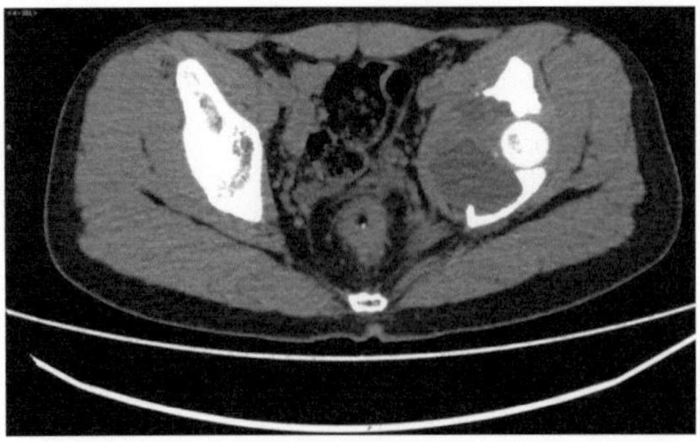

Fig. 36.3 Axial CT image of the bony pelvis in soft tissue window

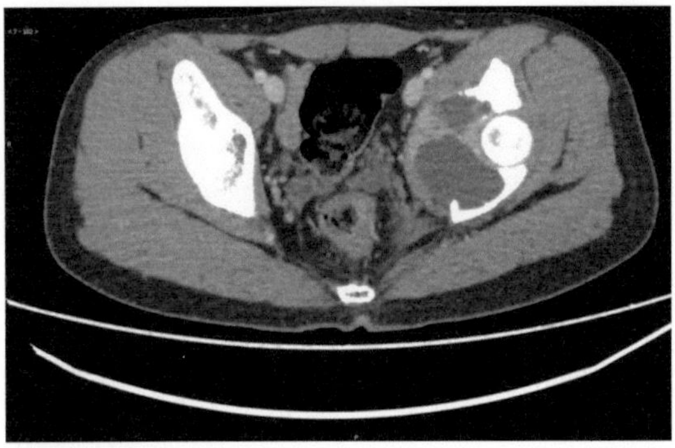

Fig. 36.4 Axial post-contrast CT image of the bony pelvis in soft tissue window

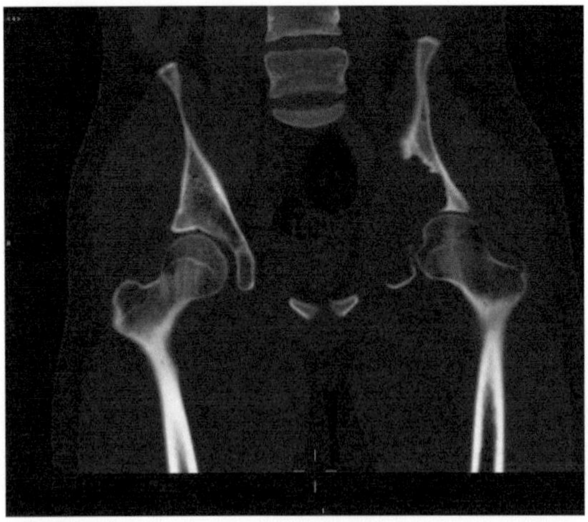

Fig. 36.5 Coronal CT image of the bony pelvis in bone window

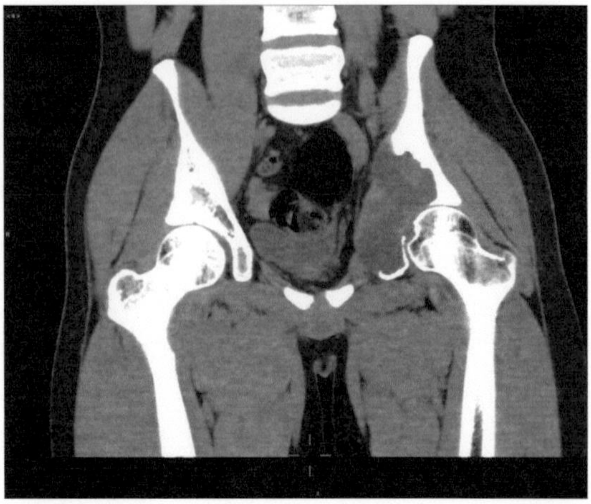

Fig. 36.6 Coronal CT image of the bony pelvis in soft tissue window

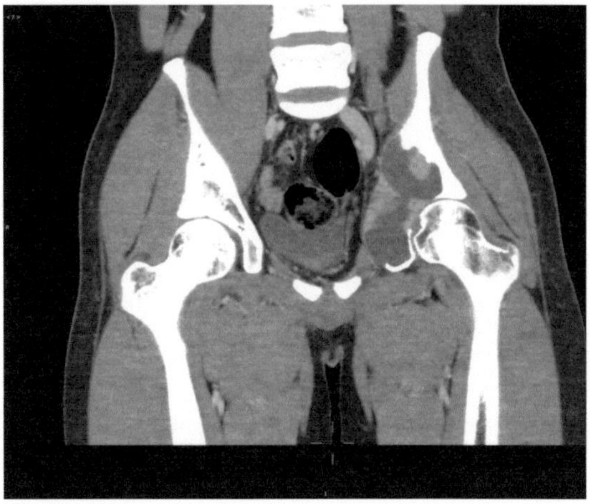

Fig. 36.7 Coronal post-contrast CT image of the bony pelvis in soft tissue window

36.3.3 MR Imaging (Figs. 36.8, 36.9, 36.10, and 36.11)

MR images of the bony pelvis demonstrated irregular and expansile bone lytic destruction of the left acetabulum. The lesion was well-circumscribed with high T1 signal, heterogeneous high T2 signal, and also high T2 signal on

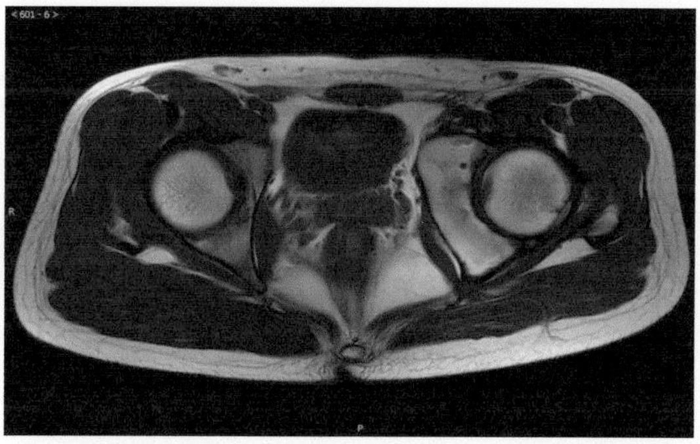

Fig. 36.8 Axial T1-weighted MR image of the bony pelvis

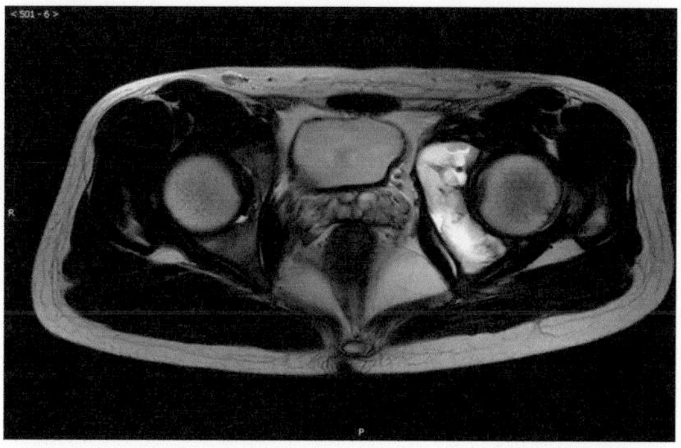

Fig. 36.9 Axial T2-weighted MR image of the bony pelvis

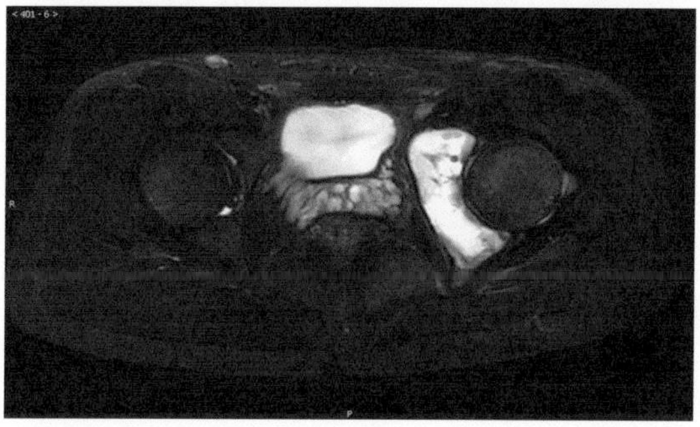

Fig. 36.10 Axial fat-suppressed T2-weighted MR image of the bony pelvis

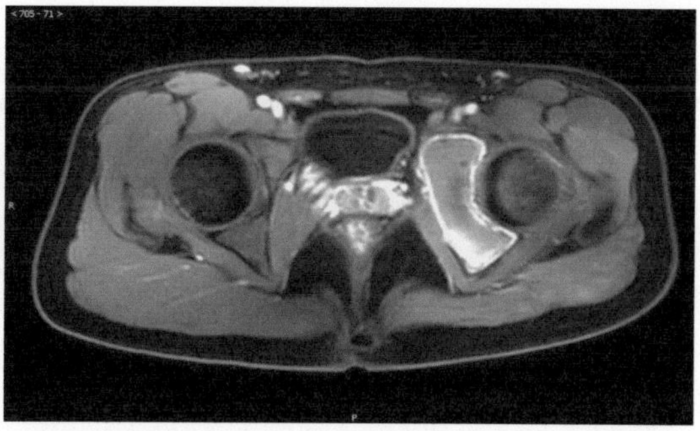

Fig. 36.11 Axial post-contrast fat-suppressed T1-weighted MR image of the bony pelvis

fat-suppressed sequences. Avid enhancement noted along the peripheral and septations with internal large area of non-enhancement.

36.4 Description and Discussion from Residents

The radiograph showed lytic and expansile bone destruction around the left ilium, acetabulum, and pubic bone with clear margin. Mild peripheral sclerosis noted along the lateral, superior and inferior margins of the lesion with cortical destruction internally, and no periosteal reaction or soft tissue mass. CT images showed expansile and lytic bone destruction with focal sclerosis, some septations, and internal inhomogeneous densities with low and iso-density nodules. The soft tissue mass appeared extruding beyond the cortex focally. The iso density nodules showed avid enhancement and low-density areas showed no enhancement. Our diagnosis and differential diagnosis include giant cell tumor of bone (GCT), aneurysmal bone cyst (ABC), and chondrogenic tumors. MR images showed high signal of the lesion on both T1- and T2-weighted sequences with internal punctate low signal and peripheral circular enhancement. The high T1 signal could represent subacute hemorrhage or protein-rich mucus component. Circular low T2 signal noted in the peripheral on T2-weighted images, making hemorrhage more likely of the high T1 signal. Our consideration is GCT, with ABC, chondromyxoid fibroma in the differential diagnosis. Given the lack of obvious calcification, we didn't include other chondrogenic tumor in the consideration.

36.5 Analysis and Comments from Professor Cheng Xiao-Guang

The patient was a male adolescent. The radiograph demonstrated apparent expansile bone destruction of the left acetabulum with peripheral sclerosis laterally and not obvious in the medial aspect. CT images showed the lateral margin of the lesion well with indistinct cortex internally and changes of focal lifting of the periosteum from the expansion. No apparent calcification or ossification noted internally. The overall densities of the lesion were lower than the peripheral muscle and fluid in the urinary bladder, suggesting predominantly fluid content of the lesion with focal solid nodules. The solid components of the lesion showed avid enhancement with no enhancement of the cystic components. Given the expansile appearance of the lesion, my differential diagnosis includes GCT and ABC. However, the patient was an adolescent, and we should be very cautious to give a diagnosis of GCT. MR images showed high T1 signal, suggesting hemorrhage of the cystic components. Walls of the cysts and solid components showed enhancements, most suggestive of ABC. However, there was no typical multicystic appearance of ABC and high density noted of the solid component, and we can't entirely exclude GCT.

36.6 Diagnosis

Chondroblastoma.

Suggested Reading

Kim J, Kumar R, Raymond AK, et al. Non-epiphyseal chondroblastoma arising in the iliac bone, and complicated by an aneurysmal bone cyst: a case report and review of the literature. Skeletal Radiol. 2010;39(6):583–7.

Laitinen MK, Stevenson JD, Evans S, et al. Chondroblastoma in pelvis and extremities- a single centre study of 177 cases. J Bone Oncol. 2019;17:100248.

Weatherall PT, Maale GE, Mendelsohn DB. Chondroblastoma: classic and confusing appearance at MR imaging. Radiology. 1994;190(2):467–74.

Unicystic Ameloblastoma: Case 37 37

37.1 Medical History

Patient is a 57-year-old female. She was found to have a mass along the right jaw for about 1 month.

37.2 Physical Examination

Focal protuberance along the right mandibular angle, palpable, about the size of an egg, with clear margin, smooth and rubbery.

37.3 Imaging Findings

37.3.1 CT Imaging (Figs. 37.1, 37.2, 37.3, 37.4, 37.5, and 37.6)

CT images of the mandible demonstrated expansile bone destruction of the right mandible angle which was well circumscribed with internal relatively homogenous densities. There was disruption of the cortex medially without associated soft tissue mass.

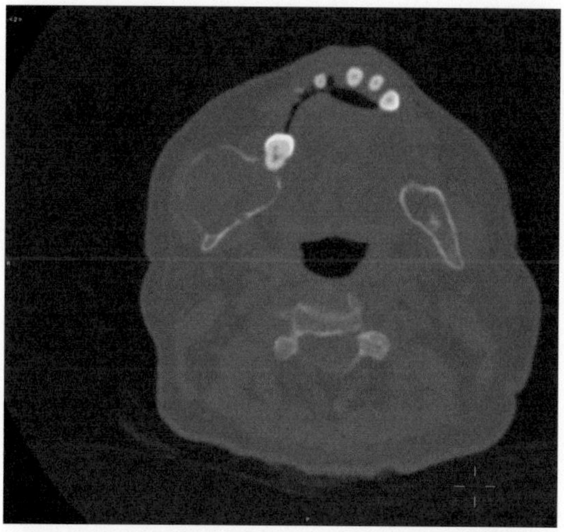

Fig. 37.1 Axial CT image of the mandible in bone window

X. Cheng et al., *Imaging of Bone Tumors in Axial Bones*,
https://doi.org/10.1007/978-981-95-2262-0_37

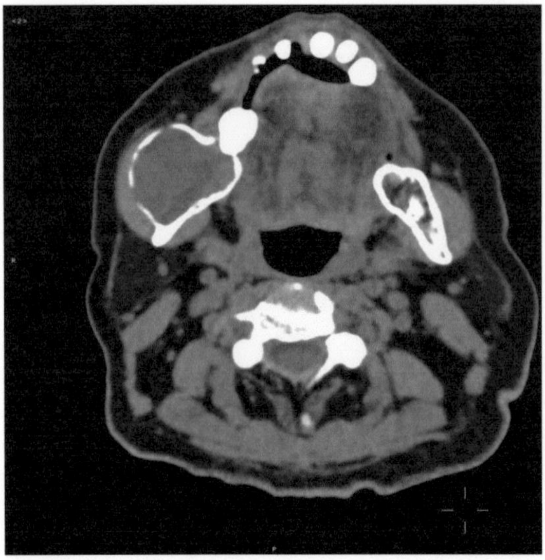

Fig. 37.2 Axial CT image of the mandible in soft tissue window

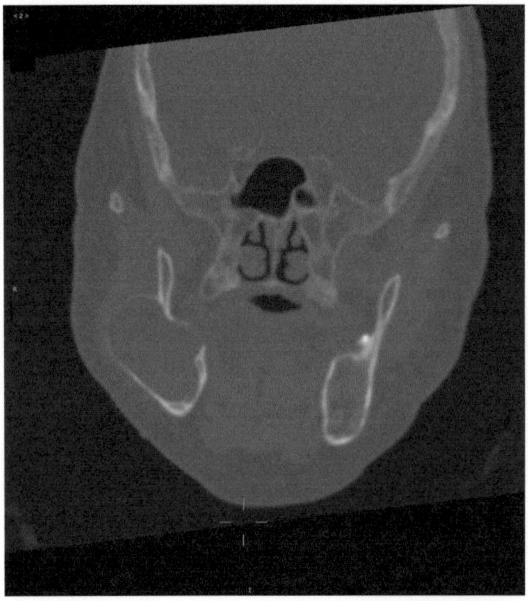

Fig. 37.3 Coronal CT image of the mandible in bone window

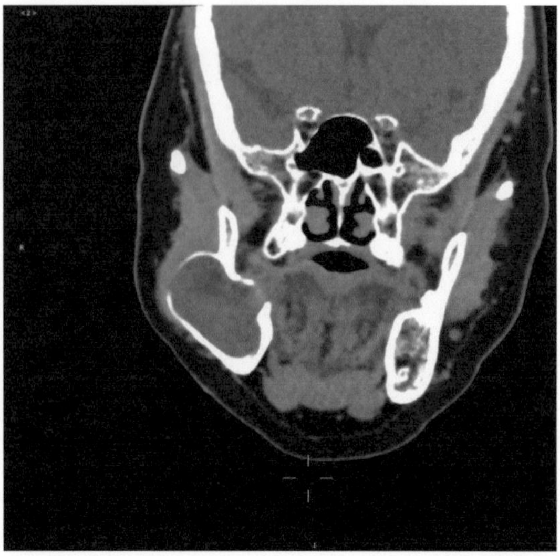

Fig. 37.4 Coronal CT image of the mandible in soft tissue window

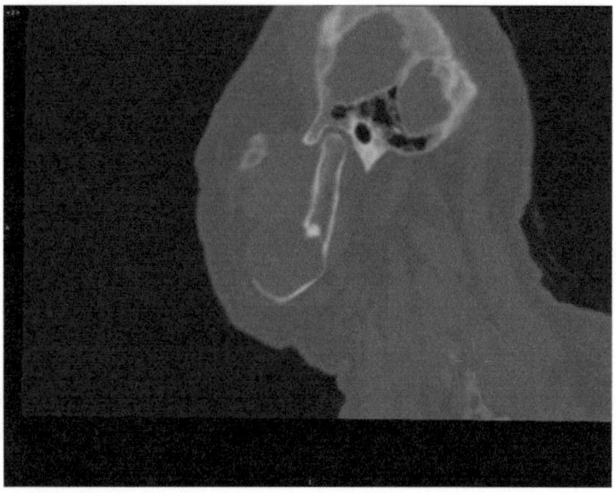

Fig. 37.5 Sagittal CT image of the mandible in bone window

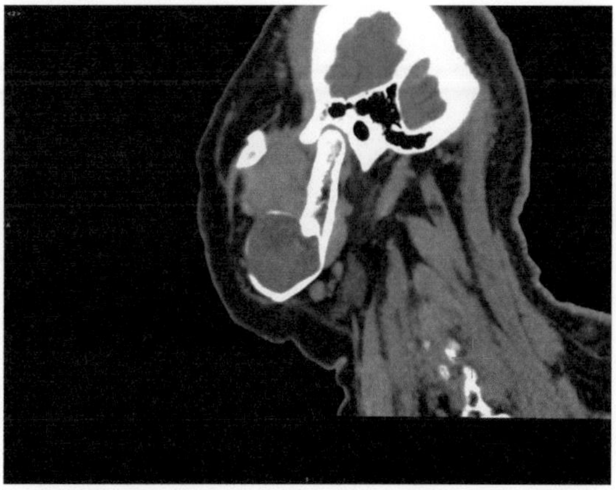

Fig. 37.6 Sagittal CT image of the mandible in soft tissue window

37.4 Description and Discussion from Residents

CT images showed expansile bone destruction of the right mandible around the angle and body with clear margin and no peripheral sclerosis. Thin bone shell noted with focal cortical disruption and no adjacent periosteal reaction or soft tissue mass. The lesion showed homogeneous densities and close relationship to the adjacent teeth with about two third of the teeth located around the lesion. Given the above findings, this is most likely a benign lesion, with our differential diagnosis centered around odontogenic cystic lesions: (1) dentigerous cyst, rarely with cortical defect, the lesion usually circles the entire tooth, not consistent with the current case; (2) radicular cyst, the tooth apex usually points to the cyst, while with the current case, the tooth apex pointed posteriorly; (3) odontogenic keratocyst, the lesion usually extends along the long axis of the mandible. With the current case, the lesion showed lateral expansion; (4) ameloblastoma is an odontogenic epithelial cell tumor. It is benign but can be locally invasive. There was focal cortical break of the current case, consistent with this entity. But there were no soft tissue changes of the current case. If there was enhancement, it would further support this diagnosis.

37.5 Analysis and Comments from Professor Cheng Xiao-Guang

CT images showed cystic expansile bone destruction along the right mandible angle with close relationship to the teeth and clear margin. Overall, my consideration is a benign lesion, likely of odontogenic disease. The preliminary discussion talked about the related differential diagnosis in detail. Additionally, the lesion could be tumor at the mandible and affected tissues surrounding the teeth, however, the first cause more likely. On the sagittal CT images, there were oval low densities along the subcutaneous region in the neck, not clear if that was related to the odontogenic disease.

(Supplement from pathologist: unicystic ameloblastoma is characteristically with close association with the teeth and with high recurrence rate. However, the World Health Organization classified it as benign tumor. Most ameloblastomas are solid neoplasm, not with cystic changes. Unicystic ameloblastoma only surrounding the teeth is rare).

37.6 Diagnosis

Unicystic ameloblastoma.

Suggested Reading

Konouchi H, Asaumi J, Yanagi Y, et al. Usefulness of contrast enhanced-MRI in the diagnosis of unicystic ameloblastoma. Oral Oncol. 2006;42(5):481–6.

Minami M, Kaneda T, Ozawa K, et al. Cystic lesions of the maxillomandibular region: MR imaging distinction of odontogenic keratocysts and ameloblastomas from other cysts. AJR Am J Roentgenol. 1996;166(4):943–9.

Navarro CM, Principi SM, Massucato EMS, et al. Maxillary unicystic ameloblastoma. Dentomaxillofac Radiol. 2004;33(1):60–2.

Neuroblastoma with Bone Metastases: Case 38

38

38.1 Medical History

Patient is an 18-year-old female. She started to experience bone pain at multiple sites without clear causes about 2 months ago, with pain around the right ribs and right iliac most severe. She was seen at the local hospital and found to have multiple bone abnormalities and received right rib biopsy.

38.2 Physical Examination

Mass around the right 8th rib, with point tenderness. Pain around the right posterior superior iliac spine.

38.3 Imaging Findings

38.3.1 Radiograph (Figs. 38.1 and 38.2)

Radiograph of the chest showed expansile bone destruction of the right 8th rib. And pelvis radiograph showed multiple areas of decreased densities in the bones.

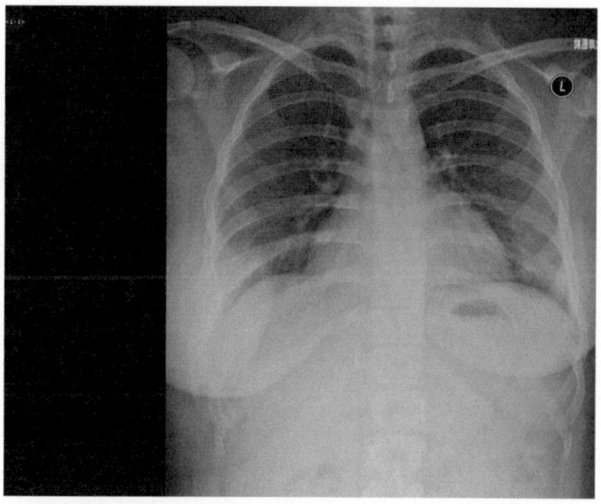

Fig. 38.1 Frontal view of the chest

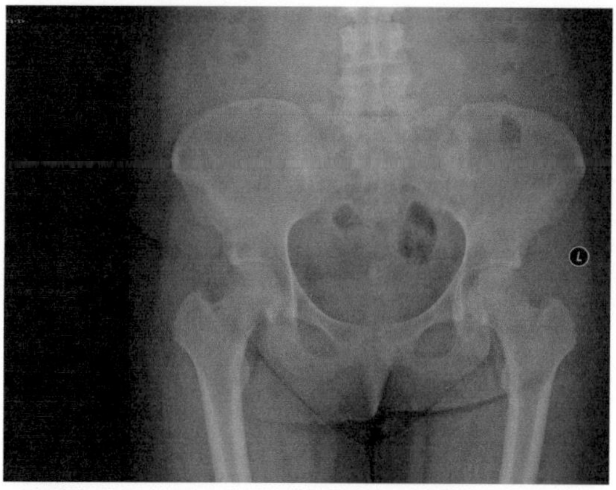

Fig. 38.2 Frontal view of the bony pelvis

X. Cheng et al., *Imaging of Bone Tumors in Axial Bones*,
https://doi.org/10.1007/978-981-95-2262-0_38

38.3.2 CT Imaging (Figs. 38.3, 38.4, 38.5, 38.6, 38.7, 38.8, 38.9, 38.10, 38.11, 38.12, and 38.13)

There was bone destruction of the right 8th rib with dense, spiculated periosteal reaction and surrounding soft tissue mass. No strong enhancement inside of the mass. There were multiple mixed bone destruction involving thoracic, lumbar spine, and sternum. Extra dura soft tissue mass in the spinal canal noted at T5–6 level.

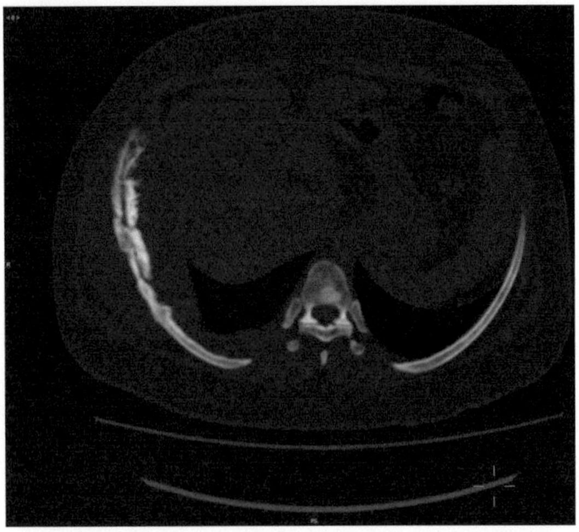

Fig. 38.3 Axial CT image of the ribs in bone window

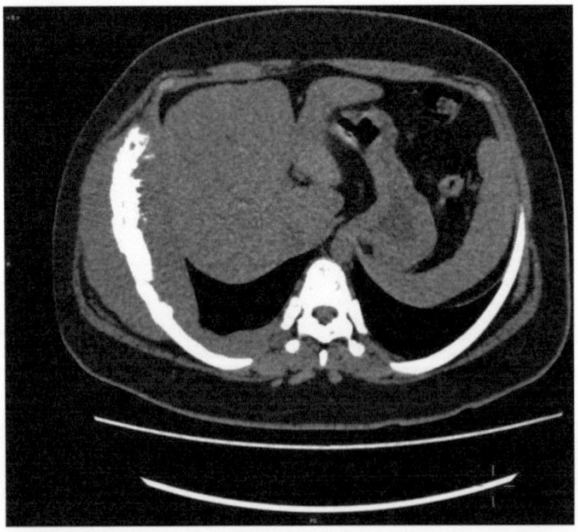

Fig. 38.4 Axial CT image of the ribs in soft tissue window

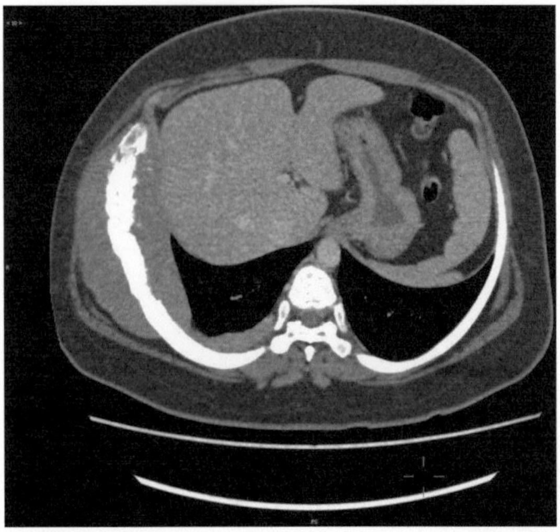

Fig. 38.5 Axial post-contrast CT image of the ribs in soft tissue window

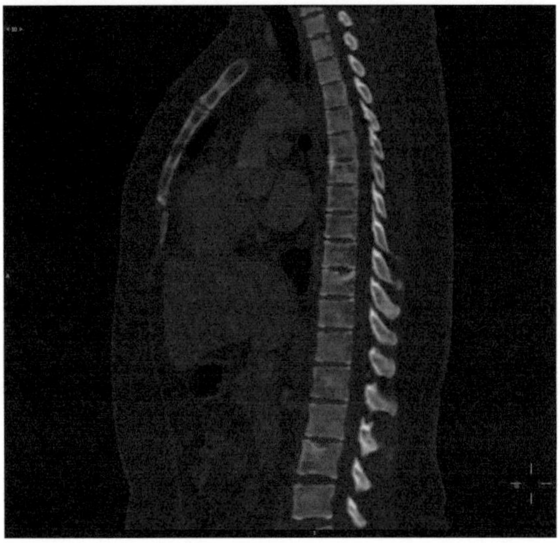

Fig. 38.6 Sagittal CT image of the thoracic spine in bone window

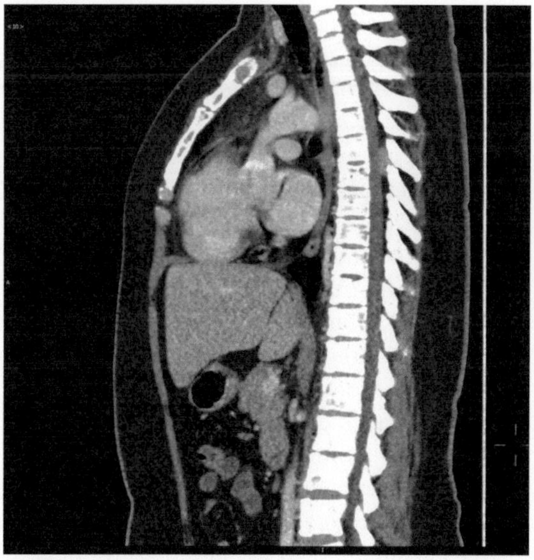

Fig. 38.7 Sagittal post-contrast CT image of the thoracic spine in soft tissue window

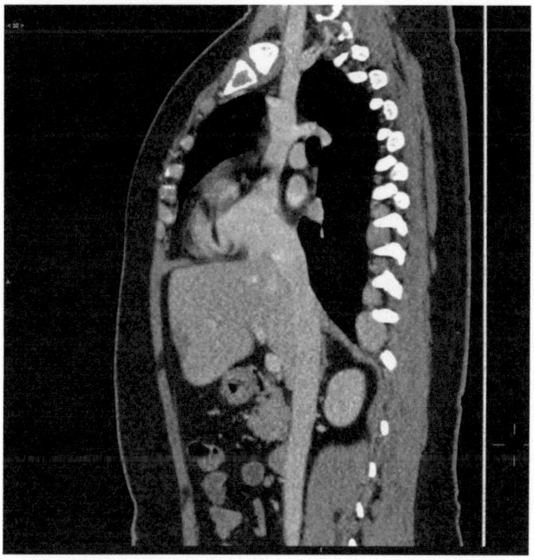

Fig. 38.8 Sagittal post-contrast CT image of the thoracic spine in soft tissue window (around the intercostal spaces)

There were multiple soft tissue masses along the intercostal spaces with avid enhancement. There were multiple areas of bone destruction in the bony pelvis, predominant lytic with heterogeneous density, with avid enhancement and ill-defined margin, without apparent periosteal reaction.

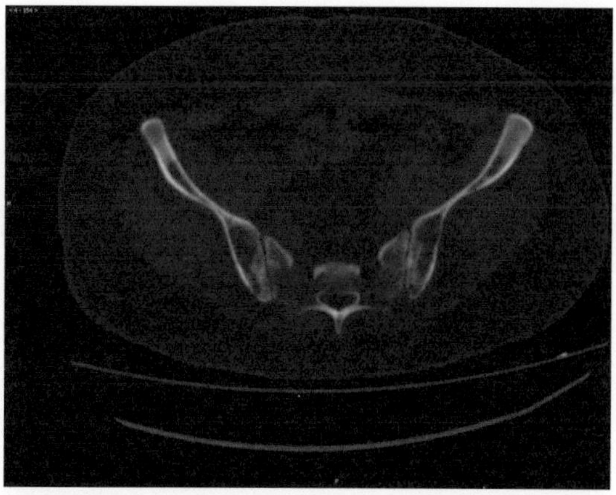

Fig. 38.9 Axial CT image of the bony pelvis in bone window

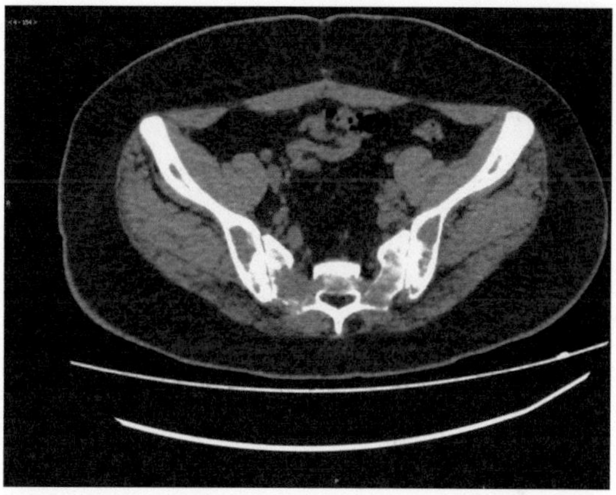

Fig. 38.10 Axial CT image of the bony pelvis in soft tissue window

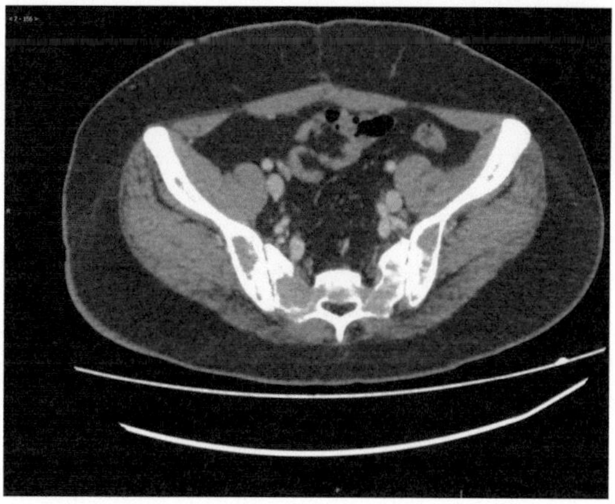

Fig. 38.11 Axial post-contrast CT image of the bony pelvis in soft tissue window

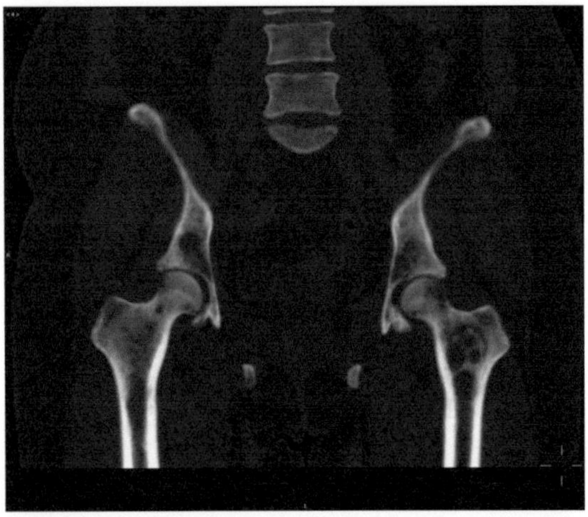

Fig. 38.12 Coronal CT image of the pelvis in bone window

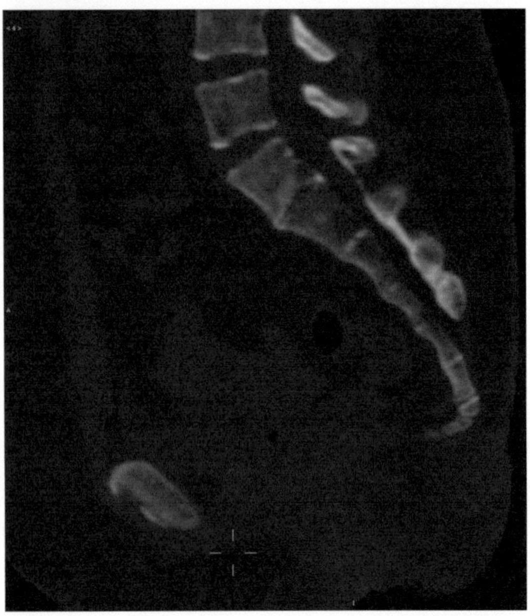

Fig. 38.13 Sagittal CT image of the pelvis in bone window

38.4 Description and Discussion from Residents

Chest radiograph demonstrated expansile changes of the right eighth rib with internal heterogeneous density and peripheral high density. Pelvis radiograph showed multiple bone destruction involving the bilateral ilia and bilateral proximal femurs. Given radiographs show multiple bone destruction, possibility of metastatic disease raised. No mass or nodule noted in the lungs on the chest CT scan. There were multiple bone destruction involving bilateral proximal humeri, clavicles, sternum, and thoracic spine vertebral bodies. There was spiculated periosteal reaction with bone destruction of right eighth rib with adjacent soft tissue mass and no apparent enhancement. Bony pelvis CT scan showed multiple bone destruction involving ilia, proximal femurs, and sacrum. There was no peripheral sclerosis along the bone destruction with avid enhancement. Multiple moth-eaten and permeated bone destruction with focal periosteal reaction and soft tissue mass, most suggestive of malignant tumor, such as multiple myeloma or other hematological malignancies. Additionally, metabolic bone disease needs to be excluded.

38.5 Analysis and Comments from Professor Cheng Xiao-Guang

The patient was a young female. Chest radiograph demonstrated expansile changes of the right eighth rib, and pelvis radiograph showed multiple bone destruction. Chest CT scan showed large bone destruction of right eighth rib with focal high density and soft tissue mass. Moderate enhancement of the soft tissue mass. Sagittal images showed multiple soft tissue masses along the spinal canal and along multiple intercostal spaces. CT scan of the bony pelvis also showed multiple bone destruction. Multiple areas of bone destruction in a young female patient, most concerning for systemic disease, such as the hematological malignancies mentioned above. However, multiple myeloma usually occurs in older patients, and the soft tissue mass of current case is big, not typical of multiple myeloma. The manifestations are more consistent with metastatic disease. The lesions along the ribs could be the primary lesions with metastatic involvement to the other sites. The diagnosis should be combined with pathology results. Please note, with multiple sites of bone destruction, hyperparathyroidism should be considered. However, there are multiple signs not consistent with that of the current case.

(From Professor Li-Hua Gong of pathology: Neuroblastoma is a primitive and undifferentiated tumor, very similar to Ewing sarcoma in properties and biological behavior, frequently accompanied with Schwannoma or malignant peripheral nerve sheath tumor. Monism could be used to explain all the pathologies.)

38.6 Diagnosis

Neuroblastoma with bone metastases.

Suggested Reading

Ishiguchi H, Ito S, Kato K, et al. Diagnostic performance of 18F-FDG PET/CT and whole-body diffusion-weighted imaging with background body suppression (DWIBS) in detection of lymph node and bone metastases from pediatric neuroblastoma. Ann Nucl Med. 2018;32(5):348–62.

Meyer JS, Siegel MJ, Farooqui SO, et al. Which MRI sequence of the spine best reveals bone-marrow metastases of neuroblastoma? Pediatr Radiol. 2005;35(8):778–85.

Undifferentiated Pleomorphic Sarcoma of Bone: Case 39

39

39.1 Medical History

Patient is a 55-year-old male. He started to experience persistent mild pain along the chest, waist, and hips without clear reason. There was no radiation and no fever. It cannot be alleviated by rest. The symptoms worsened in the last 2 months with multiple lesions in the vertebral bodies and pelvis.

39.2 Physical Examination

Not done.

39.3 Imaging Findings

39.3.1 CT Imaging (Figs. 39.1, 39.2, 39.3, 39.4, 39.5, 39.6, 39.7, 39.8, and 39.9)

There are multiple bone destruction of the thoracic, lumbar spine and bony pelvis with internal heterogeneous density with destruction of the cortex and no periosteal reaction. Mild soft tissue masses noted along the right iliac lesion and multiple vertebral bodies lesions. Heterogeneous enhancement noted with focal avid enhancement. Pathological fractures noted along T9, T12, and L3 vertebral bodies.

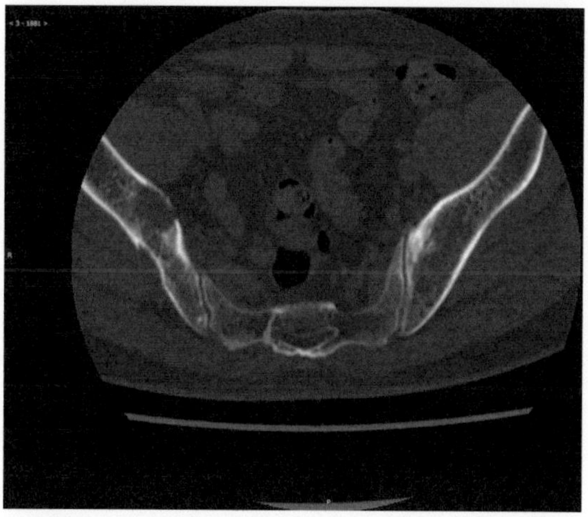

Fig. 39.1 Axial CT image of the bony pelvis in bone window

X. Cheng et al., *Imaging of Bone Tumors in Axial Bones*,
https://doi.org/10.1007/978-981-95-2262-0_39

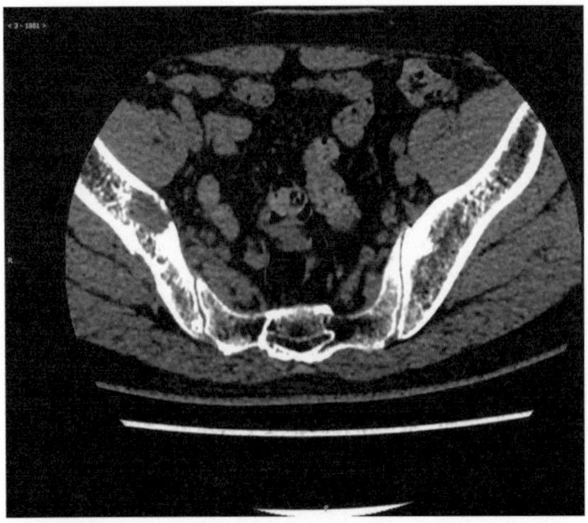

Fig. 39.2 Axial CT image of the bony pelvis in soft tissue window

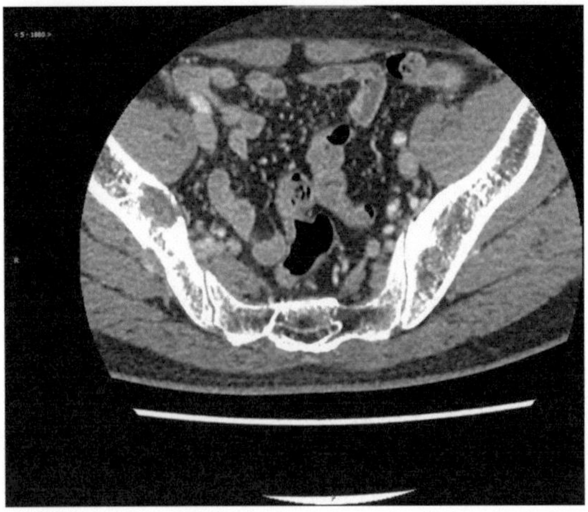

Fig. 39.3 Axial post-contrast CT image of the bony pelvis in soft tissue window

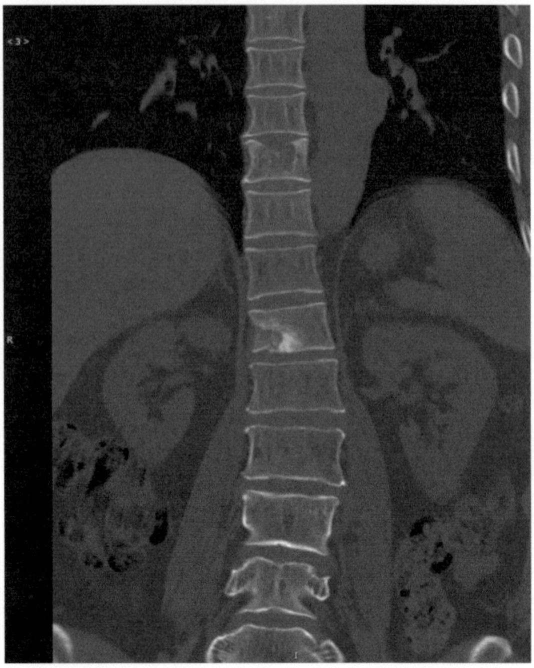

Fig. 39.4 Coronal CT image of the thoracolumbar spine in bone window

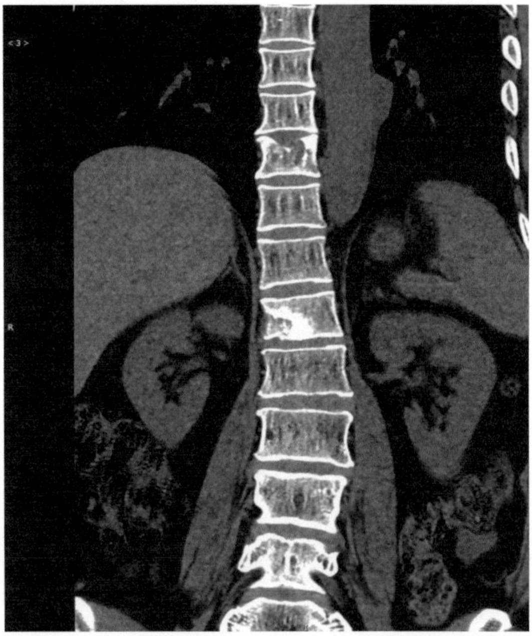

Fig. 39.5 Coronal CT image of the thoracolumbar spine in soft tissue window

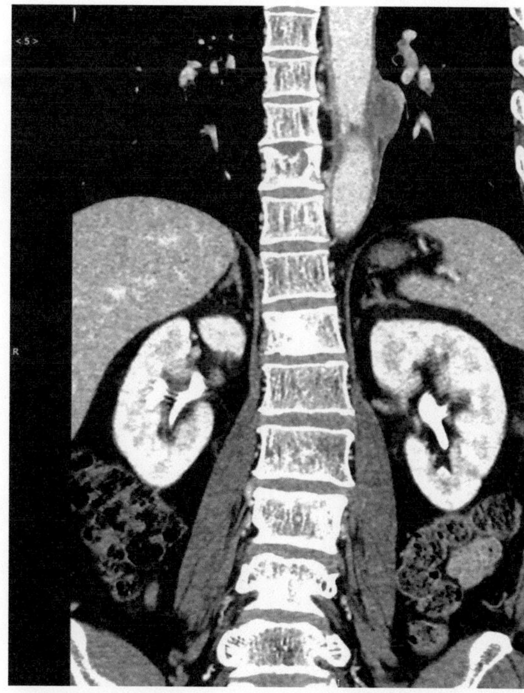

Fig. 39.6 Coronal post-contrast CT image of the thoracolumbar spine in soft tissue window

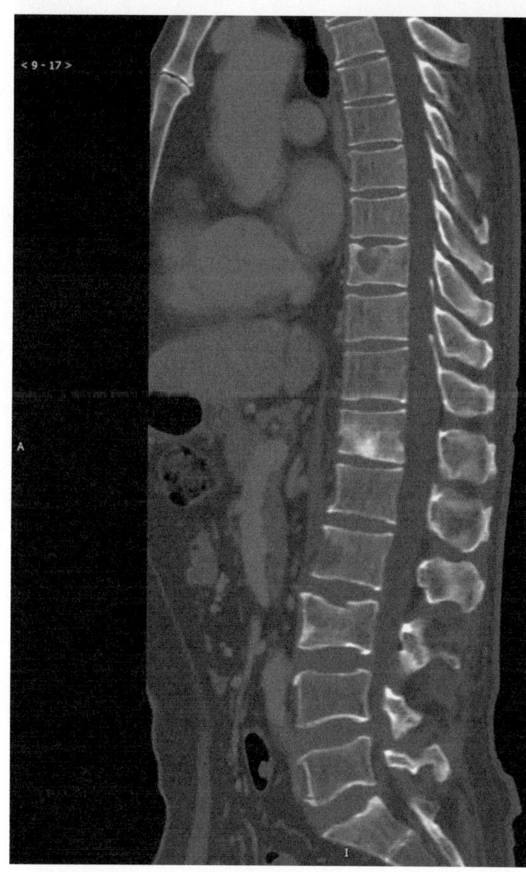

Fig. 39.7 Sagittal CT image of the thoracolumbar spine in bone window

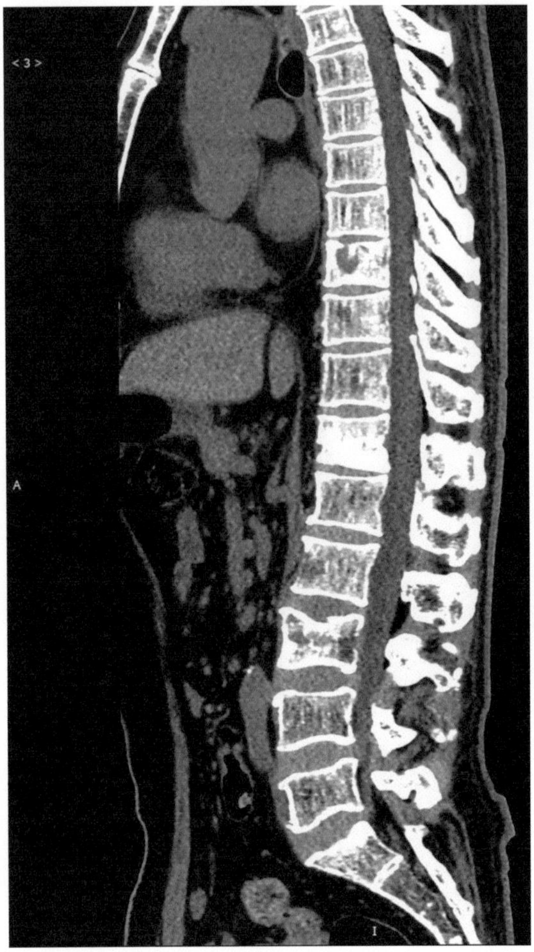

Fig. 39.8 Sagittal CT image of the thoracolumbar spine in soft tissue window

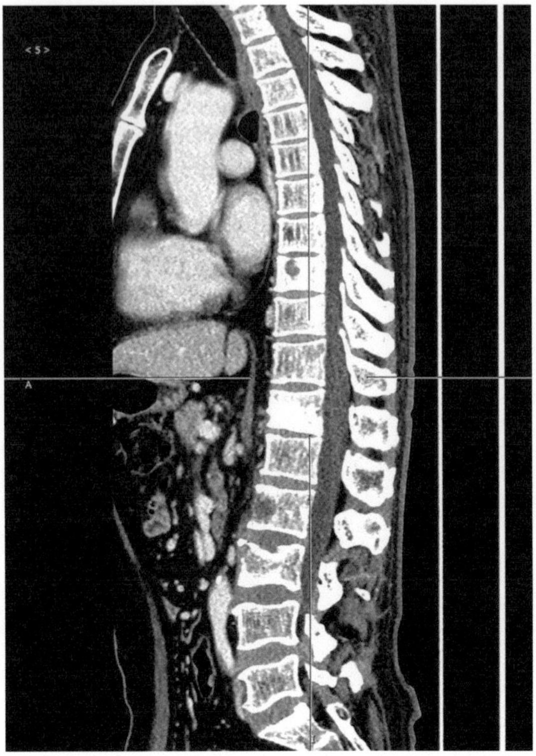

Fig. 39.9 Sagittal post-contrast CT image of the thoracolumbar spine in soft tissue window

39.4 Description and Discussion from Residents

CT images showed multiple bone destruction of the cervical, thoracic, lumbar spine and right ilium. Soft tissue attenuation slightly protruded beyond the cortical bone with clear margin. Mild peripheral sclerosis noted of some lesions. Mild enhancement noted. The lesions did not involve the posterior elements and intervertebral spaces. Given multiple lesions, differential diagnosis includes (1) malignant tumor, such as metastatic disease, multiple myeloma, hematological malignancies; (2) metabolic bone disease, such as hyperparathyroidism; and (3) benign tumor, such as eosinophilic granuloma. The patient was an older male. Osteoporosis noted in the background, the imaging findings most consistent with malignant tumor, so our top consideration is multiple myeloma. Given peripheral sclerosis along some lesions and no involvement of the posterior elements, not typical of metastatic disease, thus only included in the differential diagnosis.

39.5 Analysis and Comments from Professor Cheng Xiao-Guang

CT images showed multiple bone destruction along the spine and bony pelvis with ill-defined margin and focal peripheral sclerosis and no clear soft tissue mass. Mild enhancement noted. Compression fracture and focal increased bone densities noted on the sagittal CT images in the spine. First, hyperparathyroidism needs to be excluded. The patient was an older male; we should first consider malignant tumor, such as metastatic disease, multiple myeloma, and lymphoma. The current case does not demonstrate any characteristic imaging features.

39.6 Diagnosis

Undifferentiated pleomorphic sarcoma of bone.

Suggested Reading

Bloem JL, Reidsma II. Bone and soft tissue tumors of hip and pelvis. Eur J Radiol. 2012;81(12):3793–801.

Koplas MC, Lefkowitz RA, Bauer TW, et al. Imaging findings, prevalence and outcome of de novo and secondary malignant fibrous histiocytoma of bone. Skeletal Radiol. 2010;39(8):791–8.

Multiple Myeloma: Case 40

40

40.1 Medical History

Patient is a 53-year-old female. She started to experience low back pain after exertion about 11 months ago with soreness and discomfort and relieved by rest. About 3 months ago, pain started to radiate to the left leg without clear inciting event with self-reported improvement after massage. About 1 month ago, she started to experience low back pain and radiating to the left leg with left ribs pain without clear causes and no change after rest, with night sweats. She was seen at local hospital and diagnosed as protrusion of lumbar spine disc with no improvement after treatment.

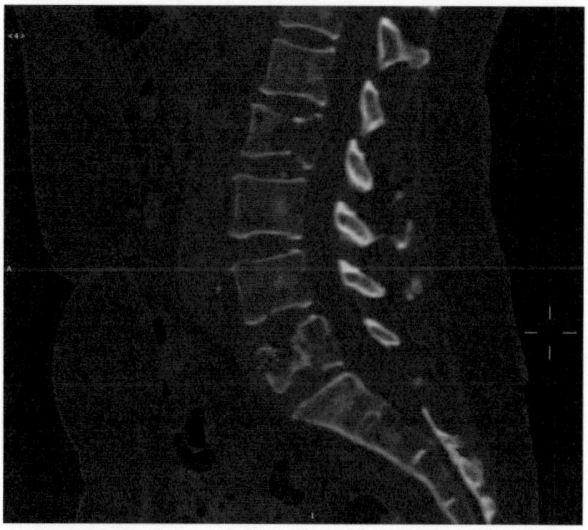

Fig. 40.1 Sagittal CT image of the lumbar spine in bone window

40.2 Physical Examination

Not done.

40.3 Imaging Findings

40.3.1 CT Imaging (Figs. 40.1, 40.2, 40.3, 40.4, 40.5, and 40.6)

There were multiple bone destruction of the thoracic, lumbar spine and bony pelvis without periosteal reaction. Some lesions showed disruption of the cortex with soft tissue mass. Avid enhancement noted within all of the lesions.

40.3.2 MR Imaging (Figs. 40.7, 40.8, 40.9, 40.10, 40.11, 40.12, 40.13, 40.14, and 40.15)

MR images demonstrated diffuse heterogeneous low T1 signal in the cervical, thoracic and lumbar spine. There were multiple areas of lytic bone destruction with low T1 and T2 signals, without internal necrosis. Pathological fractures noted of L2 and L5 vertebral bodies.

X. Cheng et al., *Imaging of Bone Tumors in Axial Bones*,
https://doi.org/10.1007/978-981-95-2262-0_40

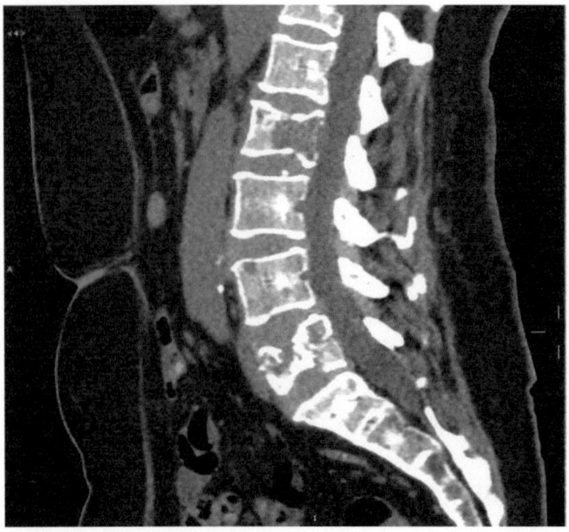

Fig. 40.2 Sagittal CT image of the lumbar spine in soft tissue window

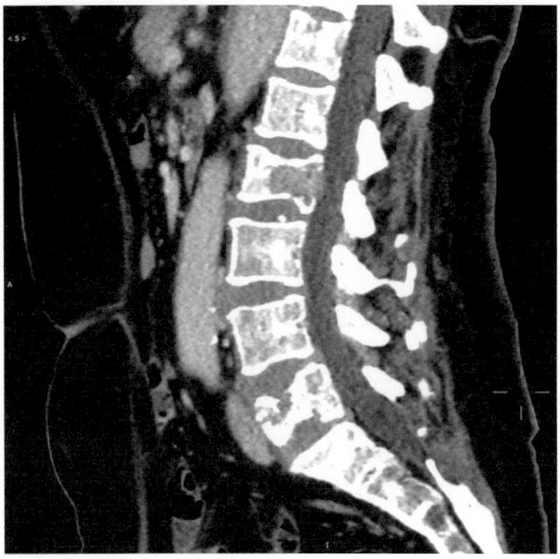

Fig. 40.3 Sagittal post-contrast CT image of the lumbar spine in soft tissue window

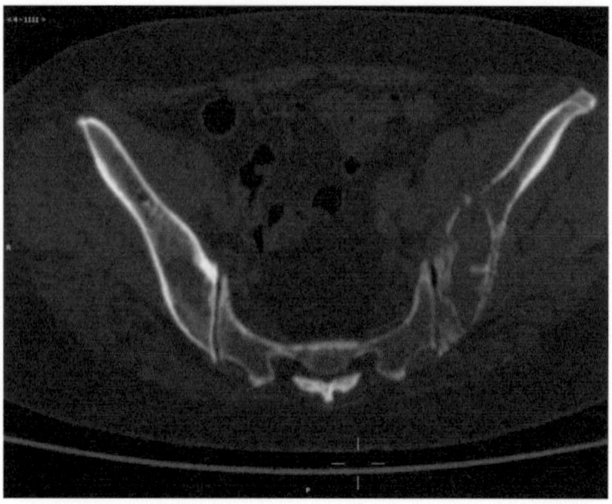

Fig. 40.4 Axial CT image of the bony pelvis in bone window

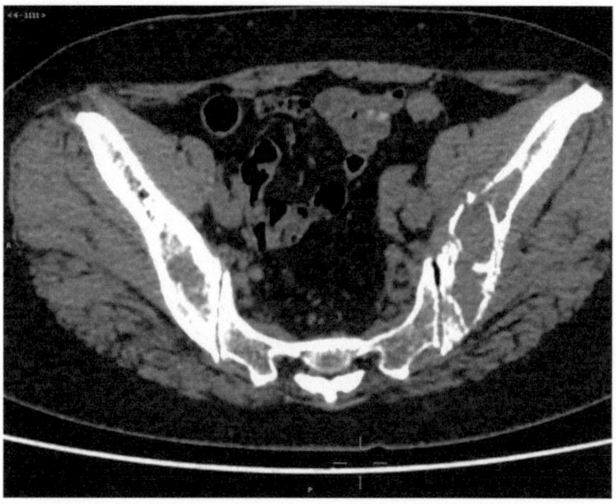

Fig. 40.5 Axial CT image of the bony pelvis in soft tissue window

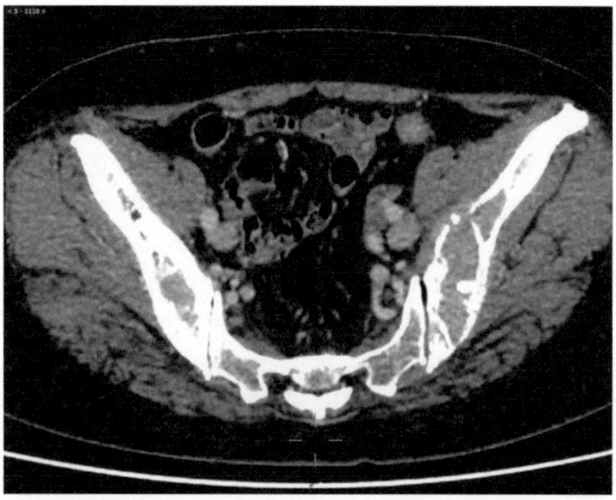

Fig. 40.6 Axial postcontrast CT image of the bony pelvis in soft tissue window

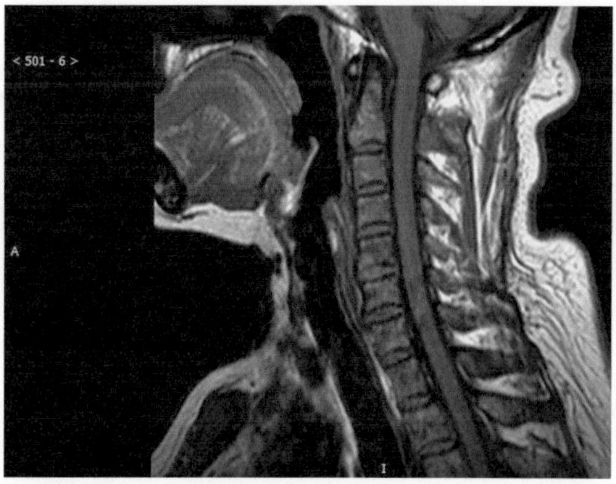

Fig. 40.7 Sagittal T1-weighted MR image of the cervical spine

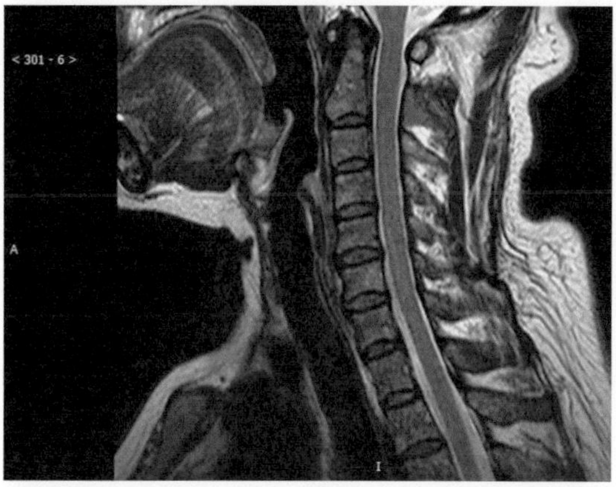

Fig. 40.8 Sagittal T2-weighted MR image of the cervical spine

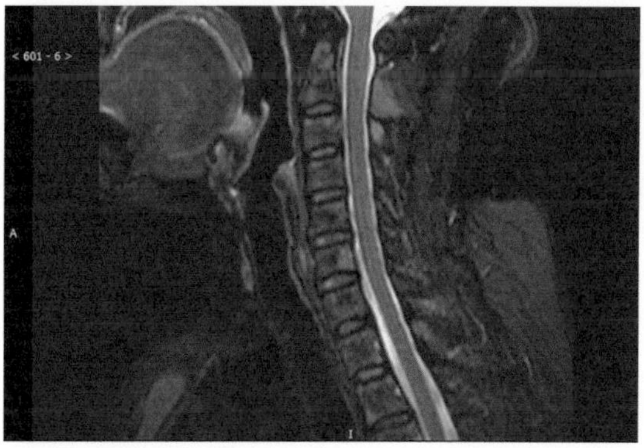

Fig. 40.9 Sagittal fat-suppressed T2-weighted MR image of the cervical spine

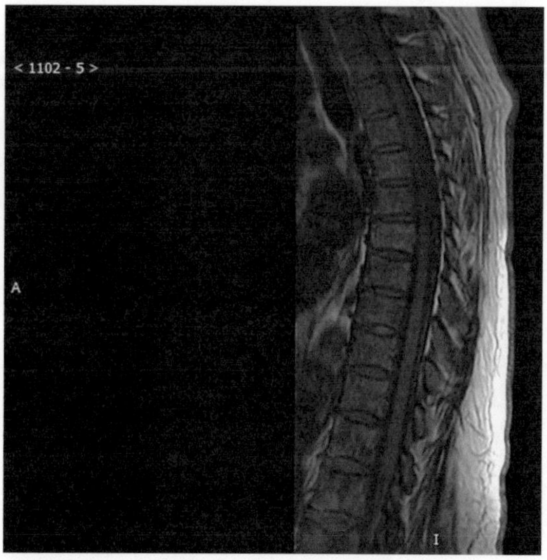

Fig. 40.10 Sagittal T1-weighted MR image of the thoracic spine

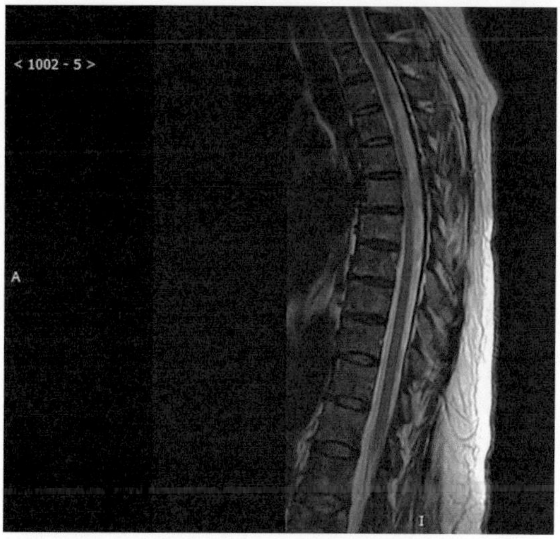

Fig. 40.11 Sagittal T2-weighted MR image of the thoracic spine

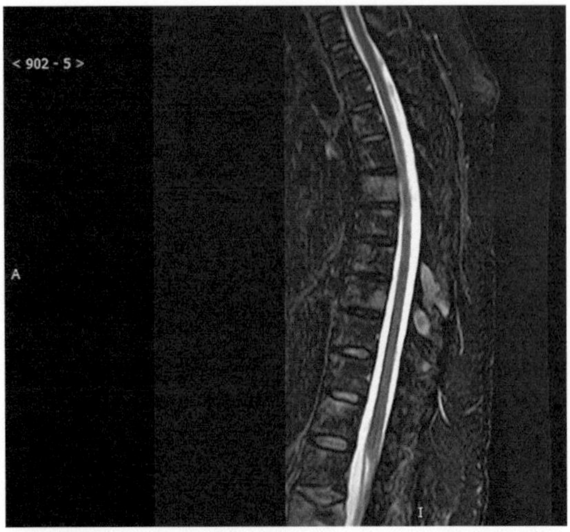

Fig. 40.12 Sagittal fat-suppressed T2-weighted MR image of the thoracic spine

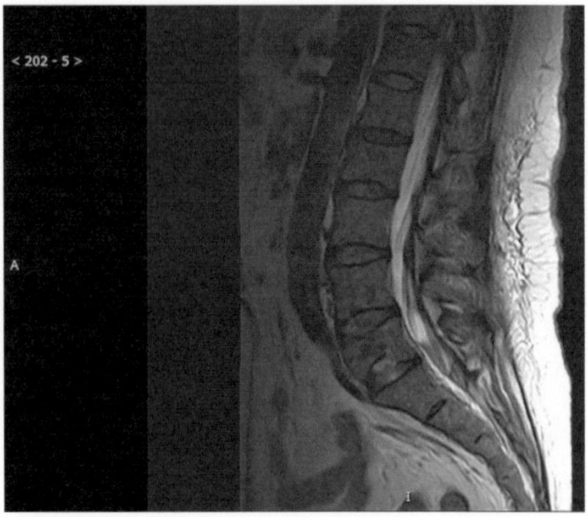

Fig. 40.14 Sagittal T2-weighted MR image of the lumbar spine

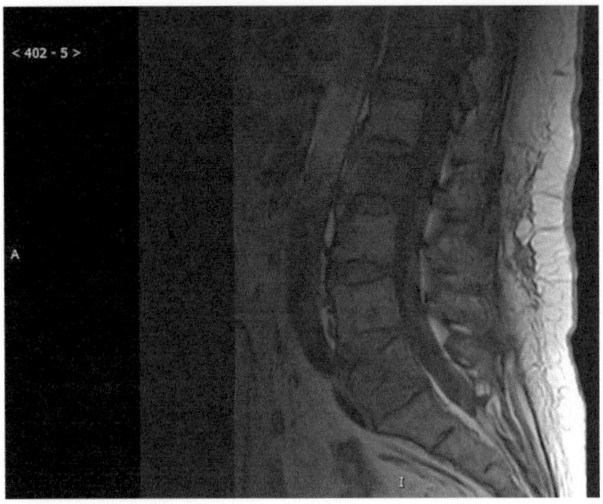

Fig. 40.13 Sagittal T1-weighted MR image of the lumbar spine

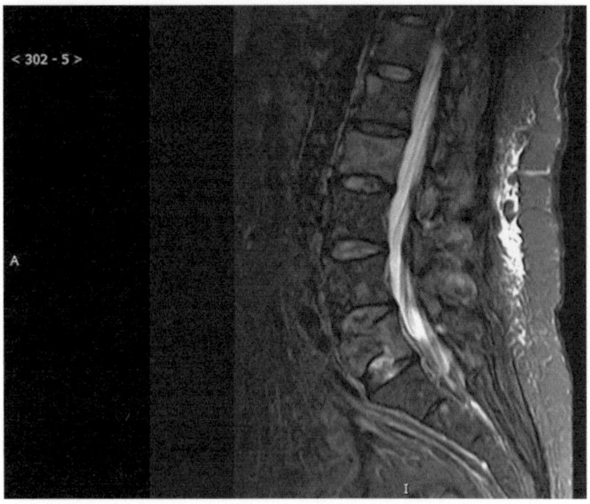

Fig. 40.15 Sagittal fat-suppressed T2-weighted MR image of the lumbar spine

40.4 Description and Discussion from Residents

CT images of the lumbar spine and bony pelvis showed multiple bone destruction involving multiple lumbar vertebral bodies, bilateral ilia, left acetabulum, and right ischium. The lesions were intramedullary with clear margin and no peripheral sclerosis with focal cortex disruption and moderate homogenous enhancement. Given patient's age, our top consideration is multiple myeloma. MR images showed L2 and L5 compression fractures with focal high T2 signal on the fat-suppressed sequences along the lumbar vertebral bodies and posterior elements, consistent with changes in multiple myeloma. Please be aware that multiple myeloma can manifest as only diffuse low T1 and T2 signal in the vertebral bodies on MR images with no clear destruction on CT images and not to miss the diagnosis.

40.5 Analysis and Comments from Professor Cheng Xiao-Guang

The patient was a middle-aged female. CT images showed multiple bone destruction, most prominent of L2 and bilateral ilia with some residual trabeculae. The lesions were relatively confined in the bones with focal cortical disruption with mild soft tissue masses protruding outside and moderate enhancement. Overall, top consideration is multiple myeloma. MR images have advantage of displaying the extent of the lesion but commonly not helpful for differentiating malignant from benign processes. There were low T1 signals of multiple vertebral bodies with relative preservation of the vertebral body morphology. Avid edema noted of L2 and L5 vertebral bodies on fat-suppressed T2-weighted images, suggesting pathological fractures. There were small rice-like high signals inside of the vertebral bodies and posterior elements, consistent with multiple myeloma, with metastatic disease in the differential diagnosis. Some myeloma cases only demonstrate as osteoporosis on X-ray and CT images without clear bone destruction. However, there is "salt and pepper" sign on MR images, as diffuse low T1 and high T2 signals on fat-suppressed sequences within the vertebral bodies.

40.6 Diagnosis

Multiple myeloma.

Suggested Reading

Huh YJ, Lee SY, Kim S, et al. Differentiation of multiple myelomas from osteolytic bone metastases: diagnostic value of tumor homogeneity on contrast-enhanced CT. Br J Radiol. 2022;95(1137):20220009.

Stanborough RO, Garner HW. Multiple myeloma: a review of atypical imaging features and other distinct plasma cell disorders that demonstrate similar imaging features. Skeletal Radiol. 2022;51(1):135–44.

Wu F, Bernard S, Fayad LM, et al. Updates and ongoing challenges in imaging of multiple myeloma: AJR expert panel narrative review. AJR Am J Roentgenol. 2021;217(4):775–85.

Chronic Lymphocytic Leukemia: Case 41

41

41.1 Medical History

Patient is a 73-year-old female. She started to experience persistent mild pain along the posterior chest without clear causes about 3 months ago and without relief by rest. The pain worsened in the last 2 weeks and examinations showed multiple lesions along T8–10 vertebral bodies.

41.2 Physical Examination

Not recorded in hospital system.

41.3 Imaging Findings

41.3.1 CT Imaging (Figs. 41.1, 41.2, 41.3, 41.4, 41.5, and 41.6)

There were suspicious increased densities at T8–10 posterior elements and decreased bone density of the T9 right transverse process with large surrounding soft tissue mass and narrowing the canal, invading T9–10 intervertebral foramen bilaterally. Avid enhancement of the soft tissue mass noted.

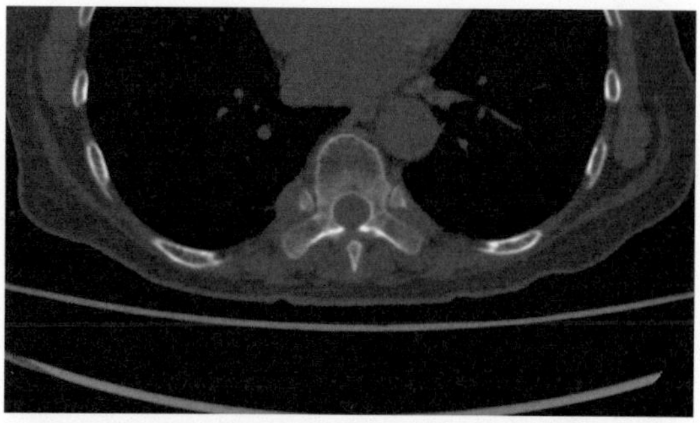

Fig. 41.1 Axial CT image of the thoracic spine in bone window

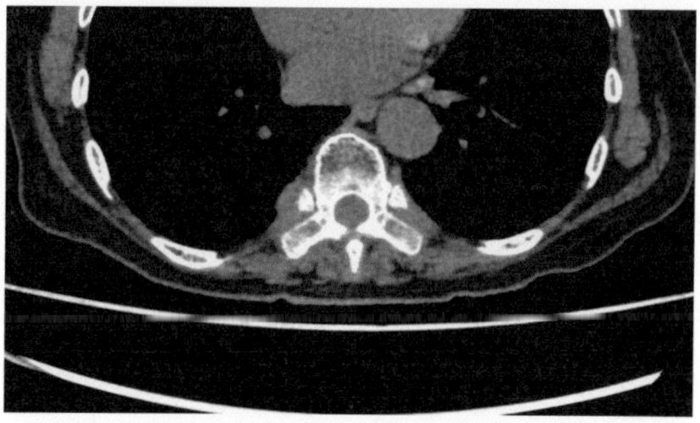

Fig. 41.2 Axial CT image of the thoracic spine in soft tissue window

X. Cheng et al., *Imaging of Bone Tumors in Axial Bones*,
https://doi.org/10.1007/978-981-95-2262-0_41

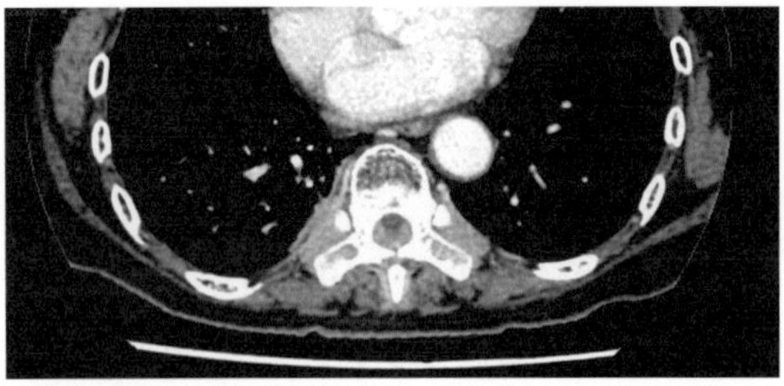

Fig. 41.3 Axial post-contrast CT image of the thoracic spine in soft tissue window

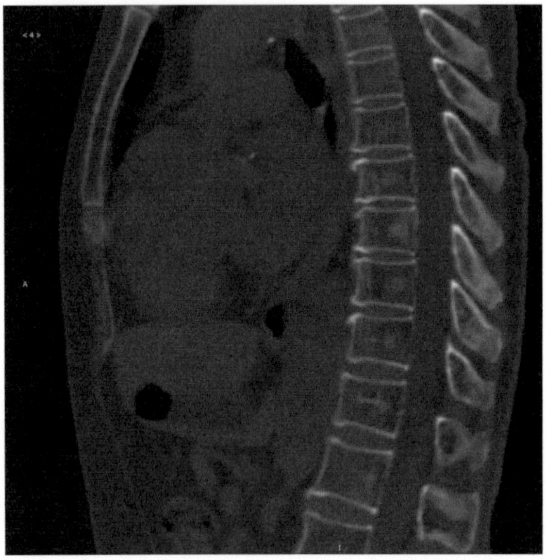

Fig. 41.4 Sagittal CT image of the thoracic spine in bone window

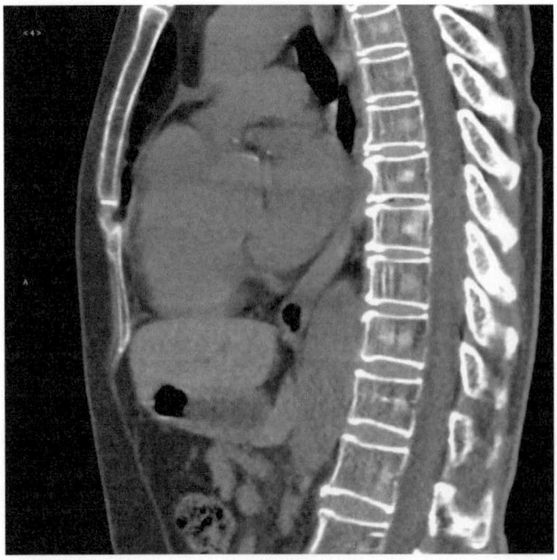

Fig. 41.5 Sagittal CT image of the thoracic spine in soft tissue window

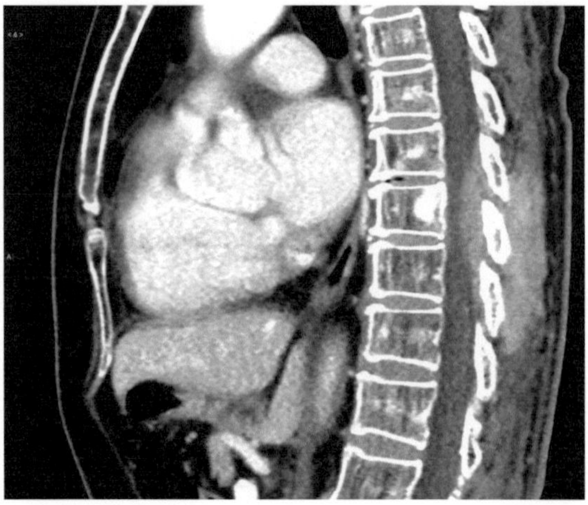

Fig. 41.6 Sagittal post-contrast CT image of the thoracic spine in soft tissue window

41.4 Description and Discussion from Residents

Patient was an older female. CT images showed suspected melting ice like bone destruction of T8–10 vertebral bodies with increased density of the posterior elements and surrounding soft tissue mass with avid enhancement. Our top consideration is small blue cell tumor, such as lymphoma.

41.5 Analysis and Comments from Professor Cheng Xiao-Guang

The patient was an older female. CT images showed bone destruction of the right T9 transverse process. No apparent bone destruction of the thoracic vertebral bodies or spinous processes noted; however, large soft tissue mass surrounded T8–10 spinous processes with avid enhancement. The soft tissue mass surrounding the spinous processes without apparent bone destruction (MRI is better at displaying bone involvement); given patient's age, top consideration is malignant tumor, such as metastatic disease, lymphoma, and primitive neuroectodermal tumor (PNET) (note: this term is no longer recommended for use; in WHO soft tissue and bone tumours classification, 5th edition, it is listed in section of

Ewing sarcoma, page 323), malignant fibrous histiocytoma (now called undifferentiated pleomorphic sarcoma).

41.6 Diagnosis

Chronic lymphocytic leukemia/small lymphocytic lymphoma.

Suggested Reading

Hanrahan CJ, Shah LM. MRI of spinal bone marrow: part 2, T1-weighted imaging-based differential diagnosis. AJR Am J Roentgenol. 2011;197(6):1309–21.

Mayerhoefer ME, Archibald SJ, Messiou C, et al. MRI and PET/MRI in hematologic malignancies. J Magn Reson Imaging. 2020;51(5):1325–35.

Navarro SM, Matcuk GR, Patel DB, et al. Musculoskeletal imaging findings of hematologic malignancies. Radiographics. 2017;37(3):881–900.

Metastatic Osteosarcoma: Case 42

42

42.1 Medical History

Patient is a 42-year-old male. He underwent resection surgery of low-grade central osteosarcoma of the left distal femur 28 months ago. Based on pathology, he did not receive chemotherapy with regular checkup. PET-CT suggested multiple bone lesions with soft tissue mass at the posterior back with surgical resection of the posterior soft tissue mass at the back.

42.2 Physical Examination

Postsurgical scar at the back.

42.3 Imaging Findings

42.3.1 CT Imaging (Figs. 42.1, 42.2, 42.3, 42.4, 42.5, 42.6, 42.7, and 42.8)

Lytic bone destruction of L3 vertebral body with pathological fracture and poorly defined margin and no peripheral sclerosis and focal cortical breakthrough and soft tissue mass. There was heterogeneous enhancement with focal avid enhancement. Space-occupying lesion of left renal inferior pole noted.

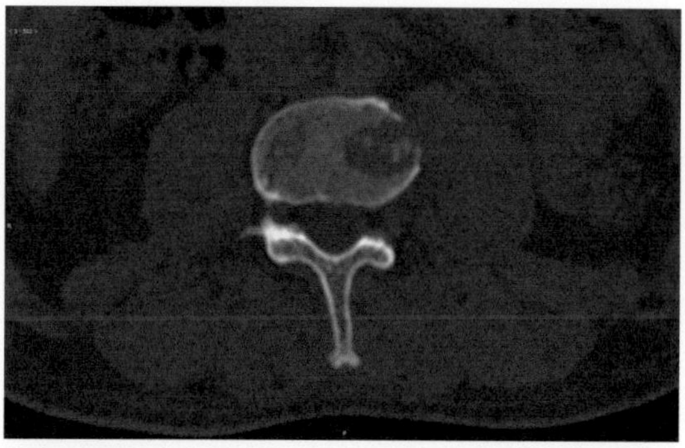

Fig. 42.1 Axial CT image of the lumbar spine in bone window (L3 level)

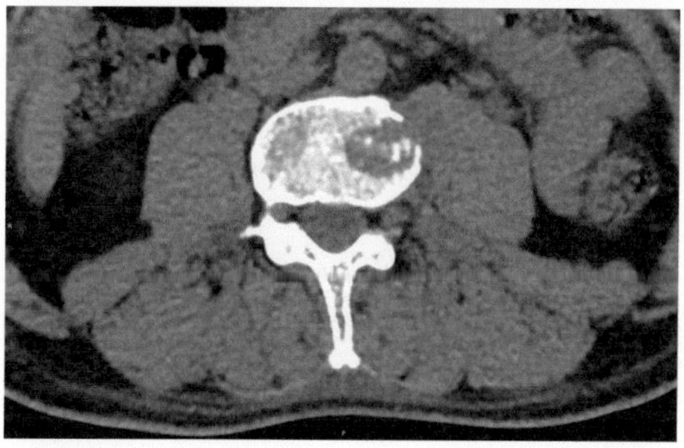

Fig. 42.2 Axial CT image of the lumbar spine in soft tissue window (L3 level)

X. Cheng et al., *Imaging of Bone Tumors in Axial Bones*,
https://doi.org/10.1007/978-981-95-2262-0_42

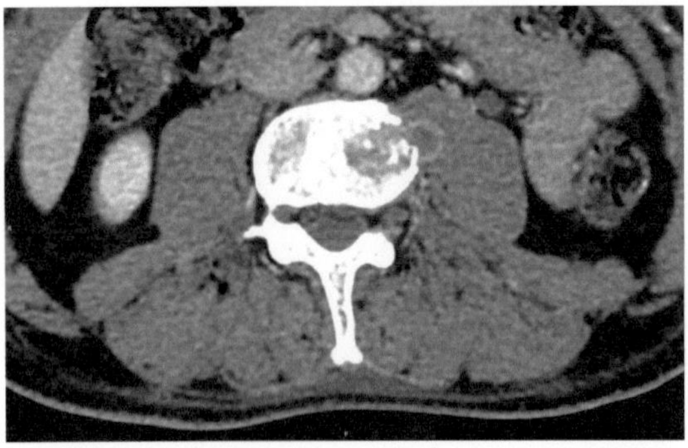

Fig. 42.3 Axial post-contrast CT image of the lumbar spine in soft tissue window (L3 level)

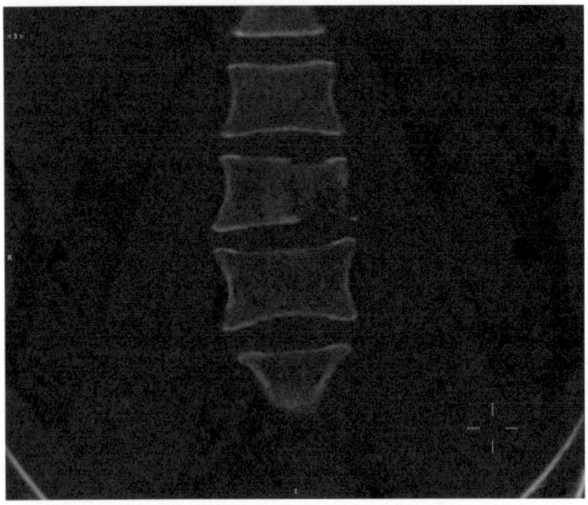

Fig. 42.4 Coronal CT image of the lumbar spine in bone window

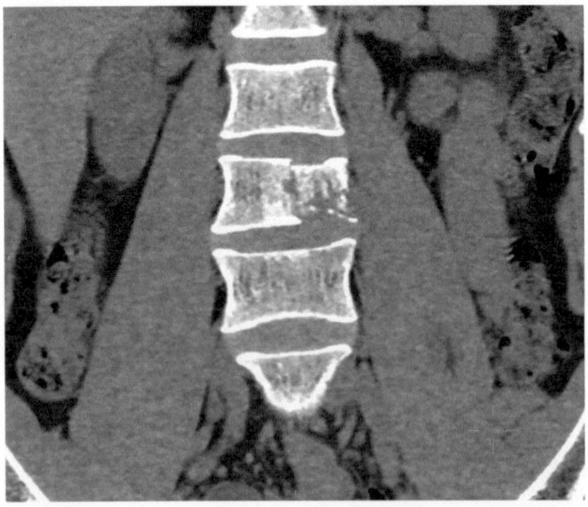

Fig. 42.5 Coronal CT image of the lumbar spine in soft tissue window

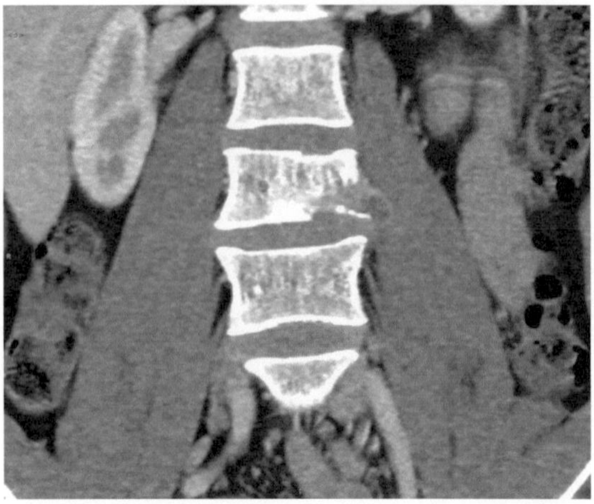

Fig. 42.6 Coronal post-contrast CT image of the lumbar spine in soft tissue window

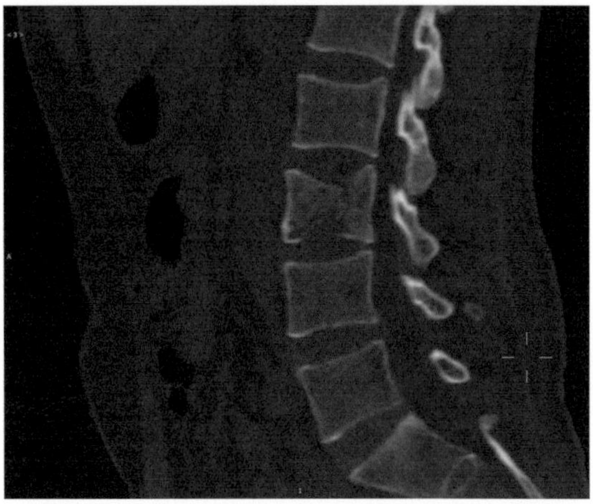

Fig. 42.7 Sagittal CT image of the lumbar spine in bone window

42.3.2 MR Imaging (Figs. 42.8, 42.9, 42.10, 42.11, 42.12, 42.13, and 42.14)

MR images demonstrated multiple foci of abnormal signal at T4, T9, L1-S1 vertebral bodies and posterior elements. There is pathological fracture of L3 vertebral body. Heterogeneous enhancement of the lesions noted.

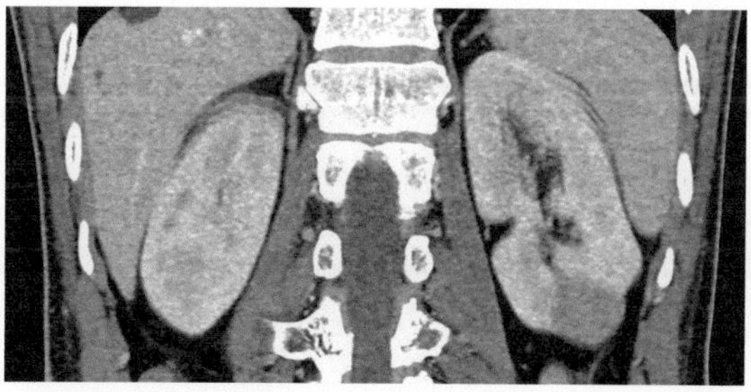

Fig. 42.8 Coronal post-contrast CT image of the kidney in soft tissue window

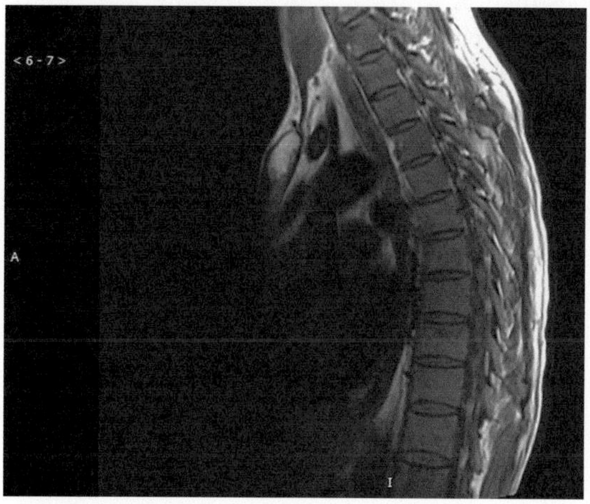

Fig. 42.9 Sagittal T1-weighted MR image of the thoracic spine

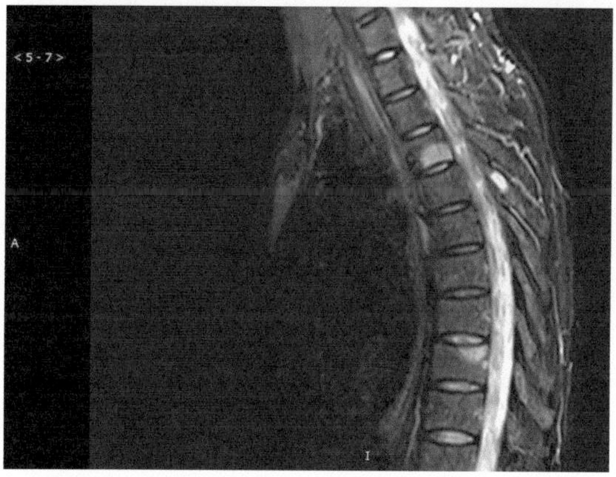

Fig. 42.10 Sagittal fat-suppressed T2-weighted MR image of the thoracic spine

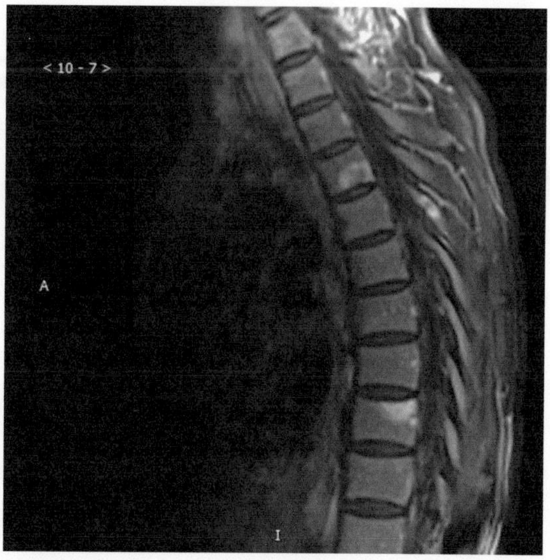

Fig. 42.11 Sagittal post-contrast fat-suppressed T1-weighted MR image of the thoracic spine

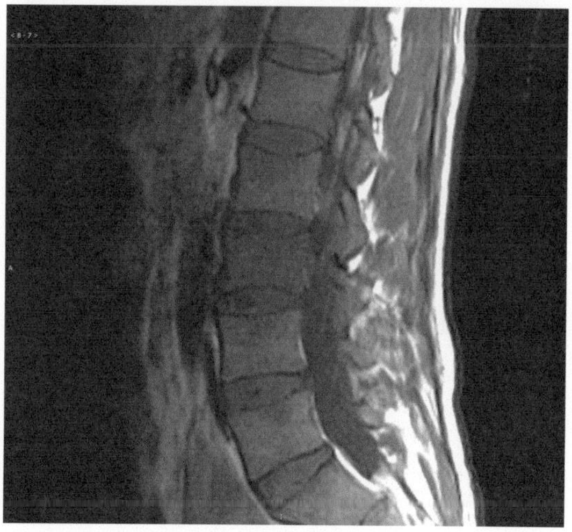

Fig. 42.12 Sagittal T1-weighted MR image of the lumbar spine

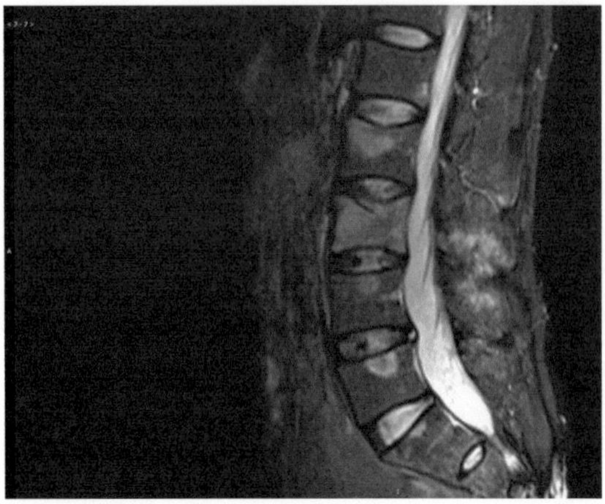

Fig. 42.13 Sagittal fat-suppressed T2-weighted MR image of the lumbar spine

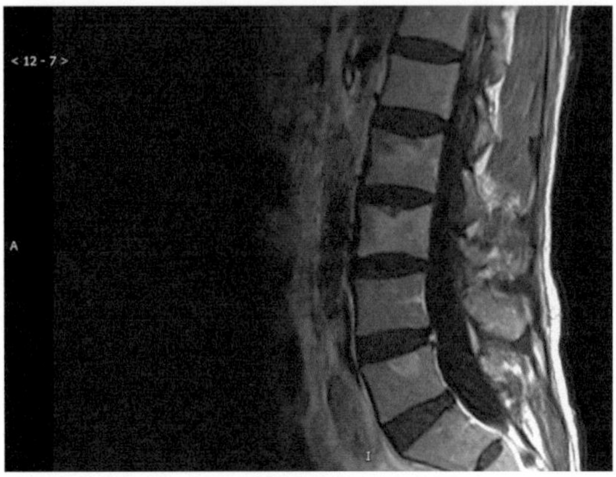

Fig. 42.14 Sagittal post-contrast fat-suppressed T1-weighted MR image of the lumbar spine

42.4 Description and Discussion from Residents

CT images showed L3 vertebral body bone destruction with pathologic fracture and indistinct margin without peripheral sclerosis and internal patchy high densities. There was focal cortical breakthrough with soft tissue mass extruding beyond the vertebral body with heterogeneous circular enhancement. There was a space-occupying lesion in the left kidney with avid enhancement. On the MR images, there were low T1 signals of multiple vertebral bodies, posterior elements, and bilateral ilia with multiple patchy high signals on fat-suppressed T2-weighted sequences. Mild enhancement noted of the lesions. Given patient's history of osteosarcoma, bone metastatic disease is our top consideration, and bone metastatic disease from renal cell carcinoma cannot be excluded.

42.5 Analysis and Comments from Professor Cheng Xiao-Guang

CT images showed L3 vertebral body bone destruction with pathologic fracture and heterogeneous enhancement of the lesion post contrast. The soft tissue mass protruded outside of the vertebral body, indicating malignant process. MR images demonstrated low T1 signals of multiple thoracic and lumbar spine vertebral bodies with multiple patchy high signals on fat-suppressed T2-weighted sequences. In most circumstances, signal of the vertebral body should be higher than the intervertebral disc on T1-weighted sequence. If the signal of the vertebral body is lower or similar to the disc, then, there is replacement of the normal fat of the vertebral body. Given patient's history, metastatic disease from osteosarcoma is my top consideration. However, given the lesion in the left kidney, osseous metastatic disease from renal cancer cannot be excluded. Multiple myeloma is in the differential diagnosis. Metastatic lesion usually has features of the primary tumor; thus, I suggest comparison. If there was more osteogenesis of the primary osteosarcoma, then usually there is osteogenesis in the metastatic lesions, vice versa.

42.6 Diagnosis

Metastatic osteosarcoma, with renal involvement.

Suggested Reading

Boyle R, Giuffre B, Bonar SF. Multifocal low-grade central osteosarcoma: a rare case. Skeletal Radiol. 2016;45(7):997–1006.

Karabulut N, Ariyürek OM, Gülsün M, et al. Renal involvement in multifocal osteosarcoma. Australas Radiol. 2002;46(1):108–10.

Metastatic Osteosarcoma: Case 43

43

43.1 Medical History

Patient is a 12-year-old girl. She complained of pain of both knees for about 3 years with some relief from rest and didn't seek treatment. She started to experience pain with restricted movement around the left shoulder about 3 months ago without relief from rest and worsening symptoms of the left shoulder lately. She had radiographs of the left humerus and demonstrated lytic bone destruction of the proximal humerus with disruption of the cortex with periosteal reaction and soft tissue mass.

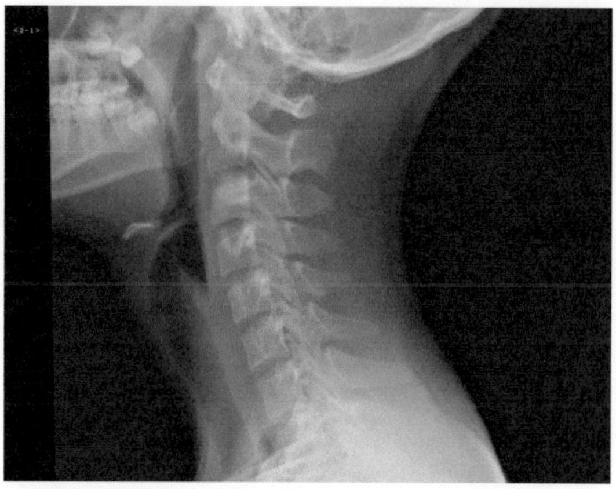

Fig. 43.1 Lateral view of the cervical spine

43.2 Physical Examination

Pain around the left upper arm proximally with increased skin temperature. There was a palpable mass, hard, mobile without clear margin and with point tenderness.

43.3 Imaging Findings

43.3.1 Radiograph (Figs. 43.1, 43.2, 43.3, 43.4, 43.5, 43.6, and 43.7)

There were focal increased densities of C2, L2 vertebral bodies. A stripe of high-density shadow noted in the soft tissues adjacent to the L2 vertebral body. Nodular high-density shadow noted along the left hila. There were diffuse high densities along the intramedullary canal of the femur, focal area with cloud-like high densities. Cortical destruction with spiculated periosteal reaction noted along the anterior distal femoral metaphysis.

43.3.2 CT Imaging (Figs. 43.8, 43.9, 43.10, 43.11, 43.12, 43.13, 43.14, 43.15, 43.16, 43.17, and 43.18)

Multiple sites of sclerotic destruction involved C3 vertebral body, right 4th rib and L2 vertebra with spiculated periosteal reaction with soft tissue mass. Within the soft tissue mass, strip-like

X. Cheng et al., *Imaging of Bone Tumors in Axial Bones*,
https://doi.org/10.1007/978-981-95-2262-0_43

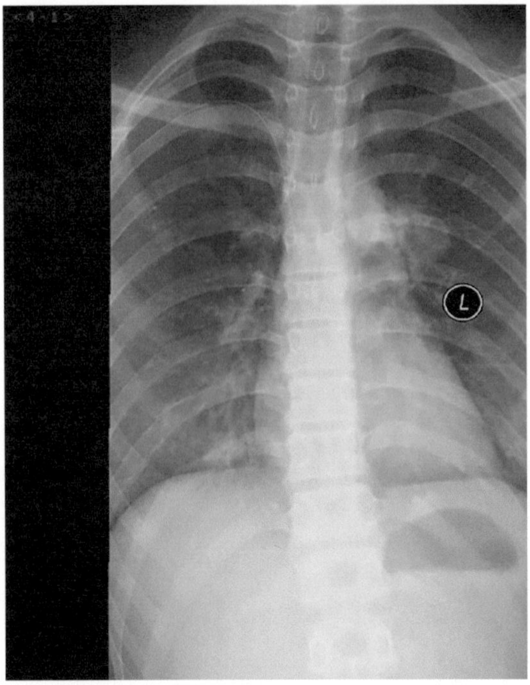

Fig. 43.2 Frontal view of the thoracic spine

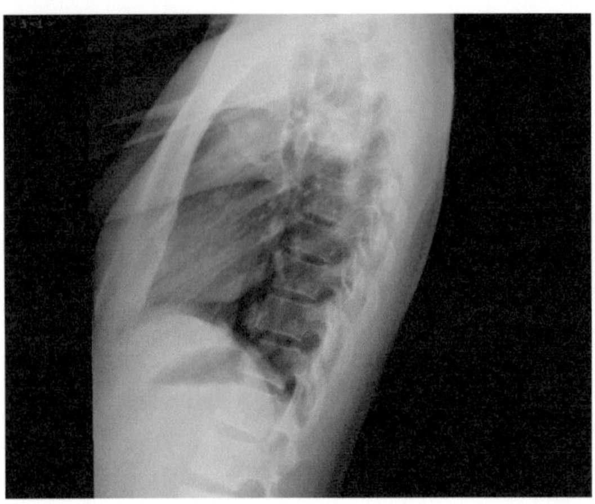

Fig. 43.3 Lateral view of the thoracic spine

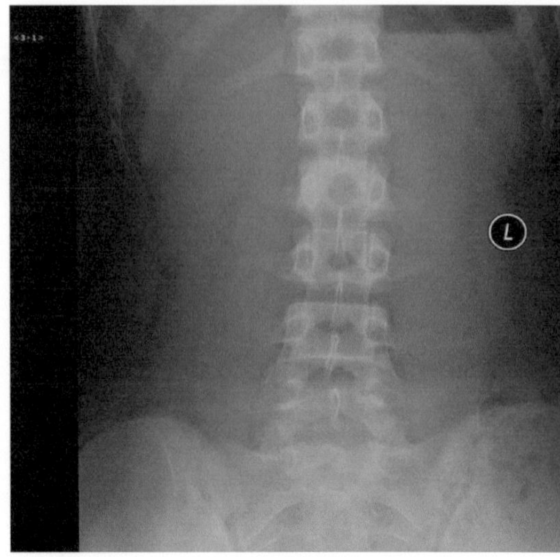

Fig. 43.4 Frontal view of the lumbar spine

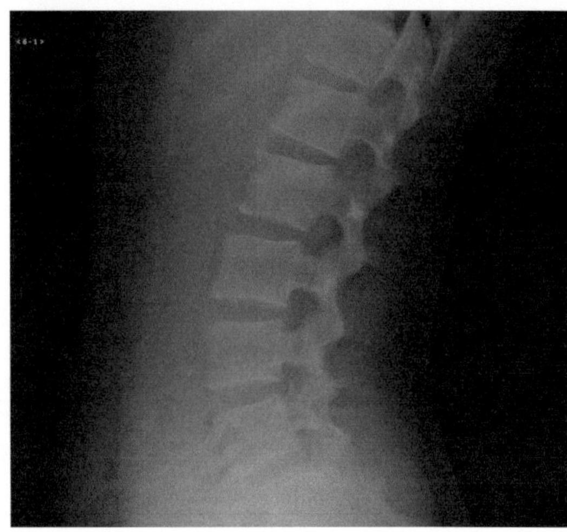

Fig. 43.5 Lateral view of the lumbar spine

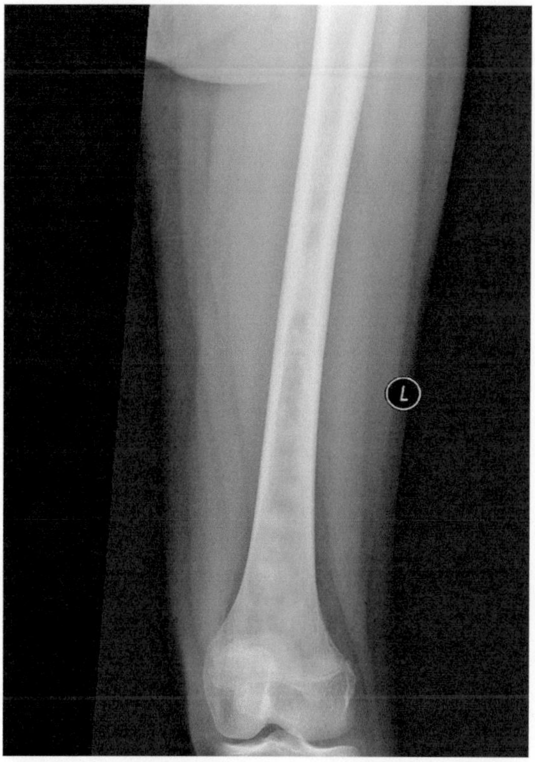

Fig. 43.6 Frontal view of the left femur

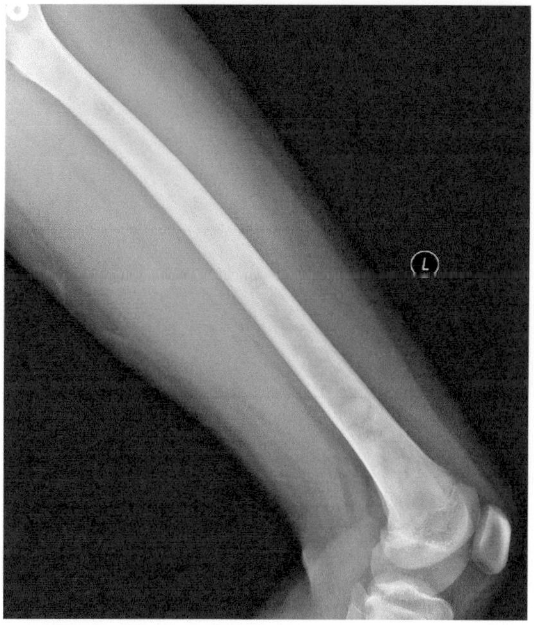

Fig. 43.7 Lateral view of the left femur

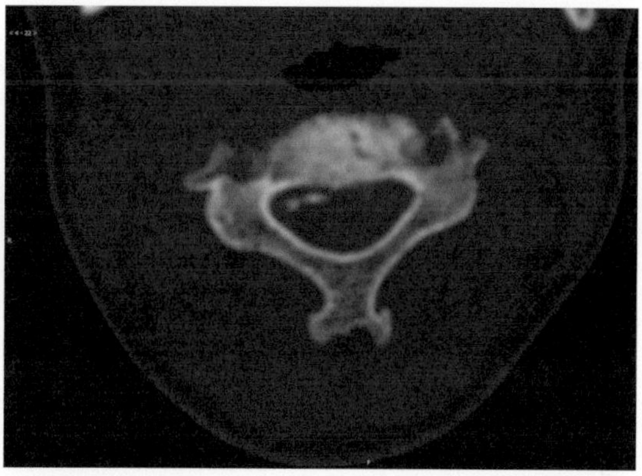

Fig. 43.8 Axial CT image of the cervical spine in bone window (C3 level)

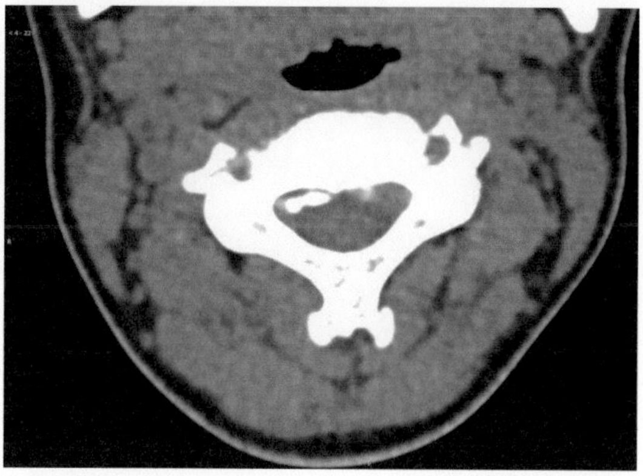

Fig. 43.9 Axial CT image of the cervical spine in soft tissue window (C3 level)

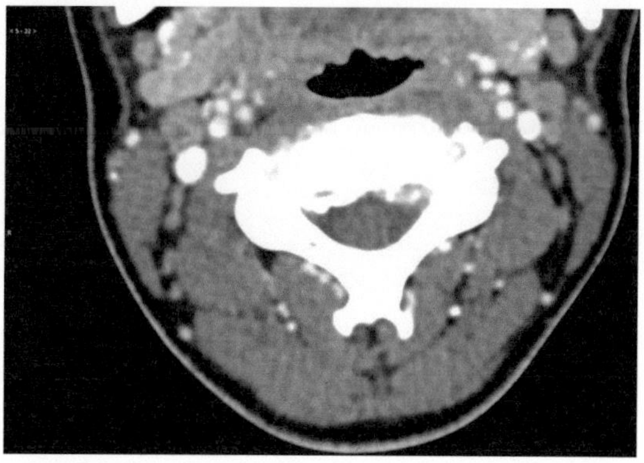

Fig. 43.10 Axial post-contrast CT image of the cervical spine in soft tissue window (C3 level)

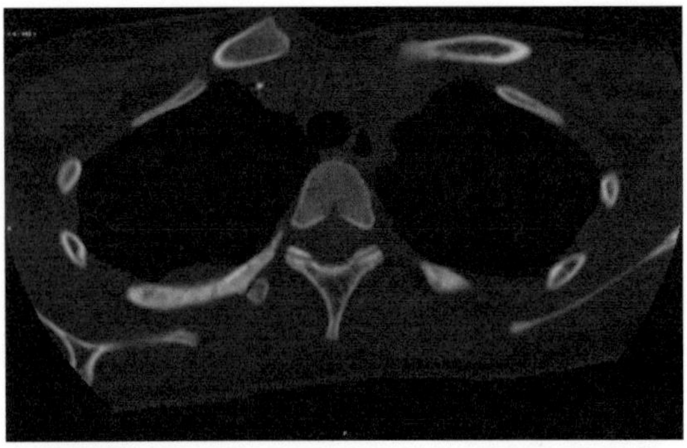

Fig. 43.11 Axial CT image of the ribs in bone window (4th rib level)

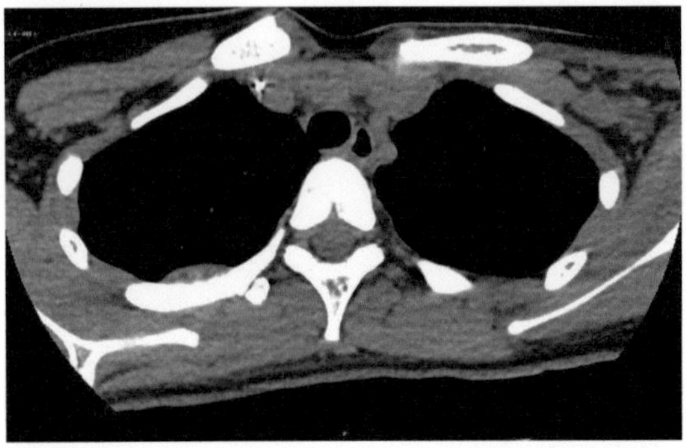

Fig. 43.12 Axial CT image of the ribs in soft tissue window (4th rib level)

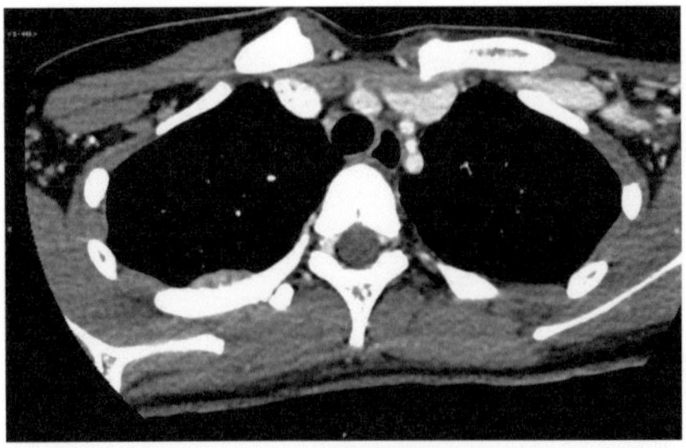

Fig. 43.13 Axial post-contrast CT image of the ribs in soft tissue window (4th rib level)

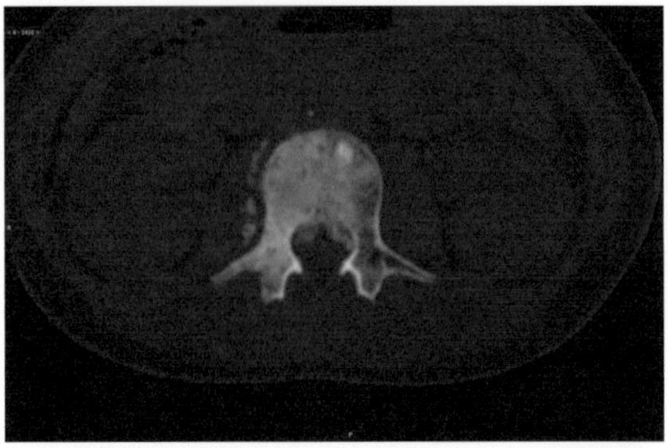

Fig. 43.14 Axial CT image of the lumbar spine in bone window (L2 level)

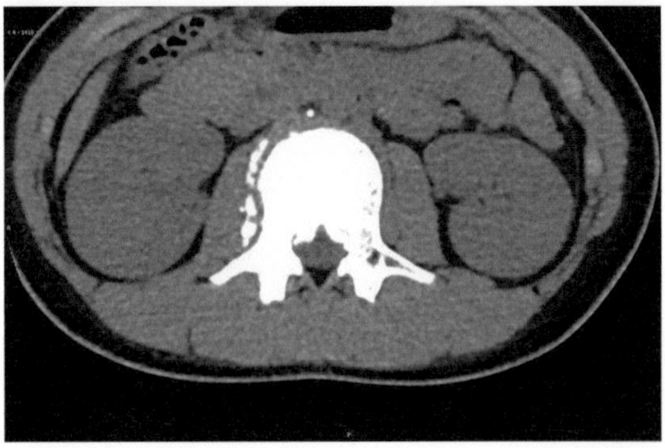

Fig. 43.15 Axial CT image of the lumbar spine in soft tissue window (L2 level)

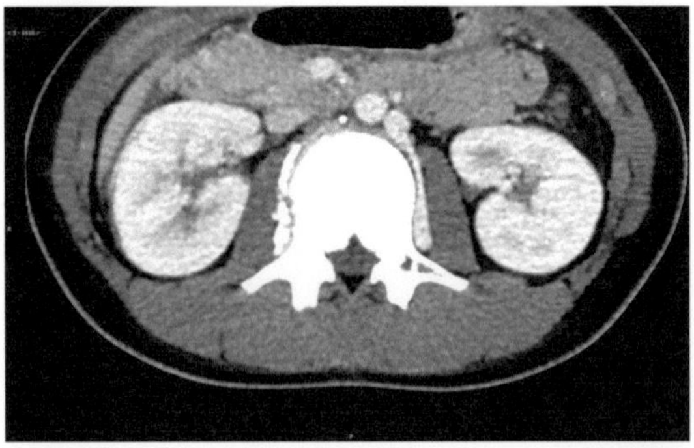

Fig. 43.16 Axial post-contrast CT image of the lumbar spine in soft tissue window (L2 level)

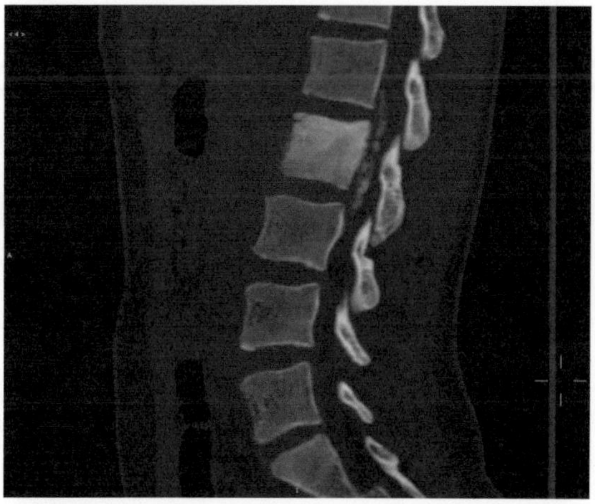

Fig. 43.17 Sagittal CT image of the lumbar spine in bone window

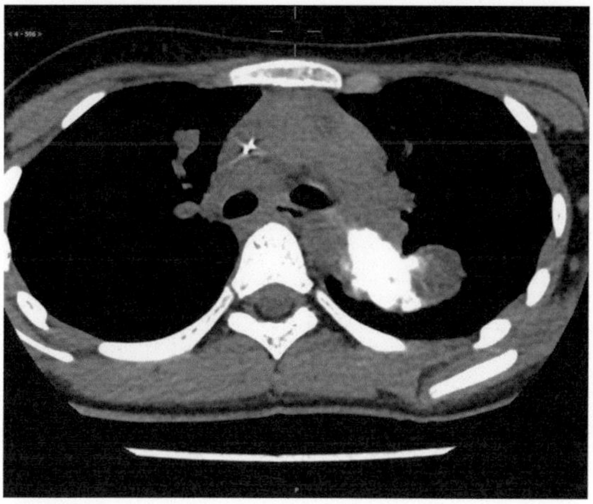

Fig. 43.18 Axial CT image of the chest in mediastinal window

and punctate osteogenesis noted with avid enhancement of the soft tissue area. The mass from L2 posteriorly compressed the canal. Multiple masses or nodules noted in the lung with mineralization internally.

43.4 Description and Discussion from Residents

The patient is a child. Radiographs showed increased bone density of C3, L2. There were high densities in the intramedullary cavity of the distal left femur with nodular shape. The current case showed involvement of multiple bones, likely of metastatic disease. CT images showed heterogeneous high densities of C3, L2, ribs and left femur with cloud-like osteogenesis and focal soft tissue mass, most suggestive of multicentric osteosarcoma. Multiple nodular and patchy densities in the lung with prominent blood vessels along the lumbar spine, indicating high malignancy of the lesion. Given multiple bone involvements, differential diagnosis is metastatic disease.

43.5 Analysis and Comments from Professor Cheng Xiao-Guang

Radiographs showed increased densities of multiple bones. Increased bone density of multiple vertebral bodies, ribs, left femur with surrounding soft tissue changes and multiple ossifications in the lung noted on the CT images. Given patient's age, my consideration is multicentric osteosarcoma or osteosarcoma with multiple metastatic diseases. It is challenging to differentiate these two diagnoses. If patient is older, sclerotic metastatic disease should be considered.

43.6 Diagnosis

Metastatic osteosarcoma, bone metastases with pulmonary metastases

Note: By definition, multicentric osteosarcoma is not accompanied by pulmonary metastatic disease or other visceral metastatic disease.

Suggested Reading

Hopper KD, Moser RP Jr, Haseman DB, et al. Osteosarcomatosis. Radiology. 1990;175(1):233–9.

Nguyen JC, Baghdadi S, Pogoriler J, et al. Pediatric osteosarcoma: correlation of Imaging findings with histopathologic features, treatment, and outcome. Radiographics. 2022;42(4):1196–213.

Fibrous Dysplasia: Case 44

44

44.1 Medical History

Patient is a 50-year-old female. Multiple bone lesions were found during a health check-up. She was seen at the outpatient clinic of our hospital.

44.2 Physical Examination

No abnormalities.

44.3 Imaging Findings

44.3.1 CT Imaging (Figs. 44.1, 44.2, 44.3, 44.4, 44.5, 44.6, 44.7, 44.8, 44.9, and 44.10)

Multiple expansile bone destruction occurred in the thoracic, lumbar, sacral spine with marginal sclerosis with local cortical thinning and interruption, without clear soft tissue mass. Most lesions contained ground glass-like high densities. No significant enhancement was noted.

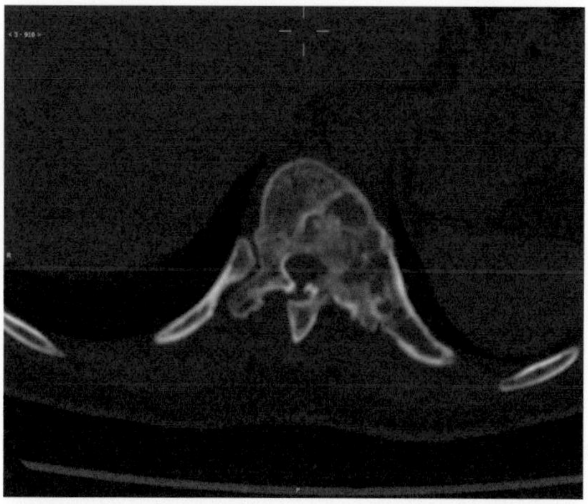

Fig. 44.1 Axial CT image of the thoracic spine in bone window (T10 level)

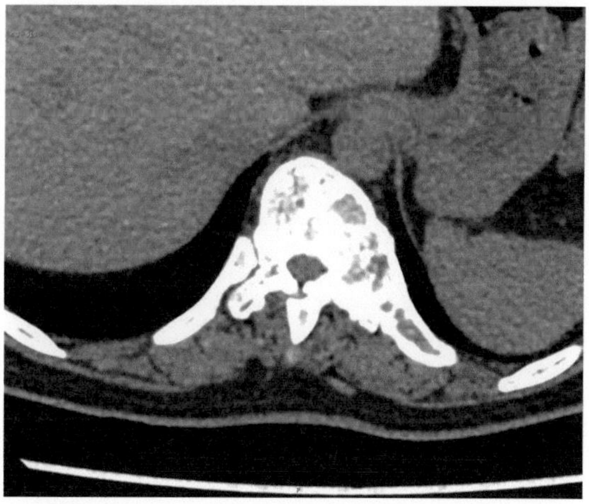

Fig. 44.2 Axial CT image of the thoracic spine in soft tissue window (T10 level)

X. Cheng et al., *Imaging of Bone Tumors in Axial Bones*,
https://doi.org/10.1007/978-981-95-2262-0_44

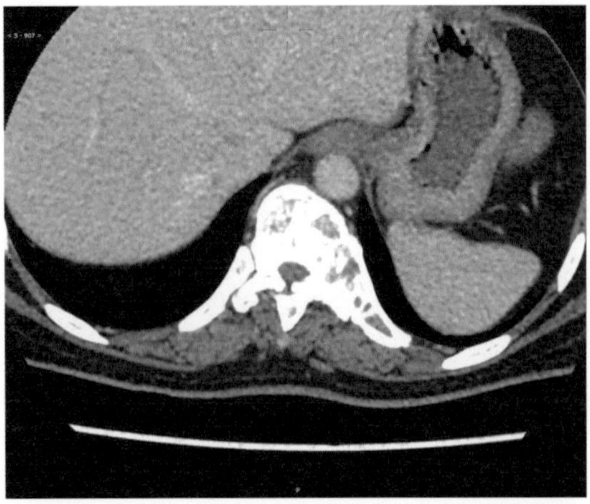

Fig. 44.3 Axial post-contrast CT image of the thoracic spine in soft tissue window (T10 level)

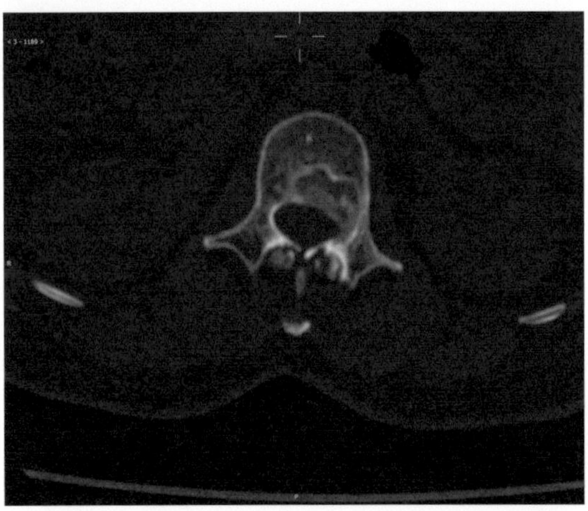

Fig. 44.4 Axial CT image of the lumbar spine in bone window (L1 level)

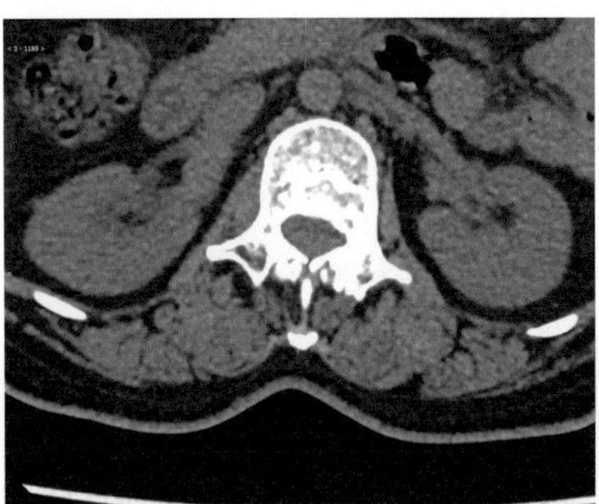

Fig. 44.5 Axial CT image of the lumbar spine in soft tissue window (L1 level)

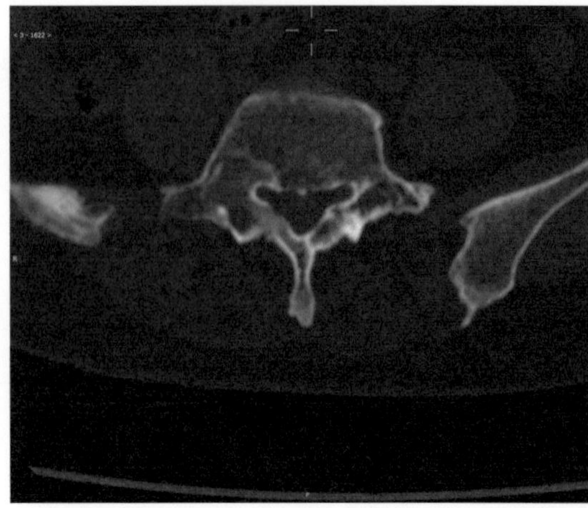

Fig. 44.6 Axial CT image of the lumbar spine in bone window (L5 level)

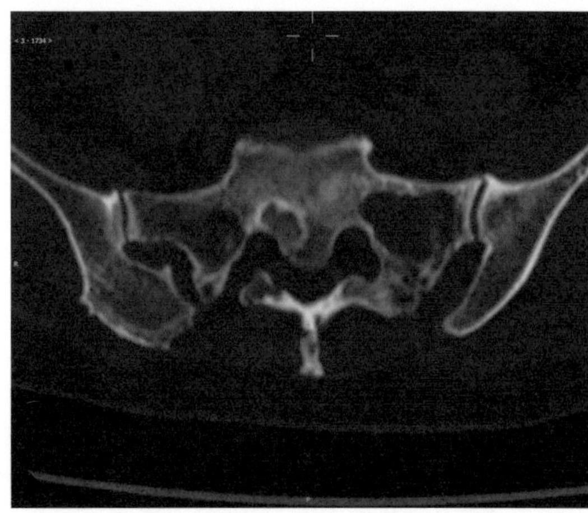

Fig. 44.7 Axial CT image of the sacrum in bone window (S1 level)

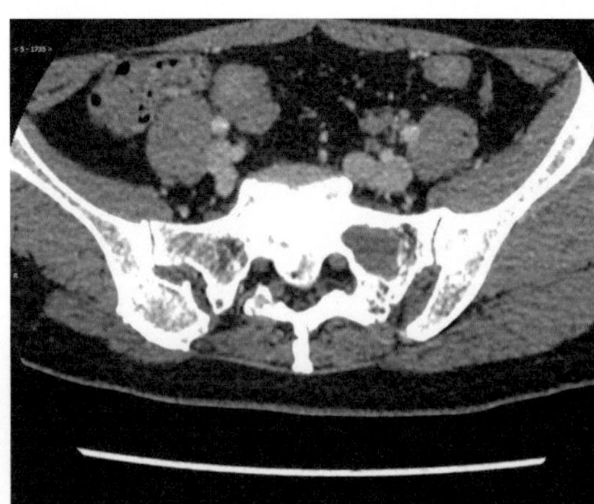

Fig. 44.8 Axial post-contrast CT image of the sacrum in soft tissue window (S1 level)

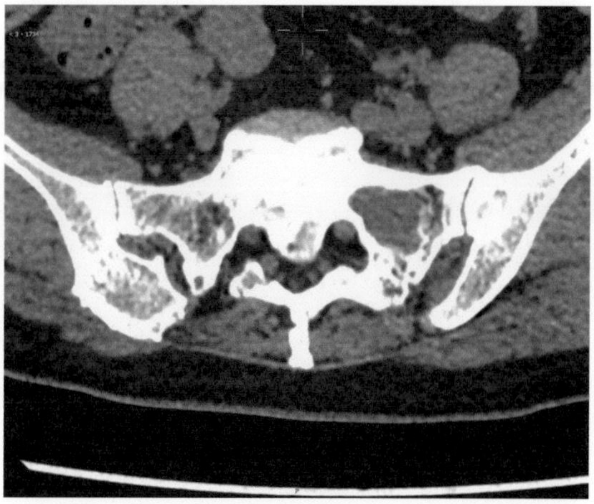

Fig. 44.9 Axial CT image of the sacrum in soft tissue window (S1 level)

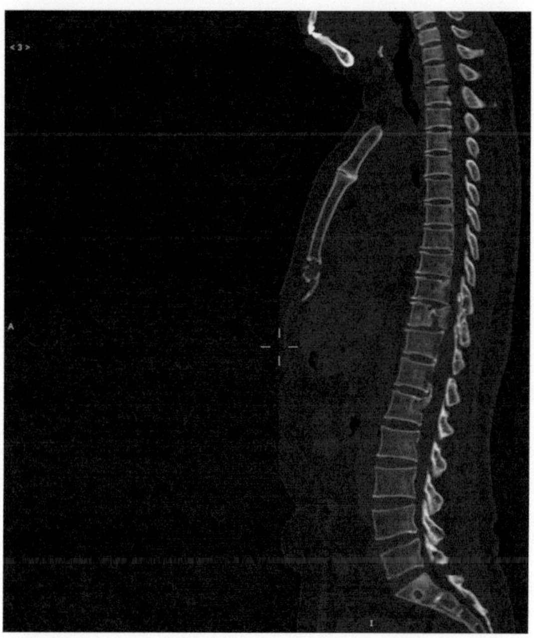

Fig. 44.10 Sagittal CT image of the spine in bone window

44.4 Description and Discussion from Residents

The patient was a middle-aged female. CT images showed multiple bone destruction of thoracic, lumbar spines and sacrum, left ribs, involving vertebral bodies and posterior elements with focal mild expansion, clear margin, and peripheral sclerosis. Ground glass-like high densities noted inside of the lesion without soft tissue mass and no apparent enhancement. Given the above findings, we favor benign process. Our top consideration is polyostotic fibrous dysplasia. If patient with additional skin changes, endocrine pathology, McCune-Albright syndrome should be considered. Metabolic bone disease is in the differential diagnosis. The osseous structures show preserved morphology without apparent osteoporosis of the current case, thus, not considered here.

44.5 Analysis and Comments from Professor Cheng Xiao-Guang

The patient is a middle-aged female. CT images showed multiple bone destruction along the axial skeleton of thoracic, lumbar spine, and sacrum. Ground glass opacity noted in most of the lesions with peripheral sclerosis. My top consideration is polyostotic fibrous dysplasia. Given the wide involvement of the current case with relative older age of the patient, I would include metastatic disease in the differential diagnosis. Additionally, metabolic bone disease should be included in the differential diagnosis, such as hyperparathyroidism from renal failure, and amyloidosis. Both kidneys appeared normal on the scan of current studies; thus renal osteodystrophy can be excluded.

44.6 Diagnosis

Fibrous dysplasia, polyostotic.

Suggested Reading

Ariyaratne S, Jenko N, Iyengar KP, et al. Primary benign neoplasms of the spine. Diagnostics (Basel). 2023;13(12):2006.

Park SK, Lee IS, Choi JY, et al. CT and MRI of fibrous dysplasia of the spine. Br J Radiol. 2012;85(1015):996–1001.

Primary Hyperparathyroidism: Case 45

45

45.1 Medical History

Patient is a 32-year-old female. She started to suffer from pain at bilateral hip without radiation about 2 months ago and with relief after rest. Sometimes, she also felt sick and vomit.

45.2 Physical Examination

Not done.

45.3 Imaging Findings

45.3.1 Radiograph (Fig. 45.1)

There are multiple ovoid lesions with decreased bone density along bilateral iliac wings and acetabulum with mild peripheral sclerosis. There is also bone absorption along the auricular surface of both iliac.

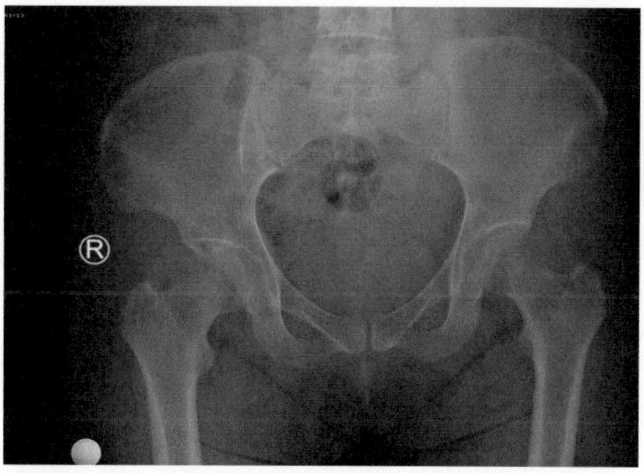

Fig. 45.1 Frontal view of the pelvis

45.3.2 CT Imaging (Figs. 45.2, 45.3, 45.4, 45.5, 45.6, 45.7, 45.8, 45.9, 45.10, 45.11, 45.12, 45.13, 45.14, 45.15, and 45.16)

There is fuzziness along the cortex and bone trabeculae. Bone destruction, mainly as lytic destruction, noted along facial bones, right 1st, 7th, 9th ribs

X. Cheng et al., *Imaging of Bone Tumors in Axial Bones*,
https://doi.org/10.1007/978-981-95-2262-0_45

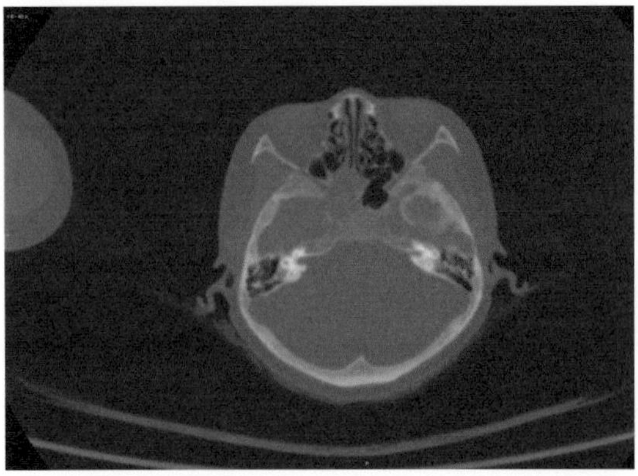

Fig. 45.2 Axial CT image of the craniofacial bone in bone window

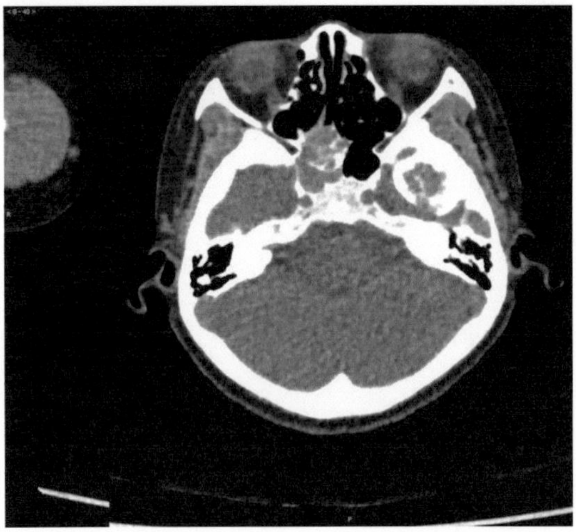

Fig. 45.3 Axial CT image of the craniofacial bone in soft tissue window

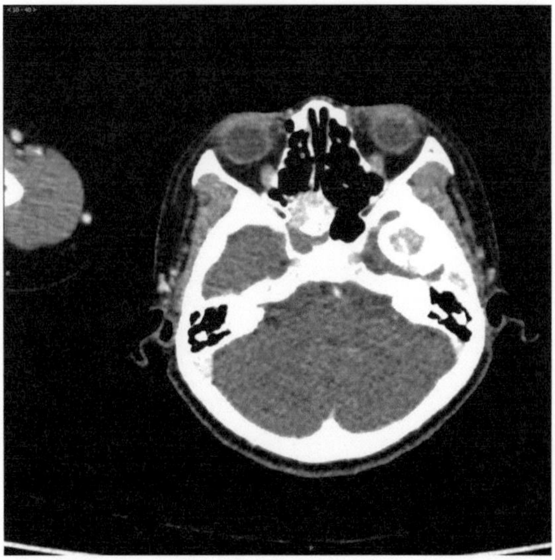

Fig. 45.4 Axial post-contrast CT image of the craniofacial bone in soft tissue window

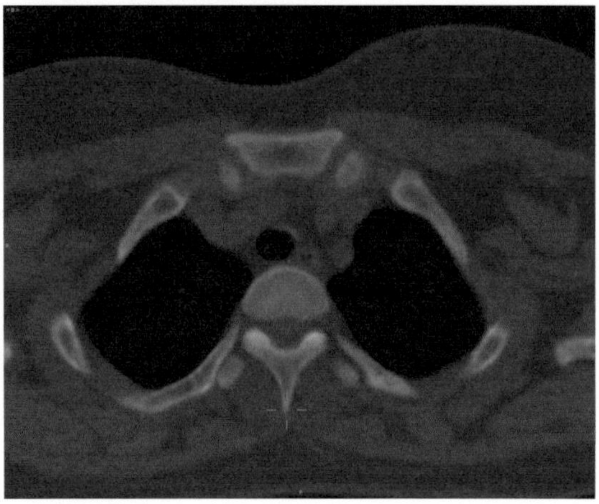

Fig. 45.5 Axial CT image of the ribs in bone window (1st rib level)

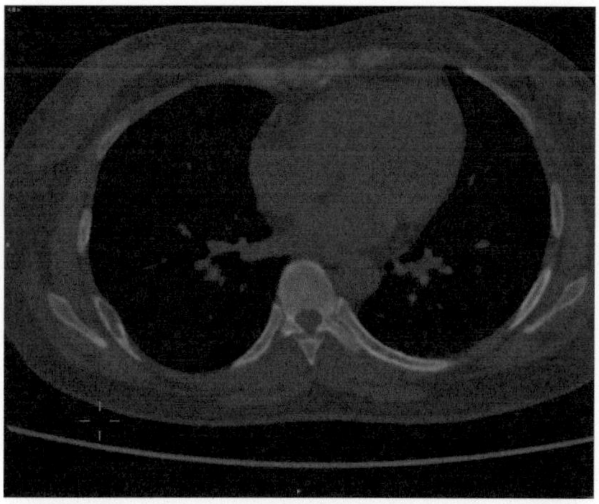

Fig. 45.6 Axial CT image of the ribs in bone window (7th rib level)

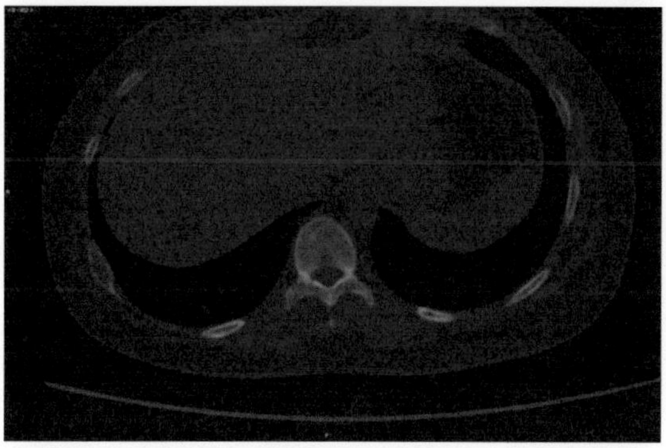

Fig. 45.7 Axial CT image of the ribs in bone window (9th rib level)

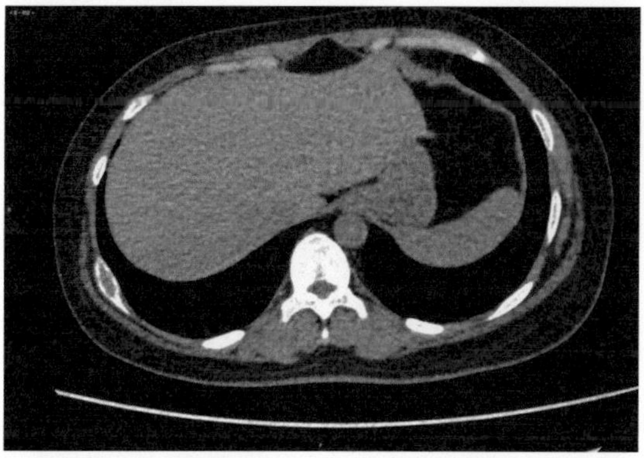

Fig. 45.8 Axial CT image of the ribs in soft tissue window (9th rib level)

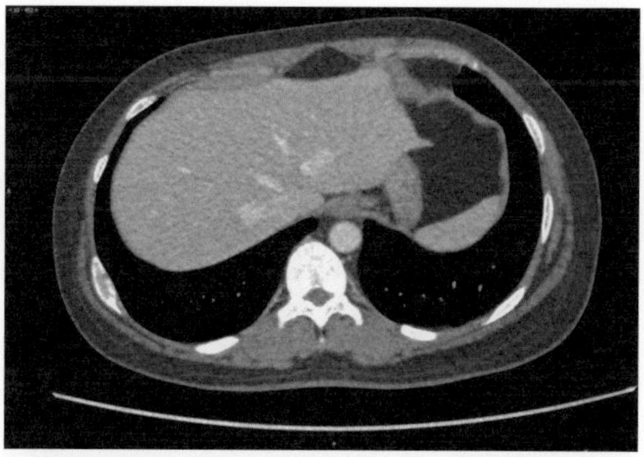

Fig. 45.9 Axial post-contrast CT image of the ribs in soft tissue window (9th rib level)

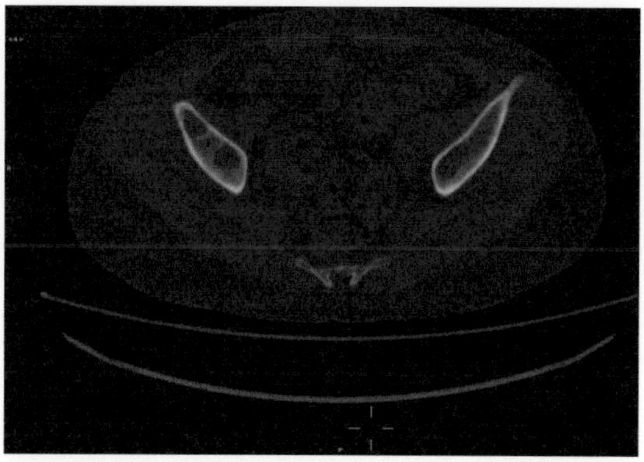

Fig. 45.10 Axial CT image of the bony pelvis in bone window

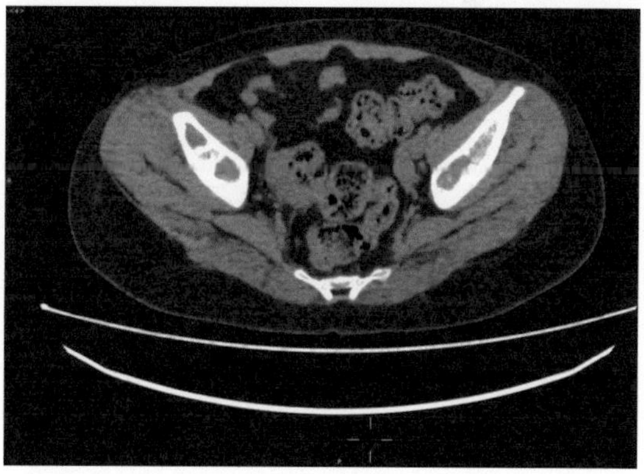

Fig. 45.11 Axial CT image of the bony pelvis in soft tissue window

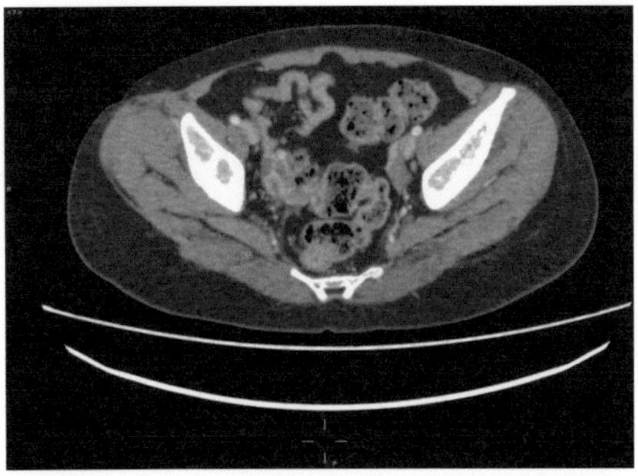

Fig. 45.12 Axial post-contrast CT image of the bony pelvis in soft tissue window

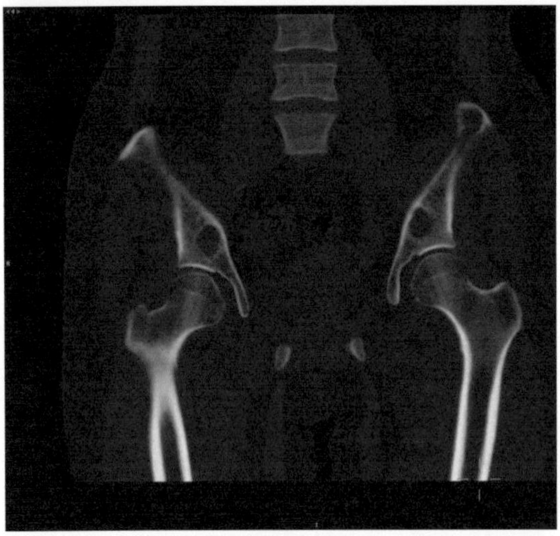

Fig. 45.13 Coronal CT image of the bony pelvis in bone window

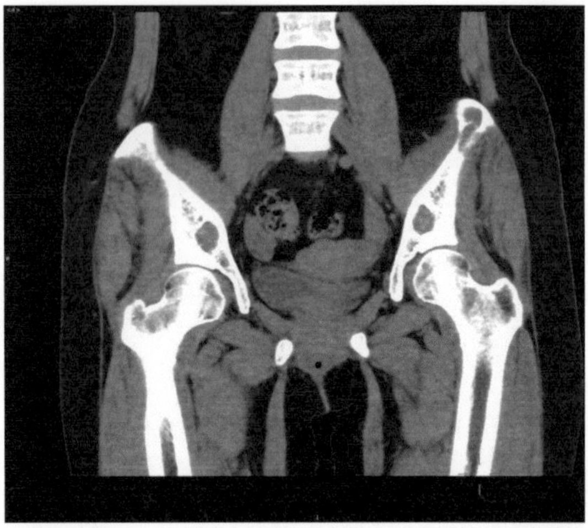

Fig. 45.14 Coronal CT image of the bony pelvis in soft tissue window

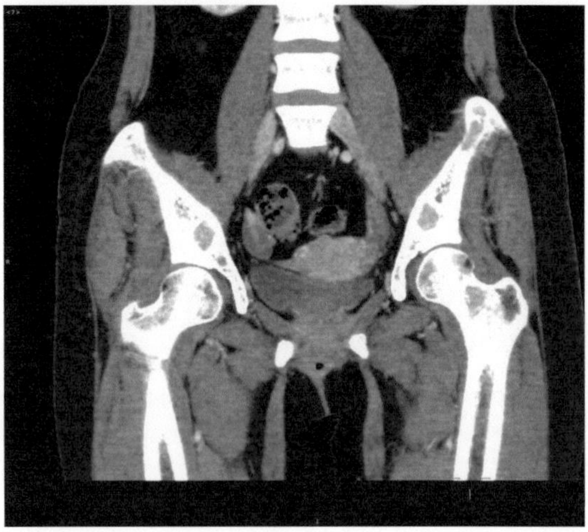

Fig. 45.15 Coronal post-contrast CT image of the bony pelvis in soft tissue window

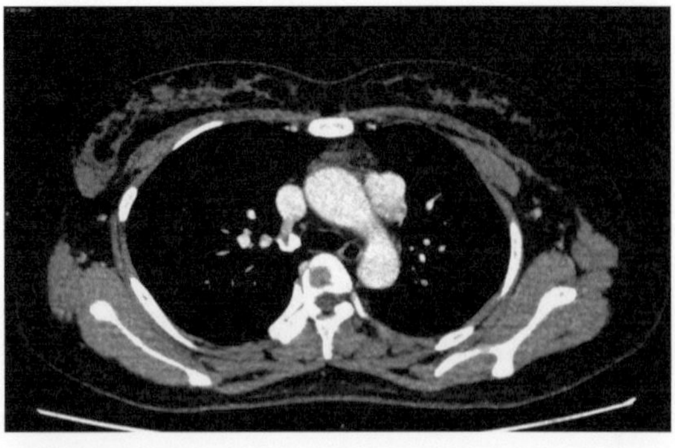

Fig. 45.16 Axial post-contrast CT image of the chest in mediastinal window

and bony pelvis, with clear margin and peripheral mild sclerosis with apparent enhancement. There is soft tissue mass along the anterior mediastinum.

45.4 Description and Discussion from Residents

The patient is a young female. Radiograph showed suspicious decreased bone density along both acetabula. CT images showed expansile bone destruction along ethmoid and sphenoid sinuses junction and left temporal bone with internal high density with clear margin and peripheral sclerosis. There was also expansile bone destruction along multiple ribs with peripheral sclerosis. Multiple lytic destruction noted along the iliac with heterogeneous internal density and avid enhancement of the above lesions. Multiple bone destruction in a young female, we have the following differential diagnosis: (1) tumor, such as lymphoma, other hematological malignancies and eosinophilic granuloma. (2) Metabolic bone disease, such as hyperparathyroidism, often with associated background of osteoporosis.

45.5 Analysis and Comments from Professor Cheng Xiao-Guang

The patient is a young female. Radiograph showed normal bone mineralization without evidence of osteoporosis. CT images showed expansile changes along the sinus and left temporal bone with internal high densities; multiple bone destruction in the bony pelvis with clear margin and limited to the cortex without soft tissue mass. Avid enhancement noted. Current case is of multiple widespread bone destruction in a young female, my top consideration is hyperparathyroidism. However, no apparent background of osteoporosis noted, combining results from serum calcium, phosphorus and parathyroid hormone level would be helpful for reaching the diagnosis. Given the imaging findings along the craniofacial bones, differential diagnosis includes fibrous dysplasia, osteomalacia from phosphaturic mesenchymal tumor.

45.6 Diagnosis

Primary hyperparathyroidism (ectopic parathyroid adenoma).

Suggested Reading

Ayadi C, Lanjery S, Andour H, et al. Multiple brown tumors in primary hyperparathyroidism. Radiol Case Rep. 2022;17(11):4239–43.

Hong WS, Sung MS, Chun KA, et al. Emphasis on the MR imaging findings of brown tumor: a report of five cases. Skeletal Radiol. 2011;40(2):205–13.

Jacquet-Francillon N, Prevot N. Brown tumors in nuclear medicine: a systematic review. Ann Nucl Med. 2023;37(5):255–70.

Renal Osteodystrophy with Tertiary Hyperparathyroidism: Case 46

46

46.1 Medical History

Patient is a 31-year-old male. He has renal failure with dialysis therapy for 8 years. ECT showed whole-body metabolic bone abnormalities with vertebral body destruction of T5 and T10 with compression to the spinal canal.

46.2 Physical Examination

Decreased skin feeling below the xiphoid process of the sternum. Right lower extremity muscle strength level III; left lower extremity muscle strength level III.

46.3 Imaging Findings

46.3.1 Radiograph (Figs. 46.1 and 46.2)

There was diffuse osteoporosis with changes of osteomalacia. Sclerosis bands with fuzzy border were seen along the end plates of the thoracic vertebral bodies; bone absorption noted along bilateral sacroiliac joints and pubic symphysis; mild expansile lytic bone changes of the right proximal femur with cortical thinning.

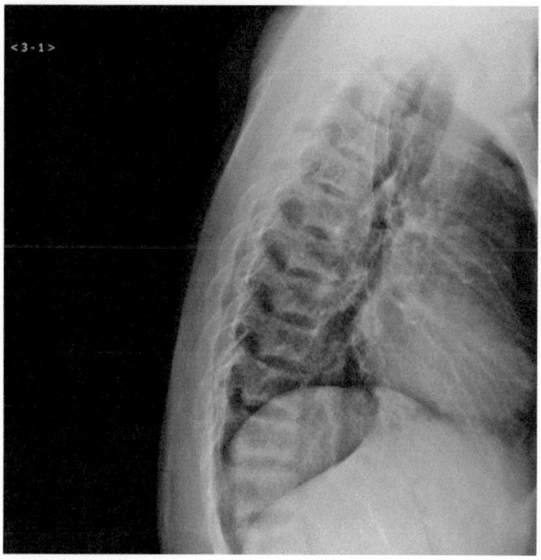

Fig. 46.1 Lateral view of the thoracic spine

46.3.2 CT Imaging (Figs. 46.3, 46.4, 46.5, 46.6, 46.7, 46.8, 46.9, 46.10, and 46.11)

There is heterogeneous of bone density of multiple bones with fuzzy trabeculae and increased bone densities along superior and inferior end plates of the vertebral bodies of the spine (rugger-jersey spine sign). Multiple lytic bone destruction of vertebral bodies, posterior elements, and ster-

X. Cheng et al., *Imaging of Bone Tumors in Axial Bones*,
https://doi.org/10.1007/978-981-95-2262-0_46

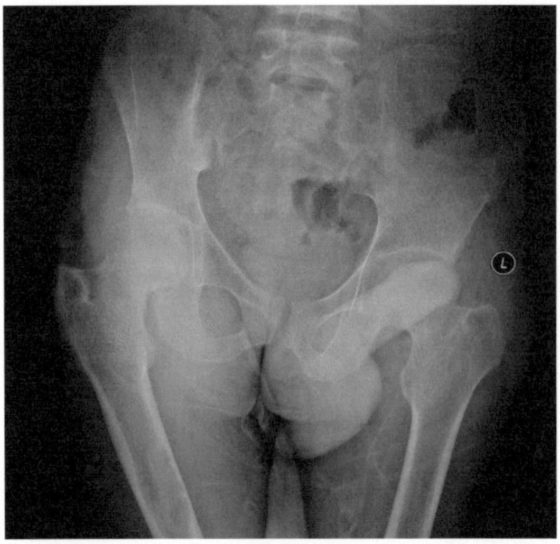

Fig. 46.2 Frontal view of the pelvis

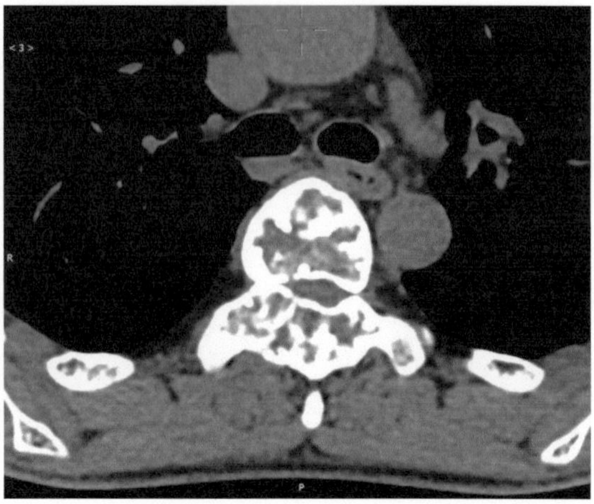

Fig. 46.4 Axial CT image of the thoracic spine in soft tissue window (T5 level)

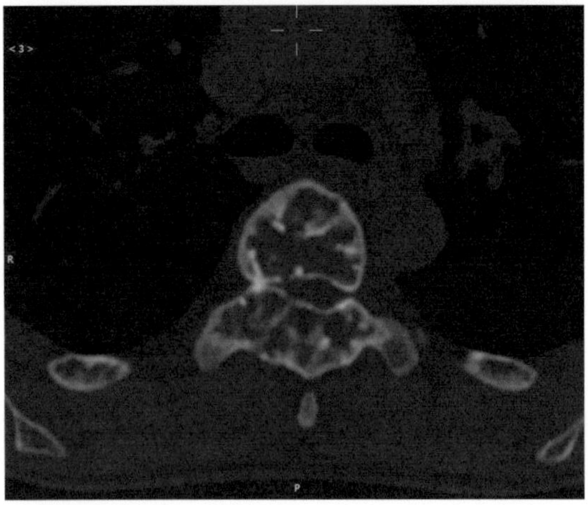

Fig. 46.3 Axial CT image of the thoracic spine in bone window (T5 level)

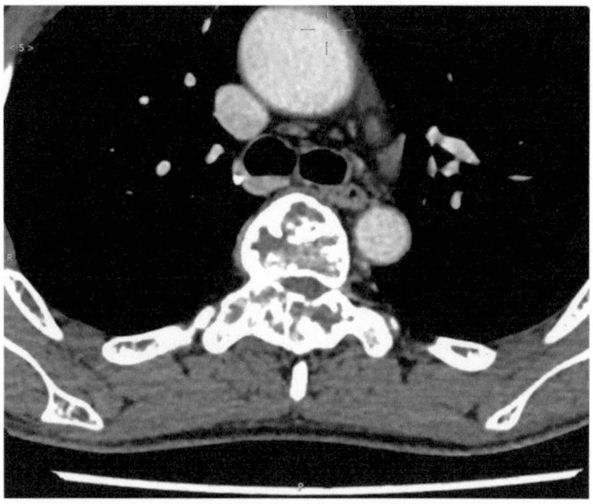

Fig. 46.5 Axial post-contrast CT image of the thoracic spine in soft tissue window (T5 level)

num with focal mild expansion with clear margin and peripheral sclerosis with avid enhancement.

46.3.3 MR Imaging (Figs. 46.12, 46.13, and 46.14)

Multiple thoracic spine vertebral bodies showed biconcave changes with linear sclerosis along the end plates. Bone destruction along vertebral bodies and spinous processes of T5, T8–11 with low T1-weighted, and high fat-suppressed T2-weighted signals with heterogeneous enhancement. There was narrowing of the spinal canal along T5, T9, and T10 levels with spinal cord edema at T9 and T10 levels.

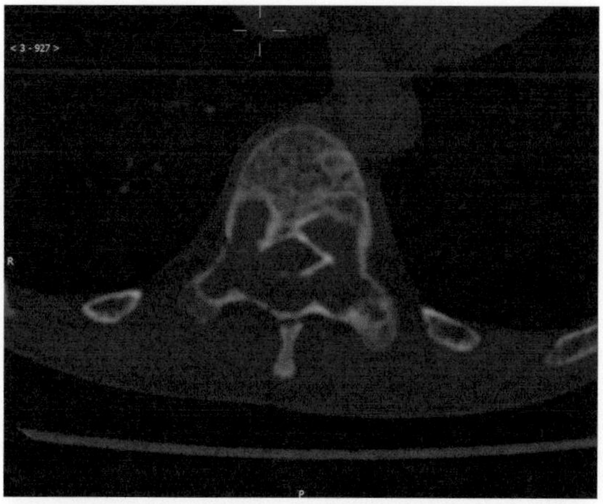

Fig. 46.6 Axial CT image of the thoracic spine in bone window (T10 level)

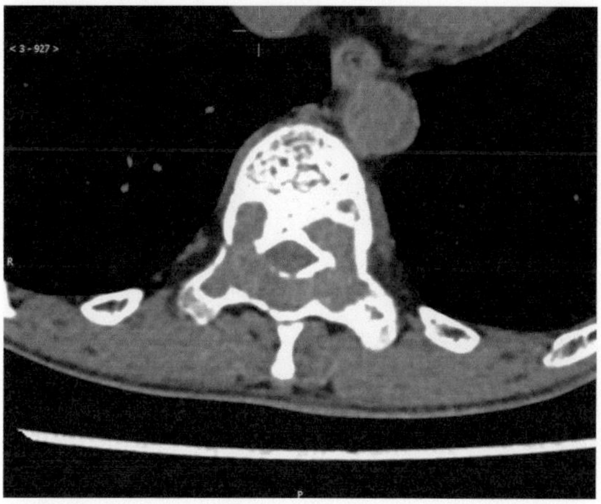

Fig. 46.7 Axial CT image of the thoracic spine in soft tissue window (T10 level)

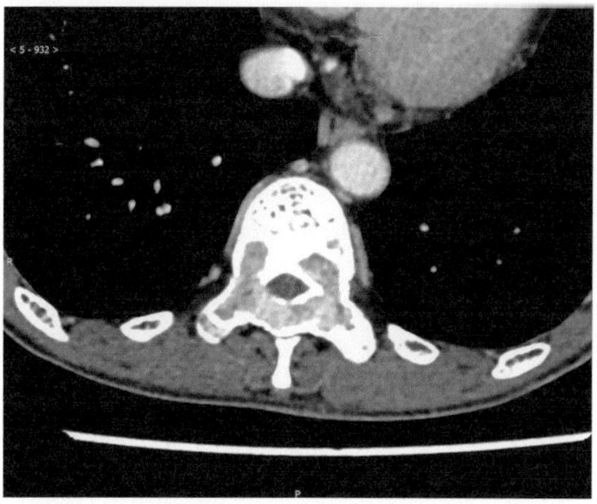

Fig. 46.8 Axial post-contrast CT image of the thoracic spine in soft tissue window (T10 level)

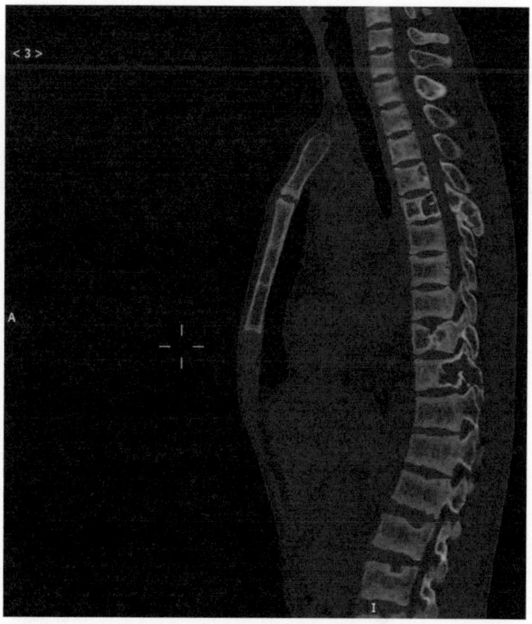

Fig. 46.9 Sagittal CT image of the thoracic spine in bone window

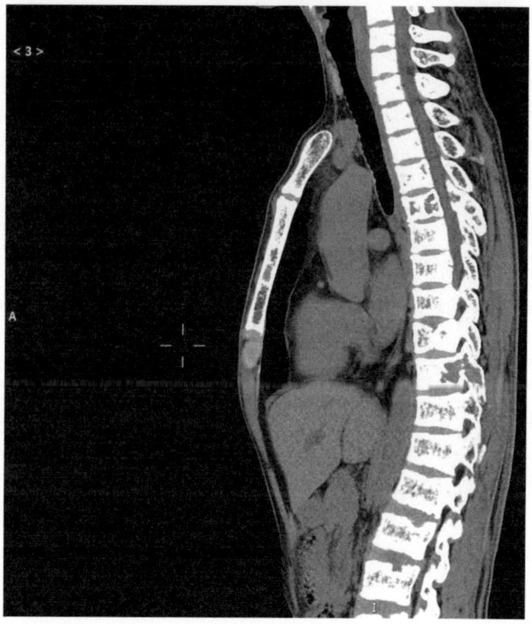

Fig. 46.10 Sagittal CT image of the thoracic spine in soft tissue window

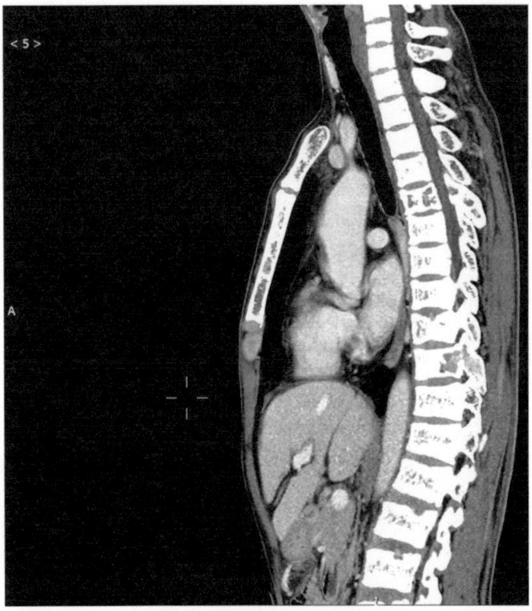

Fig. 46.11 Sagittal post-contrast CT image of the thoracic spine in soft tissue window

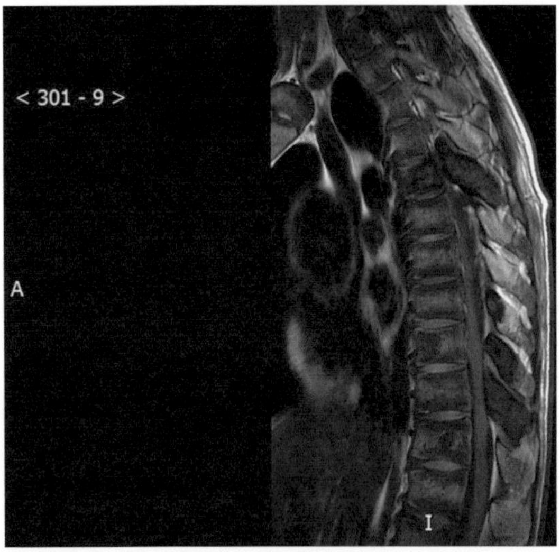

Fig. 46.12 Sagittal T1-weighted MR image of the thoracic spine

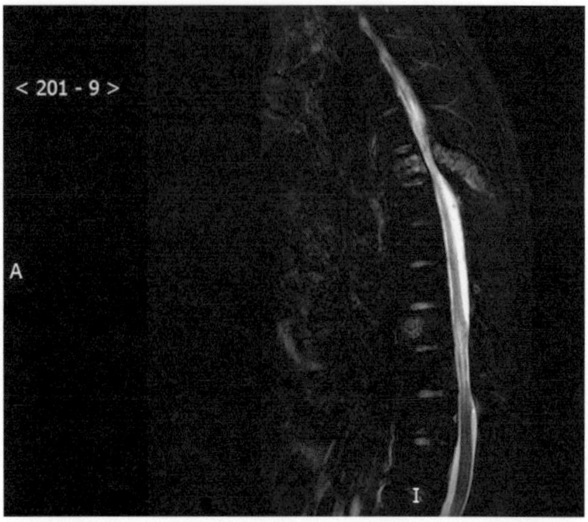

Fig. 46.13 Sagittal STIR weighted MR image of the thoracic spine

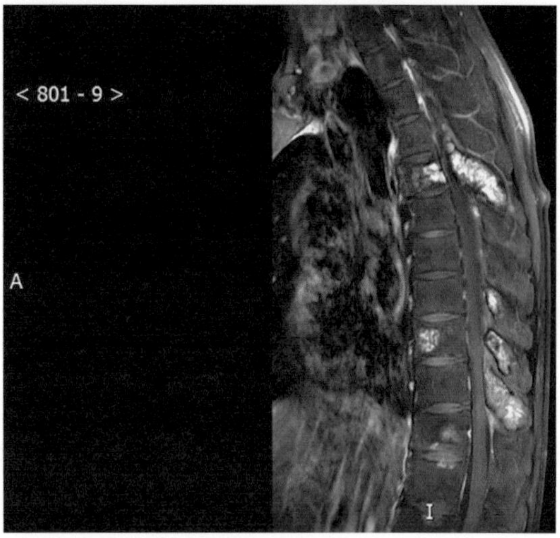

Fig. 46.14 Sagittal post-contrast fat-suppressed T1-weighted MR image of the thoracic spine

46.4 Description and Discussion from Residents

The patient is a young male. Radiographs showed osteoporosis of the vertebral bodies and pelvis. Increased bone densities along superior and inferior portions of the vertebral bodies as "rugger-jersey spine" noted. Expansile changes noted of the right femur with thinning of the cortex. The disease affected multiple sites of the whole body. CT images showed multiple lytic bone destruction involving sternum, thoracic, lumbar spine vertebral bodies, posterior elements with focal expansion and peripheral sclerosis, and internal residual bone crest. Given the presence of renal failure, our consideration is renal osteodystrophy with hyperparathyroidism with brown tumor. Additionally, amyloid in dialysis patients can have similar bone destructive changes. MR images showed mild expansion of the vertebral lesions with high fat-suppressed T2-weighted signal. Focal areas in some lesions showed no high signal, which likely reflects hemorrhage. Avid heterogeneous enhancement noted. Parathyroid hormone level checked: 1811 pg/ml. Overall, the case is consistent with renal osteodystrophy with hyperparathyroidism. Similar bone destruction if only involves single vertebral body, solidary plasmacytoma of bone, and giant cell tumor of the bone should be included in the differential diagnosis.

46.5 Analysis and Comments from Professor Cheng Xiao-Guang

The patient is a young male with renal disease and dialysis therapy. Radiographs showed decreased bone densities of multiple vertebral bodies with "rugger-jersey spine" sign and bone destruction of the right proximal femur. Please note when evaluating the pelvis radiograph in a patient with renal osteodystrophy, we should be alert of identifying insufficiency fracture of the femoral neck. CT images showed background of renal osteodystrophy with lytic bone destruction of multiple vertebral bodies and posterior elements. Sclerosis along the end plates of the vertebral bodies and expansile changes of the bone destruction noted on MR images. My consideration is hyperparathyroidism from renal osteodystrophy and additionally, amyloid arthropathy can be seen in dialysis patient.

46.6 Diagnosis

Renal osteodystrophy with tertiary hyperparathyroidism.

Suggested Reading

Ferrari C, Lavelli V, Santo G, et al. ^{18}F-fluorocholine PET/CT, Tc-99m-MIBI and TC-99m-MDP SPECT/CT in tertiary hyperparathyroidism with renal osteodystrophy. Diagnostics (Basel). 2020;10(10):851.

Lafage-Proust MH. Bone and chronic kidney disease. Semin Musculoskelet Radiol. 2023;27(4):463–70.

Whitehouse RW, Ahmad G, Kirwadi A, et al. Imaging of chronic kidney disease-mineral and bone disorder. Radiol Clin North Am. 2022;60(4):547–59.

47 Skeletal Fluorosis: Case 47

47.1 Medical History

Patient was a 57-year-old female. She had suffered from arthralgia from multiple joints about 20 years with involving neck, back, right shoulder, both knees, and both heels. It was accompanied by morning stiffness with restricted activities. She lost the ability to stand up about 12 years ago and had left femoral fracture about 5 years ago when getting on to the bed. Dorsal edema with swelling of both feet started about 1 year ago and more on the right. Edema and swelling of the both lower legs started about 3 months ago. Lab works showed alkaline phosphatase (AKP) 214 U/L, calcium 2.38 mmol/L, phosphorus 0.55 mmol/L, 24-hour urine calcium 4.392 mmol, urine phosphatase 16 mmol, urine fluorine 4.963 mg/L.

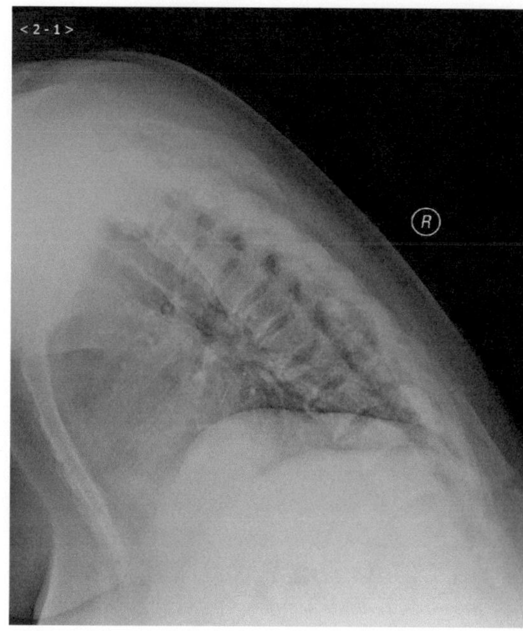

Fig. 47.1 Lateral view of the thoracic spine

47.2 Physical Examination

Not done.

47.3 Imaging Findings

47.3.1 Radiograph (Figs. 47.1 and 47.2)

There was forced position with increased densities of the spine and fuzziness of the facet joints with ossifications along the anterior longitudinal ligament, interspinous ligament, and supraspinal ligament at some segments. There were increased bone densities in the bony pelvis with thickened cortex and blurred trabeculae and ossifications along the tendon and ligament attachments. There were narrowed joint spaces of the hips with productive changes along the acetabulum.

X. Cheng et al., *Imaging of Bone Tumors in Axial Bones*,
https://doi.org/10.1007/978-981-95-2262-0_47

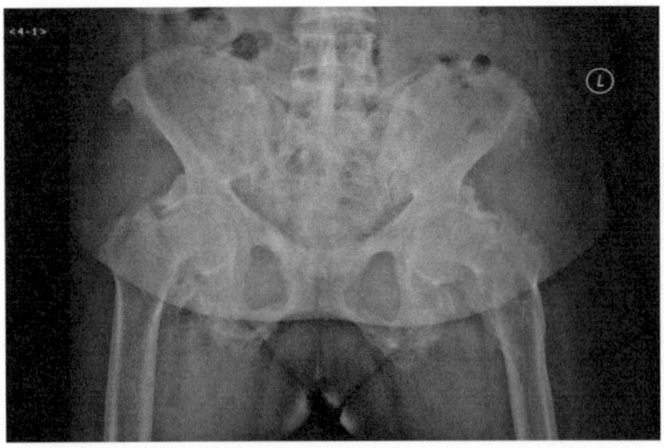

Fig. 47.2 Frontal view of the pelvis

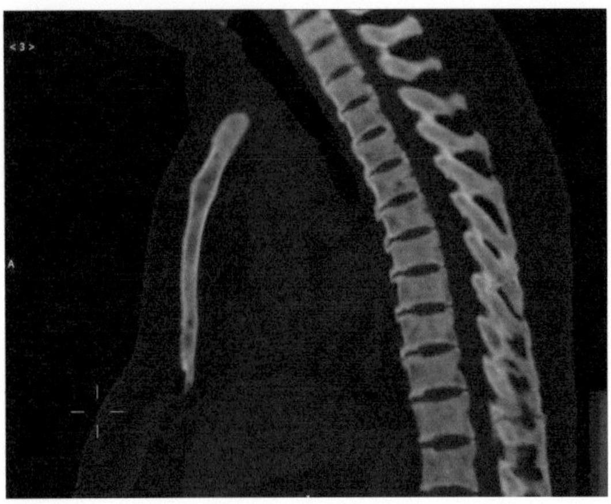

Fig. 47.3 Sagittal CT image of the thoracic spine in bone window

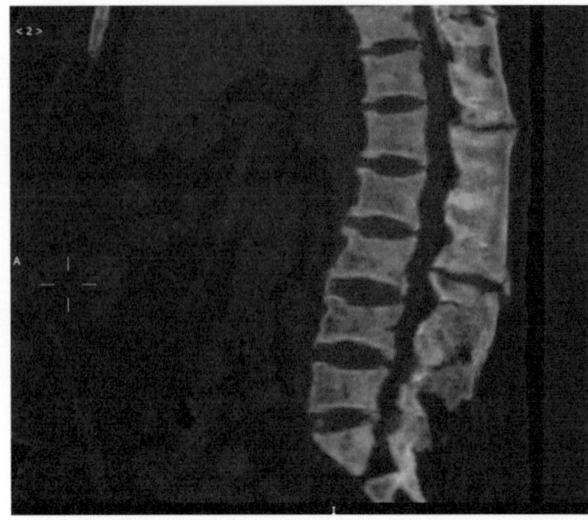

Fig. 47.4 Sagittal CT image of the lumbar spine in bone window

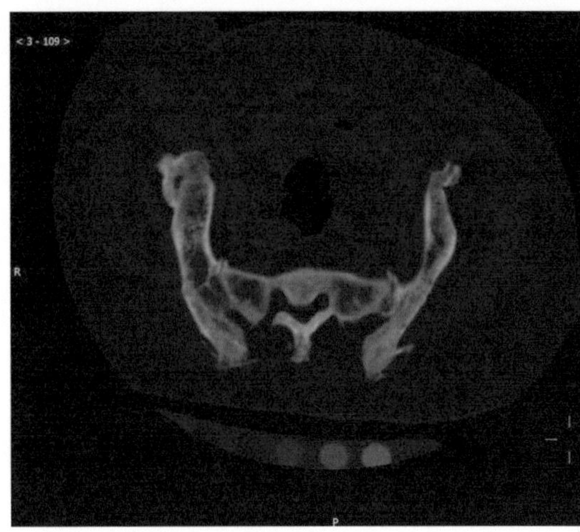

Fig. 47.5 Axial CT image of the pelvis through sacroiliac joints in bone window

47.3.2 CT Imaging (Figs. 47.3, 47.4, 47.5, and 47.6)

There were heterogeneous increased bone densities of multiple bones with trabecular blurring or haziness. Diffuse ossification noted along anterior longitudinal ligament, interspinous ligament, and supraspinal ligament along the thoracic and lumbar spines. Ossifications were also noted along tendon and ligament attachments around the bony pelvis.

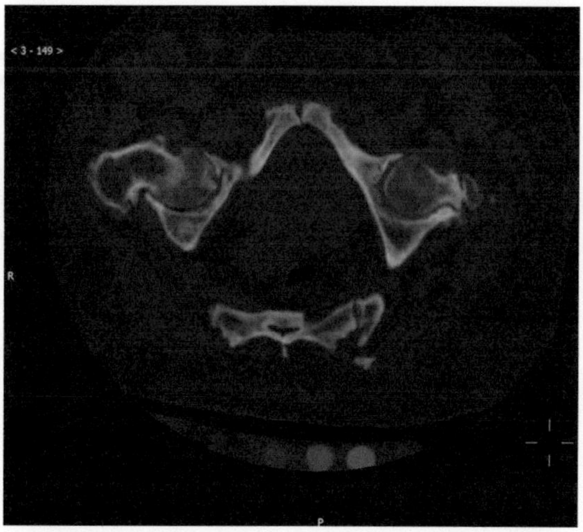

Fig. 47.6 Axial CT image of the pelvis through hips in bone window

47.4 Description and Discussion from Residents

The patient was an older female, with long medical history. Radiographs showed diffuse increased bone density of the thoracic spine and pelvis; multiple ossifications noted along interspinous ligament along the thoracic spine and at the tendon attachments around the bony pelvis and around bilateral hip joints; decreased joint spaces of the both hips and sacroiliac joints. Diffuse increased bone density of multiple bones, ossifications along the attachments of tendons and ligaments, and focal fracture were noted on the CT images. The above constellation of findings is most suggestive of metabolic bone disease. Lab works showed normal levels of calcium and phosphorus with increased urine fluorine; thus, our top consideration is skeletal fluorosis, with osteopetrosis and renal osteodystrophy in the differential diagnosis. However, "sandwich vertebrae" is usually present in those entities.

47.5 Analysis and Comments from Professor Cheng Xiao-Guang

Overall, the presentation of the current case is whole-body metabolic bone disease. Radiographs showed diffuse increased bone density, decreased joint spaces of the facet joints, and ossification of the interspinous ligament. CT images demonstrated the abnormalities in more details: diffuse increased bone density, fusion of the small joints, ossifications along the tendons and ligaments, and characteristic of skeletal fluorosis. Given the presence of ossification of the ligament, renal osteodystrophy can be excluded. Skeletal fluorosis was more common in the past. Origin of the fluorosis are usually from two sources: increased level of fluoride in the drinking water and food pollution. After prevention and treatment, the prevalence has significantly decreased. Diagnosis of skeletal fluorosis needs to combine medical history, clinical presentation, lab works, and imaging findings. Given increased urine fluorine, the diagnosis is skeletal fluorosis.

47.6 Diagnosis

Skeletal fluorosis.

Suggested Reading

Sellami M, Riahi H, Maatallah K, et al. Skeletal fluorosis: don't miss the diagnosis! Skeletal Radiol. 2020;49(3):345–57.

Wang Y, Yin Y, Gilula LA, et al. Endemic fluorosis of the skeleton: radiographic features in 127 patients. AJR Am J Roentgenol. 1994;162(1):93–8.

Osteopetrosis: Case 48

48

48.1 Medical History

Patient is a 26-year-old male. He had left hip pain after exercise about 5 years ago with restricted activity. There was relief of symptoms after symptomatic treatment. The pain around the left hip worsened about 1 year ago after playing basketball.

48.2 Physical Examination

Not done.

48.3 Imaging Findings

48.3.1 Radiograph (Figs. 48.1, 48.2, 48.3, 48.4, 48.5, 48.6, 48.7, 48.8, 48.9, and 48.10)

There were diffuse increased bone densities with narrowing of the medullary cavity. "Sandwich vertebrae" sign noted. Intervertebral disc space is preserved. There was enlargement of the distal femurs bilaterally.

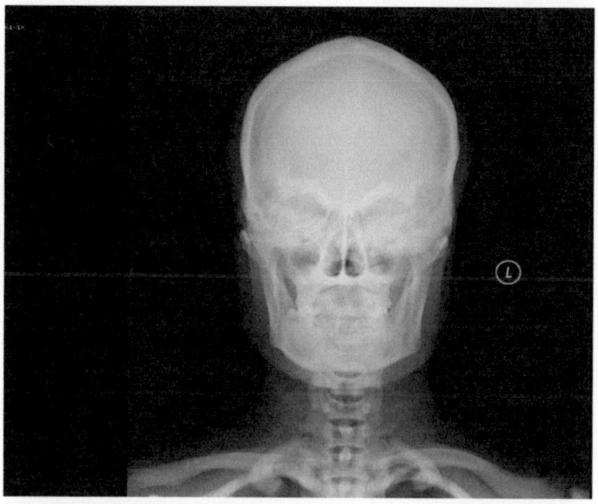

Fig. 48.1 Frontal view of the skull

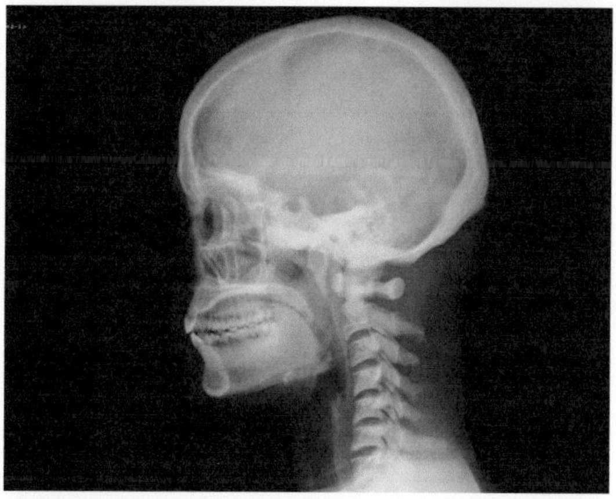

Fig. 48.2 Lateral view of the skull

X. Cheng et al., *Imaging of Bone Tumors in Axial Bones*,
https://doi.org/10.1007/978-981-95-2262-0_48

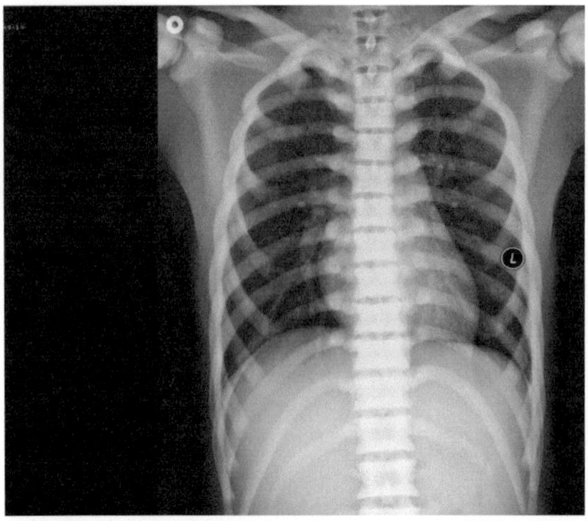

Fig. 48.3 Frontal view of the thoracic spine

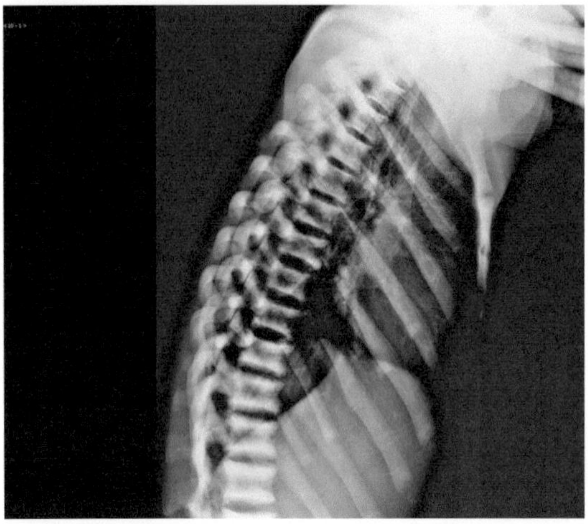

Fig. 48.4 Lateral view of the thoracic spine

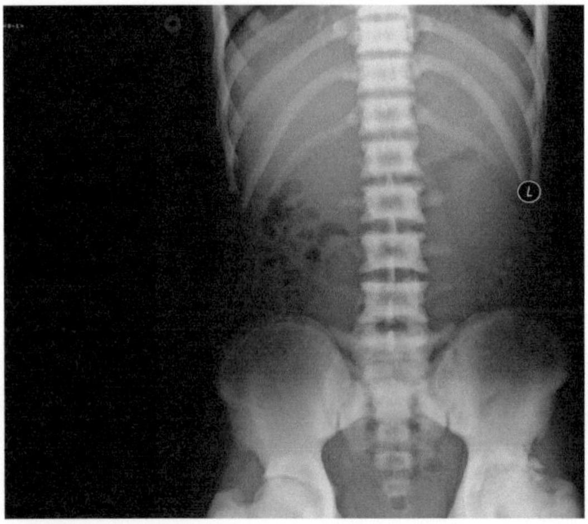

Fig. 48.5 Frontal view of the lumbar spine

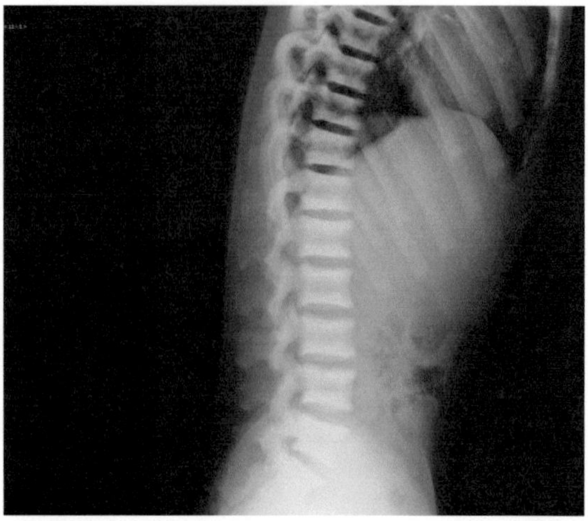

Fig. 48.6 Lateral view of the lumbar spine

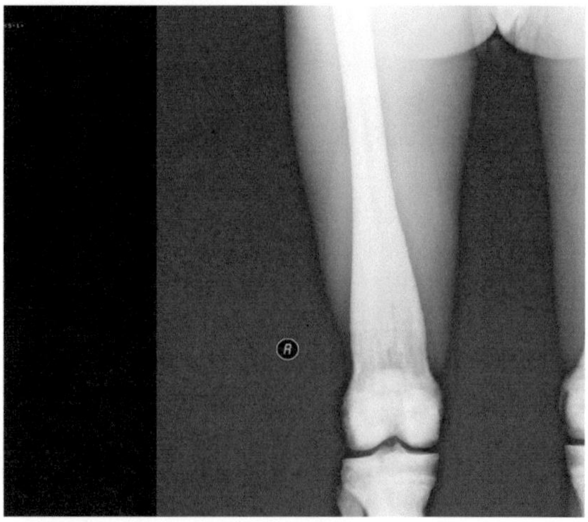

Fig. 48.7 Frontal view of the right femur

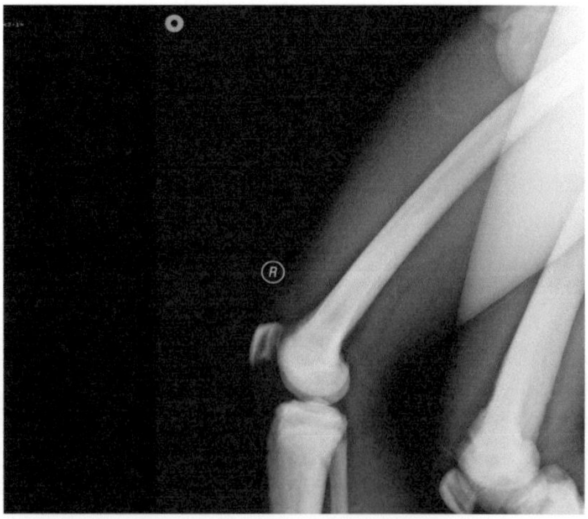

Fig. 48.8 Lateral view of the right femur

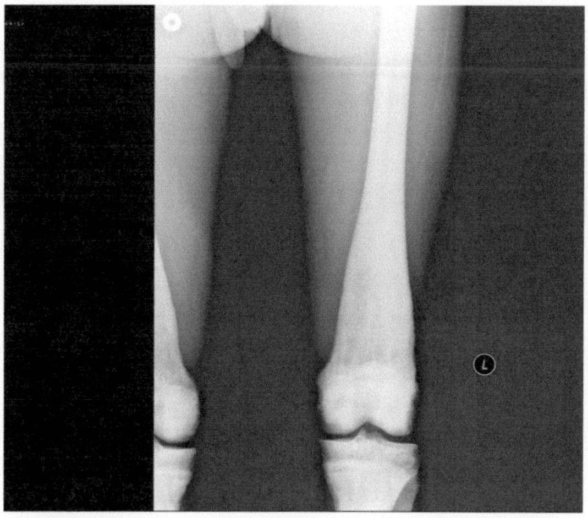

Fig. 48.9 Frontal view of the left femur

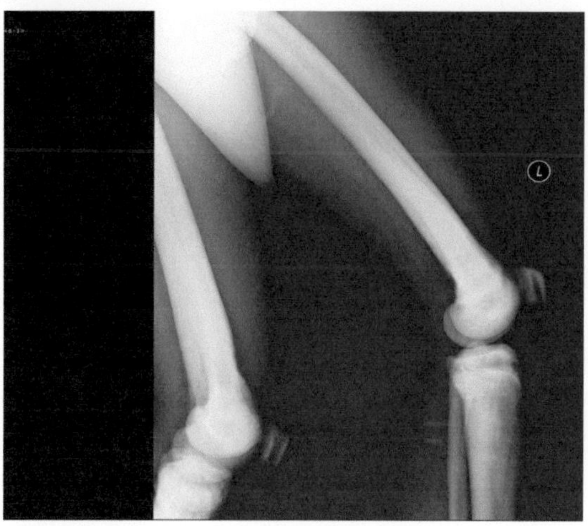

Fig. 48.10 Lateral view of the left femur

48.3.2 CT Imaging (Figs. 48.11 and 48.12)

There were diffuse increased bone densities of the bony pelvis and bilateral femurs with fuzziness about the medullary cavity. There was linear low-density shadow along the roof of the left acetabulum with extensive productive changes along the acetabulum and femoral head with multiple subchondral cysts.

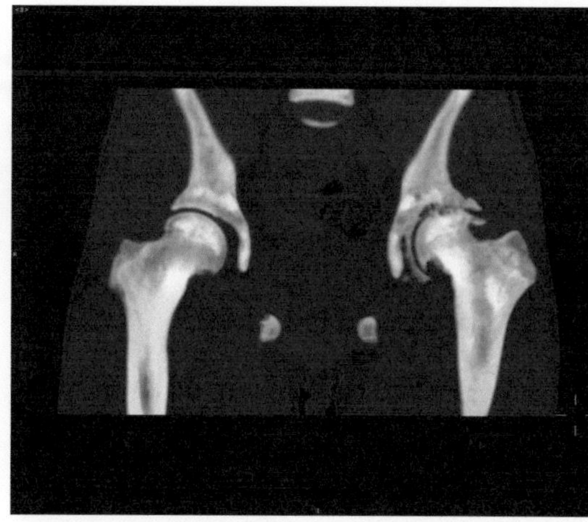

Fig. 48.11 Coronal CT image of the bony pelvis through both hips in bone window

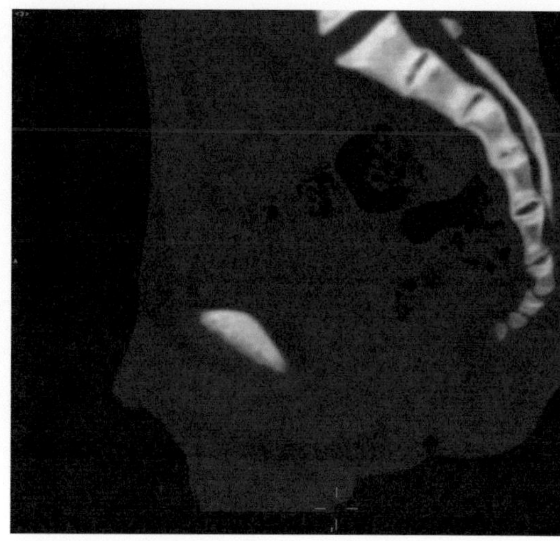

Fig. 48.12 Sagittal CT image of the sacrum in bone window

48.4 Description and Discussion from Residents

Radiographs showed symmetric increased bone density of the skull, bony pelvis, femurs, and ribs with thickening of the cortex, narrowing of the medullary cavity with fuzziness. Increased densities along the endplates of the vertebral bodies with central low density were typical of "sandwich vertebrae" sign. CT images showed increased bone density, cortical thickening, and apparent narrowing of the medullary cavity. The above findings are characteristic of osteopetrosis.

48.5 Analysis and Comments from Professor Cheng Xiao-Guang

The patient was a young male. There was diffuse increased bone density with thickened cortex, narrowed medullary cavity with "sandwich vertebrae" sign, all typical of osteopetrosis. The main pathogenesis of osteopetrosis is from dysfunction of the osteoclasts, leading to limited bone resorption and accumulation of bone; thus, the bone structure is relatively fragile, and patient is prone to fall with fracture. There is no good treatment nowadays.

48.6 Diagnosis

Osteopetrosis.

Suggested Reading

Calder AD, Arulkumaran S, D'Arco F. Imaging in osteopetrosis. Bone. 2022;165:116560.

Stoker DJ. Osteopetrosis. Semin Musculoskelet Radiol. 2002;6(4):299–305.

49 Paget Disease of Bone: Case 49

49.1 Medical History

Patient is a 44-year-old male. He found to have bowing of the both lower extremities in the last 5 years with pain around the knee, not related to activities and occasional left shoulder pain in the last 2 years.

49.2 Physical Examination

Anterior bowing deformities of the bilateral femurs and bilateral tibias.

49.3 Imaging Findings

49.3.1 Radiograph (Figs. 49.1, 49.2, 49.3, 49.4, 49.5, 49.6, 49.7, and 49.8)

There was mild bone expansion of the left temporal bone, left region of mandible, left proximal humerus, right iliac, and left proximal femur with thickening of the cortex and coarsening of the trabeculae with focal lucent regions. There was bowing of bilateral femurs and tibias with cortical thickening.

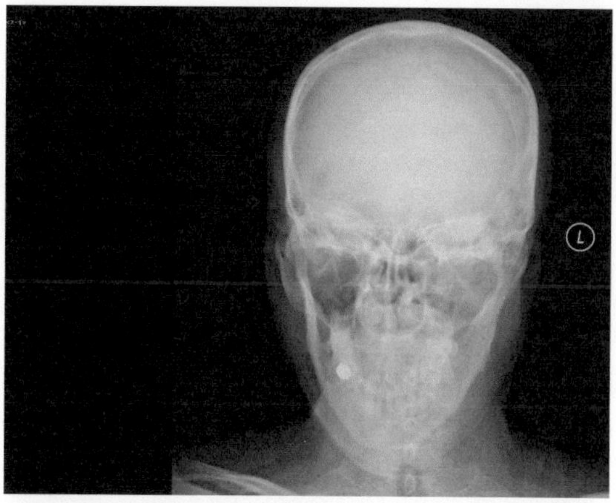

Fig. 49.1 Frontal view of the skull

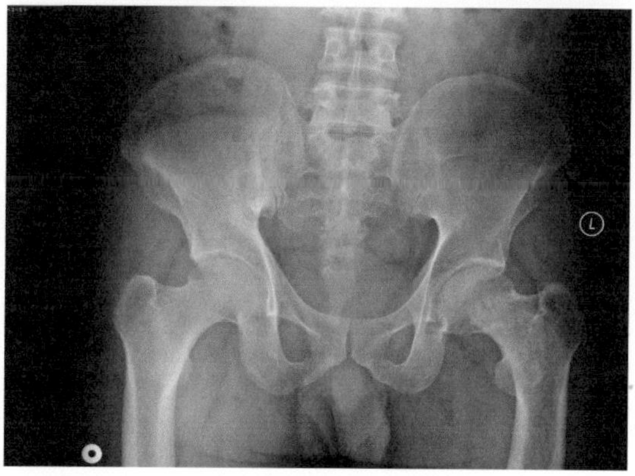

Fig. 49.2 Frontal view of the bony pelvis

X. Cheng et al., *Imaging of Bone Tumors in Axial Bones*,
https://doi.org/10.1007/978-981-95-2262-0_49

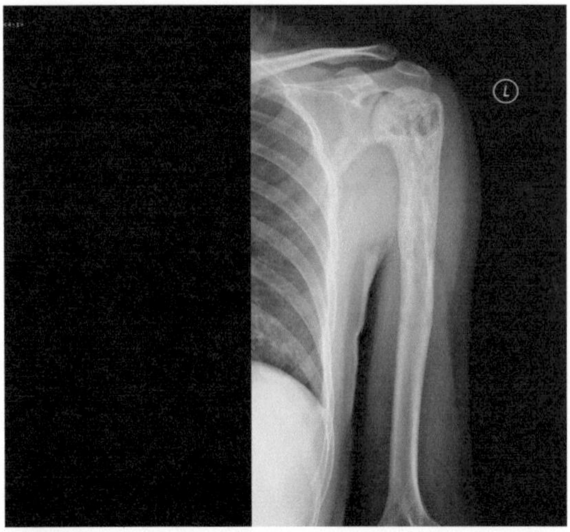

Fig. 49.3 Frontal view of the left humerus

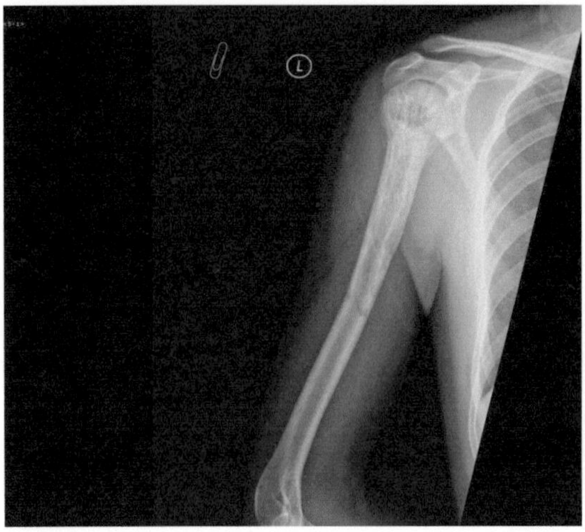

Fig. 49.4 Lateral view of the left humerus

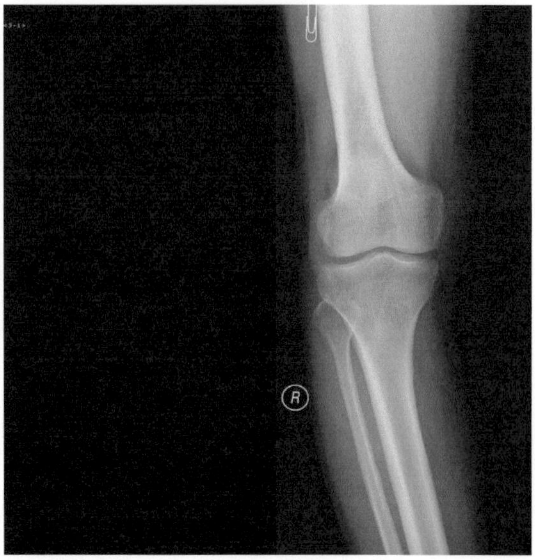

Fig. 49.5 Frontal view of the right knee

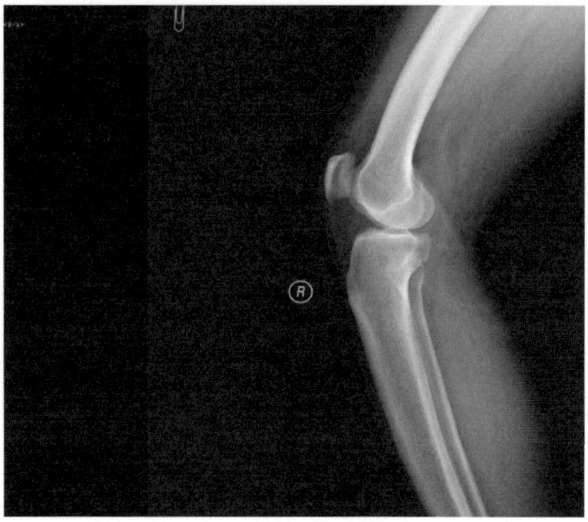

Fig. 49.6 Lateral view of the right knee

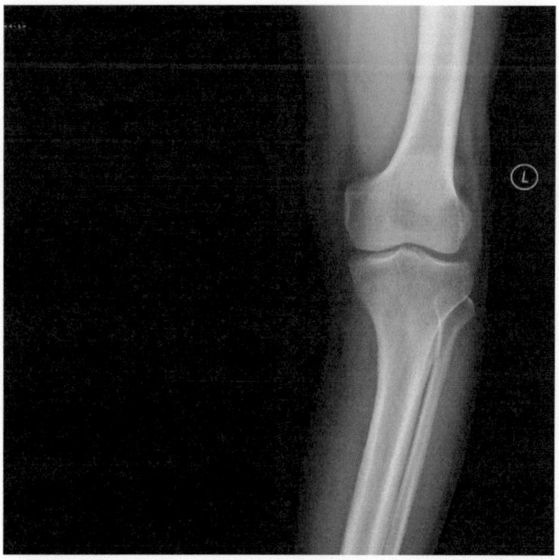

Fig. 49.7 Frontal view of the left knee

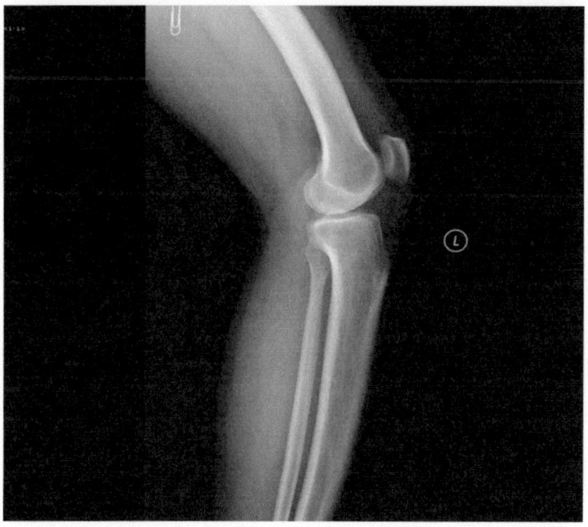

Fig. 49.8 Lateral view of the left knee

49.4 Description and Discussion from Residents

Patient was a middle-aged male. There was slightly higher density on the left maxillary sinus. There was bone expansion of the left mandible and frontal facial bones with increased densities. There was deformity of the proximal left humerus with thickened cortex and coarsened trabeculae with not clear margin between the cortex and medullary cavity, without periosteal reaction or soft tissue mass. There was mild expansion of the left proximal femur with heterogeneous high densities and internal patchy low densities. There was mild anterior bowing of both femurs and tibias. The cortices of both tibias were thickened with decreased densities along the anterior cortex, without apparent abnormalities in the medullary cavity. As for multiple bone involvements of current case, the differential diagnosis includes fibrous dysplasia and Paget disease. With fibrous dysplasia, patient usually presents with a younger age with changes along the cortex as thickening or thinning, but very rarely presents with intracortical stratification as of current case and sclerosis usually more apparent than the current case. Thus, our top consideration is Paget disease.

49.5 Analysis and Comments from Professor Cheng Xiao-Guang

The patient is a middle-aged male, with multiple bone involvements. Bone expansion noted of the proximal humerus with thickening of the cortex and coarsened trabeculae, consistent with Paget disease. Clinical presentation of Paget disease is usually bone pain, with lab works showing apparent elevated alkaline phosphatase level. Treatment with bisphosphonate is usually with good results.

49.6 Diagnosis

Paget disease of bone.

Suggested Reading

Lalam RK, Cassar-Pullicino VN, Winn N. Paget disease of bone. Semin Musculoskelet Radiol. 2016;20(3):287–99.

Lombardi A, Yui Aihara AY, Fernandes ARC, et al. Imaging of Paget's disease of bone. Radiol Clin North Am. 2022;60(4):561–73.

Smith SE, Murphey MD, Motamedi K, et al. From the archives of the AFIP. Radiologic spectrum of Paget disease of bone and its complications with pathologic correlation. Radiographics. 2002;22(5):1191–216.

50 SAPHO Syndrome: Case 50

50.1 Medical History

Patient is a 51-year-old female. She had intermittent back pain without clear causes started about 11 years ago. Symptoms worsened with activities or cold weather with dry mouth and dry eyes. She had no fever, rash, acne, palmoplantar pustulosis, or joint swelling with pain. In the recent 5 years, the symptoms worsened with right sternoclavicular pain about half year ago.

50.2 Physical Examination

Not recorded in hospital system.

50.3 Imaging Findings

50.3.1 CT Imaging (Figs. 50.1, 50.2, 50.3, 50.4, 50.5, 50.6, and 50.7)

There was bone expansion with sclerosis around the right sternoclavicular joint and junction of the sternal manubrium and body, especially around the proximal clavicle. Cystic changes noted at subchondral bones with preserved joint space. Bone sclerosis noted along the first sternocostal connections. There were multiple areas of bone sclerosis along the anterior corners and endplates of the thoracic spine with fuzzy border.

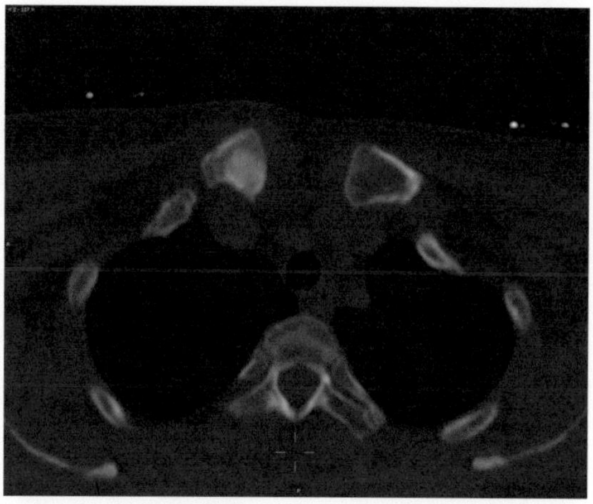

Fig. 50.1 Axial CT image of the chest through sternoclavicular joints in bone window

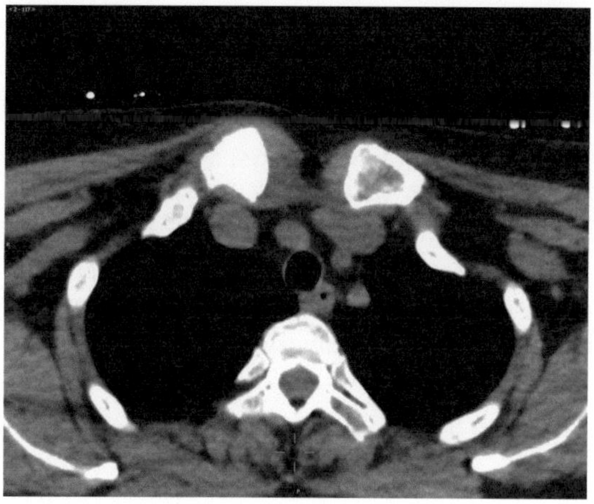

Fig. 50.2 Axial CT image of the chest through sternoclavicular joints in soft tissue window

X. Cheng et al., *Imaging of Bone Tumors in Axial Bones*,
https://doi.org/10.1007/978-981-95-2262-0_50

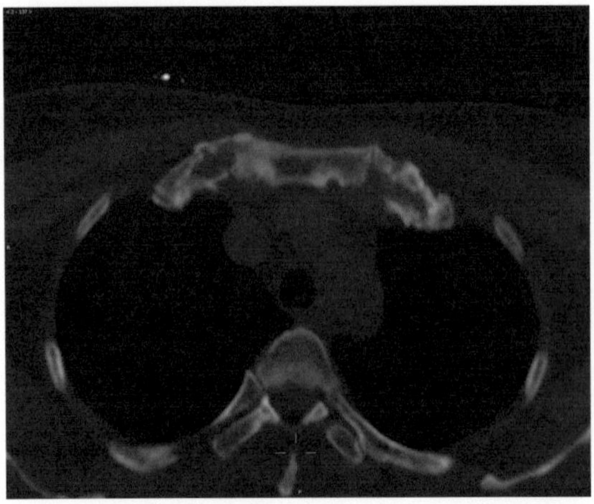

Fig. 50.3 Axial CT image of the chest through first sternocostal junctions in bone window

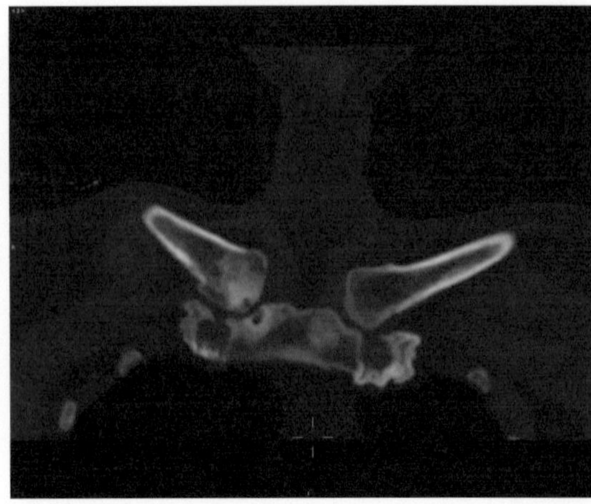

Fig. 50.5 Coronal CT image of the chest through sternoclavicular joints in bone window

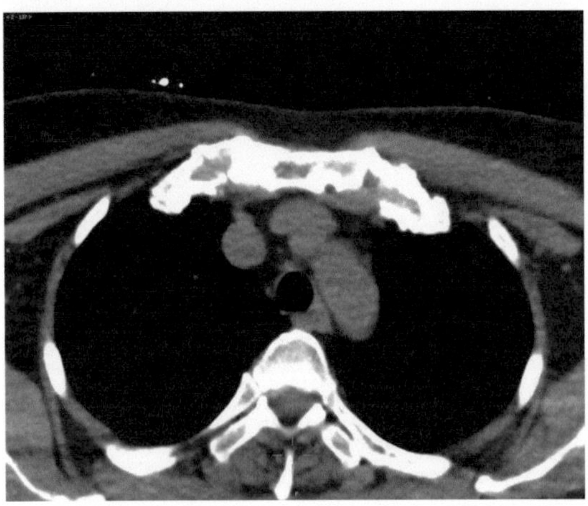

Fig. 50.4 Axial CT image of the chest through first sternocostal junctions in soft tissue window

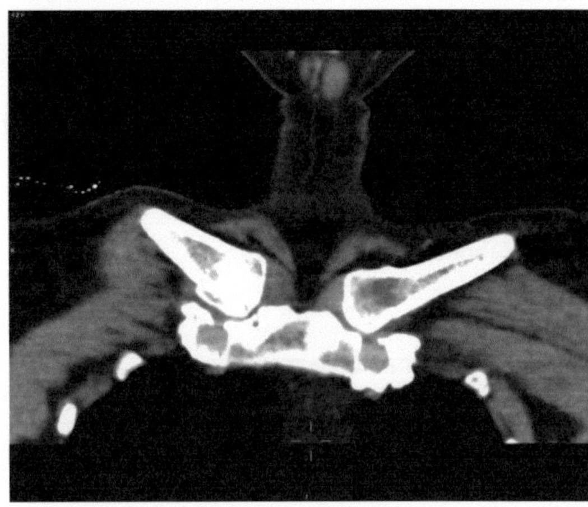

Fig. 50.6 Coronal CT image of the chest through sternoclavicular joints in soft tissue window

50.3.2 MR Imaging (Figs. 50.8, 50.9, 50.10, and 50.11)

MR images demonstrated preserved sacroiliac joint spaces with fuzziness along the joint with extensive marrow edema along the joints.

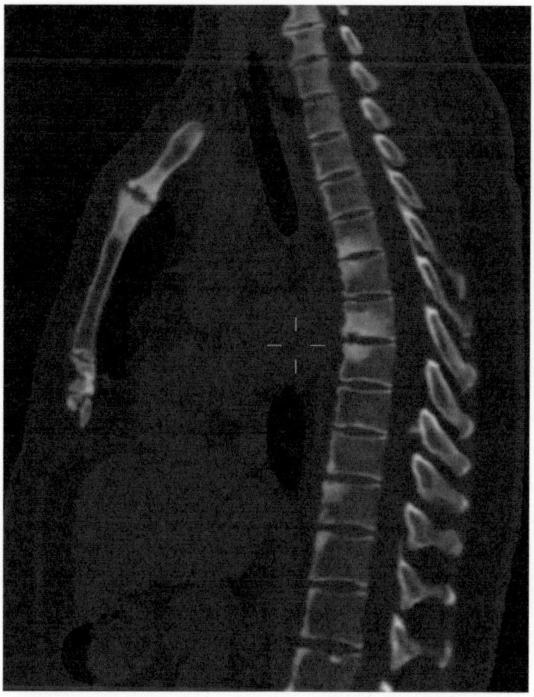

Fig. 50.7 Sagittal CT image of the thoracic spine in bone window

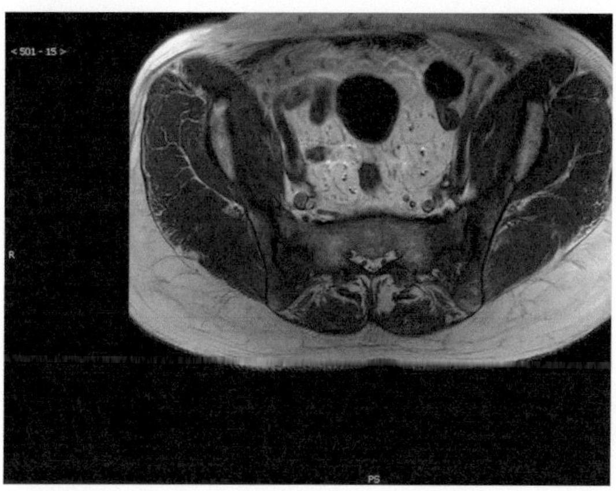

Fig. 50.8 Axial T1-weighted MR image of the sacroiliac joints

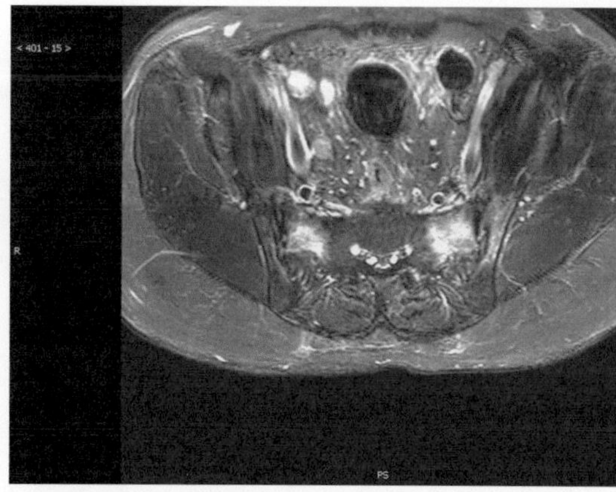

Fig. 50.9 Axial fat-suppressed T2-weighted MR image of the sacroiliac joints

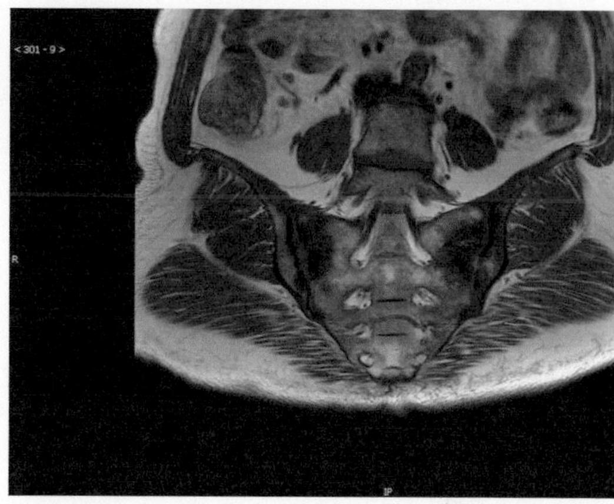

Fig. 50.10 Coronal T1-weighted MR image of the sacroiliac joints

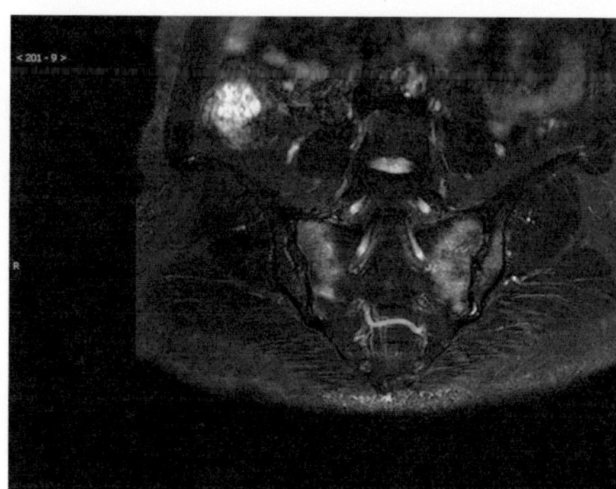

Fig. 50.11 Coronal fat-suppressed T2-weighted MR image of the sacroiliac joints

50.4 Description and Discussion from Residents

CT images showed inflammatory changes along the right sternoclavicular joint, first sternocostal junctions, and sternal manubrium-body junction with focal apparent sclerosis. Focal scleroses along multiple endplates of the cervical and thoracic spines as endplate inflammatory changes were shown. Female patient with multiple bones of osteitis-like changes and apparent involvement of the sternoclavicular joint, suggesting SAPHO syndrome, needs further correlation with clinical presentation and lab works. Bilateral sacroiliitis noted on the MR images. Given the involvement of multiple joints with inflammation, our top consideration is SAPHO syndrome.

50.5 Analysis and Comments from Professor Cheng Xiao-Guang

Patient is a middle-aged female. CT scan images showed increased density around the junction of sternal manubrium and body with narrowed space. There were apparent inflammatory arthropathy changes of the first sternocostal joints and right sternoclavicular joint. Endplate inflammation changes of multiple thoracic vertebral bodies were noted, with segmental distribution, with "corner" sign. Bilateral symmetrical edema along the sacroiliac joints noted on MR images. Middle-aged female with inflammatory sclerosis of multiple joints and vertebral endplates; top consideration is SAPHO syndrome. This patient did not present with rash, acne, or palmoplantar pustulosis. However, the five key features of SAPHO syndrome: synovitis, acne, pustulosis, hyperostosis, and osteitis don't have to present at the same time and not necessary to be all present. Thus, given the above typical imaging findings, this is my top diagnosis. Various types of seronegative spondyloarthropathy are in the differential diagnosis.

50.6 Diagnosis

SAPHO syndrome.

Suggested Reading

Laredo JD, Vuillemin-Bodaghi V, Boutry N, et al. SAPHO syndrome: MR appearance of vertebral involvement. Radiology. 2007;242(3):825–31.

McGauvran AM, Kotsenas AL, Diehn FE, et al. SAPHO syndrome: imaging findings of vertebral involvement. AJNR Am J Neuroradiol. 2016;37(8):1567–72.

MIX
Papier aus verantwortungsvollen Quellen
Paper from responsible sources
FSC® C105338

If you have any concerns about our products,
you can contact us on
ProductSafety@springernature.com

In case Publisher is established outside the EU,
the EU authorized representative is:
Springer Nature Customer Service Center GmbH
Europaplatz 3, 69115 Heidelberg, Germany

Printed by Libri Plureos GmbH
in Hamburg, Germany